Renin Angiotensin System and the Heart

Renin Angiotensin System and the Heart

Edited by
Walmor C. De Mello
Medical Sciences Campus, University of Puerto Rico, USA

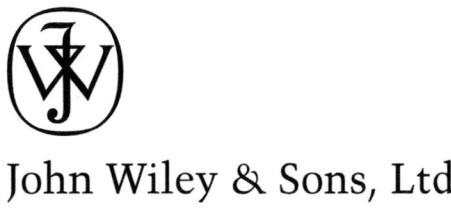

John Wiley & Sons, Ltd

Copyright © 2004 by John Wiley & Sons Ltd, The Atrium, Southern Gate, Chichester,
West Sussex PO19 8SQ, UK

Telephone (+44) 1243 779777

E-mail (for orders and customer service enquiries): cs-books@wiley.co.uk
Visit our Home Page on www.wileyeurope.com
or
www.wiley.com

All Rights Reserved. No part of this publication may be reproduced, stored in a retrieval system or transmitted in any form or by any means, electronic, mechanical, photocopying, recording, scanning or otherwise, except under the terms of the Copyright, Designs and Patents Act 1988 or under the terms of a licence issued by the Copyright Licensing Agency Ltd, 90 Tottenham Court Road, London W1T 4LP9HE, UUK, without the permission in writing of the Publisher. Requests to the Publisher should be addressed to the Permissions Department, John Wiley & Sons Ltd, The Atrium, Southern Gate, Chichester, West Sussex, PO19 8SQ, England, or emailed to permreq@wiley.co.uk, or faxed to (+44) 1243 770620.

This publication is designed to provide accurate and authoritative information in regard to the subject matter covered. It is sold on the understanding that the Publisher is not engaged in rendering professional services. If professional advice or other expert assistance is required, the services of a competent professional should be sought.

Other Wiley Editorial Offices

John Wiley & Sons, Inc., 111 River Street, Hoboken, NJ 07030, USA

Jossey-Bass, 989 Market Street, San Francisco, CA 94103-1741, USA

Wiley-VCH Verlag GmbH, Boschstr. 12, D-69469 Weinheim, Germany

John Wiley & Sons Australia Ltd, 33 Park Road, Milton, Queensland 4064, Australia

John Wiley & Sons (Asia) Pte Ltd, 2 Clementi Loop #02-01, Jin Xing Distripark, Singapore 129809

John Wiley & Sons (Canada) Ltd., 22 Worcester Road, EtobicokeRexdale, Ontario, M9W 1L1, Canada M9W 1L1

Wiley also publishes its books in a variety of electronic formats. Some content that appears in print may not be available in electronic books.

Library of Congress Cataloging-in-Publication Data

Renin angiotensin system and the heart/editor, Walmor C. De Mello.
 p. ; cm.
 Includes bibliographical references and index.
 ISBN 0-470-86292-0 (Cloth : alk. paper)
 1. Renin-angiotensin system. 2. Heart — Physiology. 3. Heart — Pathophysiology.
 [DNLM: 1. Renin-Angiotensin System — physiology. 2. Heart — drug effects.
 3. Heart Diseases — physiopathology. WG 106 R413 2004] I. De Mello, Walmor C.
 QP572.A54R466 2004
 612.1'7 — dc22   2004003362

British Library Cataloguing in Publication Data
A catalogue record for this book is available from the British Library
ISBN 0-470-86292-0

Typeset in 11/14pt Palatino by Thomson Press (India) Ltd., Chennai
Printed and bound in Great Britain by TJ International Ltd., Pads tow, Cornwall
This book is printed on acid-free paper responsibly manufactured from sustainable forestry in which at least two trees are planted for each one used for paper production.

Contents

Preface	ix
List of Contributors	xi

1 Intracellular Signaling and the Cardiac Renin Angiotensin System — 1
George W. Booz and Kenneth M. Baker

Introduction	1
Regulation of cardiac remodeling by Ang II	2
AT_1-mediated intracellular signaling	3
Paracrine/autocrine actions of Ang II	10
Intracrine actions of Ang II	10
Summary	11
References	12

2 Cardiac Physiology and the Renin Angiotensin System: Lessons from Transgenic Animal Models — 19
Alisdair Ryding and John J. Mullins

Introduction	19
An overview of transgenesis	20
Transgenic evidence of a cardiac-based RAS	21
Transgenic evidence of cardiac renin uptake	23
Prorenin activity	24
Role of the RAS in cardiac hypertrophy and fibrosis	25
Conclusions and questions	26
References	26

3 Prorenin Uptake in the Heart — 31
A. H. Jan Danser

Introduction	31
How does the heart sequester circulating (pro)renin?	33
(Pro)renin receptors	34
Mannose 6-phosphate/insulin-like growth factor II receptors	36
M6P/IGFII receptor-mediated (pro)renin binding and prorenin activation	37
Does prorenin mediate direct (Ang II-independent) effects?	38
Intracellular versus extracellular angiotensin generation	40
Perspective	41
References	42

4 Role of Local Renin Angiotensin Systems in Cardiac Damage — 47
Michael Bader
- Introduction — 47
- AT_1 and cardiac hypertrophy — 49
- AT_1 and cardiac fibrosis — 52
- AT_2 in cardiac hypertrophy and fibrosis — 53
- Conclusion — 54
- References — 54

5 Cardiac Renin: *De Novo* Synthesis and Uptake — 63
Jörg Peters
- Introduction — 63
- Presence of renin in the heart — 64
- Uptake of renin into the heart — 64
- Cardiac expression of renin — 66
- Discovery of a second transcript of the rat renin gene — 67
- Differential expression of preprorenin and exon 1A renin transcripts — 69
- Possible functions of exon 1A renin — 70
- Significance of renin uptake and expression: concluding remarks — 70
- References — 71

6 The Cardiac Renin Receptors — 75
Geneviève Nguyen, Céline Burckle and Benjamin Tremey
- Introducion — 75
- The renin-binding proteins — 76
- The renin receptor — 78
- Conclusion — 80
- References — 81

7 Angiotensin II AT_2 Receptors and Cardiac Function — 85
Jun Suzuki, Takanori Kanazawa, Masaru Iwai and Masatsugu Horiuch
- Possible roles of AT_2 receptor stimulation associated with selective AT_1 receptor blockade — 85
- Expression of AT_2 receptor in cardiac tissue — 89
- Role of AT_2 receptor in cardiac structure and function — 90
- References — 95

8 The Heart: A Target for the Renin Angiotensin System. Evidence of an Intracrine System — 101
Walmor C. De Mello
- Introduction — 101
- RAS and intercellular signaling — 103
- Ang II, cell coupling and growth; an important relationship? — 107
- Evidence for an intracellular RAS — 107
- On the possible role of endogenous Ang II on heart cell communication — 108
- Aldosterone modulates the effect of Ang II — 111
- Effect of intracellular and extracellular Ang II on the inward calcium current — 112
- Acknowledgments — 113
- References — 113

9 ACE2: Its Role in the Counter-regulatory Response to Heart Failure — 119
Lawrence S. Zisman

Introduction	119
A paradigm of human heart failure: secondary activation of neurohormonal systems and a counterbalancing response	120
Angiotensin metabolites	121
Overview of peptidases	122
Carboxypeptidases	124
ACE2, a novel homolog of ACE, functions as a carboxypeptidase and angiotensinase	125
ACE2-mediated hydrolysis of biological peptides	127
Genetics and cross-species homology	127
The ACE2 knockout mouse	128
Design and characteristics of ACE2-specific inhibitors	128
Regulation of Ang-(1-7) formation in human heart failure	129
Ang II-mediated signal transduction	131
Summary	132
References	132

10 Wound Healing and the Tissue Renin Angiotensin Aldosterone System — 137
Yao Sun and Karl T. Weber

Introduction	137
Expression of tRAAS	138
Cells expressing tRAAS	144
tRAAS and wound healing	146
Summary	151
References	152

11 Trophic Effects of Aldosterone — 161
Claude Delcayre, Christophe Heymes, Paul Milliez and Bernard Swynghedauw

Introduction	161
Renal effects of aldosterone	162
Trophic effects of aldosterone	163
Results from clinical trials	167
Cardiac aldosterone production	170
References	175

12 Intracellular Angiotensin and the Actions of Intracrine Hormones — 179
Richard N. Re

Introduction	179
Intracrine angiotensin	180
Intracrine renin	183
Clinical implications	184
Intracrine physiology	184
A theory of intracrine action	188
References	190

13 Angiotensin II and Myocardial Fibrosis, Clinical Implications — 193
Begoña López, Arantxa González and Javier Díez

Introduction	193
General aspects of myocardial fibrosis	194
Role of Ang II in myocardial fibrosis	196
In vivo evidence	196
Cellular and molecular mechanisms	199
Clinical consequences	203
Therapeutic implications	207
Conclusions and perspectives	207
References	208

14 Hypertensive Heart Disease: Significance of the Renin Angiotensin System — 215
Jasmina Varagic and Edward D. Frohlich

Introduction	215
Structural and functional alterations in HHD	216
Contribution of Ang II cardiac effects to HHD	218
Cardiomyocyte hypertrophy	218
Coronary insufficiency	219
Ventricular fibrosis	220
Diastolic dysfunction	221
Cardiac RAS in development of HHD: experimental and clinical evidence	222
Pharmacological blockade of cardiac RAS	225
Acknowledgments	226
References	227

Index — 235

Preface

The finding that the heart is a target for the renin angiotensin system represents an important step in our ability to understand and prevent the cardiac abnormalities generated by pathological processes such as heart failure, essential hypertension and myocardial ischemia in which the renin angiotensin system is activated. However, the relationship between the heart and this hormonal system is deeper than that: experimental and clinical evidence has revealed that there is a local renin angiotensin system in the heart which is involved in important aspects of heart function and dysfunction.

In the present book this important subject is presented by distinguished colleagues, each one expert in his own field. Different approaches such as cell and molecular biology, transgenic animals, pharmacology and clinical studies have been used to elucidate the intricacies of this system. It is our hope that the efforts transcend the technological aspects and that we can grasp the real physiopathological meaning of the cardiac renin angiotensin system. This book represents a step in this direction.

Let us hope it can be of benefit to young investigators and to the scientific community in general.

Walmor C. De Mello
Medical Sciences Campus, UPR

List of Contributors

Michael Bader
Max-Delbrück-Center for Molecular Medicine (MDC), Robert-Rössle-Strasse 10, D-13092 Berlin-Buch, Germany

Kenneth M. Baker
The Cardiovascular Research Institute, Division of Molecular Cardiology, The Texas A&M University System Health Science Center, College of Medicine Temple, TX, USA

George W. Booz
The Cardiovascular Research Institute, Division of Molecular Cardiology, The Texas A&M University System Health Science Center, College of Medicine Temple, TX, USA

Céline Burckle
Jean-Daniel SRAER Institut National de la Santé, et de la Recherche Médicale (INSERM), Paris, France

A. H. Jan Danser
Department of Pharmacology, Erasmus Medical Center, Dr. Molewaterplein 50, The Netherlands

Walmor C. De Mello
Department of Pharmacology and Toxicology, Medical Sciences Campus, University of Puerto Rico, San Juan, Puerto Rico, USA

Claude Delcayre
Directeur de Recherches au CNRS, U572-INSERM, Hôpital Lariboisière, Paris, Cedex, France

Javier Díez
Professor of Vascular Medicine, School of Medicine; Director, Division of Cardiovascular Pathophysiology, Centre for Applied Medical Research; Vice Chairman and Head of Research, Department of Cardiology and Cardiovascular Surgery, University Clinic, University of Navarra, Pamplona, Spain

Edward D. Frohlich
Ochsner Clinic Foundation, Hypertension Research, New Orleans, LA, USA

Arantxa González
Research Fellow, Division of Cardiovascular Pathophysiology, Centre for Applied Medical Research, University of Navarra, Pamplona, Spain

Christophe Heymes
Chargé de Recherches à l'INSERM, U572-INSERM, Hôpital Lariboisière, Paris, Cedex, France

Masatsugu Horiuchi
Department of Medical Biochemistry, Ehime University School of Medicine, Shigenobu, Ehime, Japan

Masaru Iwai
Department of Medical Biochemistry, Ehime University School of Medicine, Shigenobu, Ehime, Japan

Takanori Kanazawa
Research Institute, Novartis Pharma, Tsukuba, Ibaraki, Japan

Begoña López
Senior Scientist, Division of Cardiovascular Pathophysiology, Centre for Applied Medical Research, University of Navarra, Pamplona, Spain

Paul Milliez
Chef de Clinique, AP-HP, U572-INSERM, Hôpital Lariboisière, Paris, Cedex, France

John J. Mullins
The University of Edinburgh, Molecular Physiology Laboratory, The Wilkie Building, Teviot Place, Edinburgh, UK

Geneviève Nguyen
Jean-Daniel SRAER Institut National de la Santé, et de la Recherche Médicale (INSERM), Paris, France

Jörg Peters
Physiologisches Institut, Universität Greifswald, Karlsburg, Germany

Richard N. Re
Ochsner Clinic Foundation, New Orleans, LA, USA

Alisdair Ryding
The University of Edinburgh, Molecular Physiology Laboratory, Edinburgh, UK

Yao Sun
Division of Cardiovascular Diseases, University of Tennessee Health Science Center, Memphis, TN, USA

Jun Suzuki
Department of Medical Biochemistry and Department of Internal Medicine, Ehime University School of Medicine, Shigenobu, Ehime, Japan

Bernard Swynghedauw
Directeur de Recherches à l'INSERM, U572-INSERM, Hôpital Lariboisière, Paris, Cedex, France

Benjamin Tremey
Jean-Daniel SRAER Institut National de la Santé, et de la Recherche Médicale (INSERM) Hôpital, Paris, France

Jasmina Varagic
Ochsner Clinic Foundation, Hypertension Research, New Orleans, LA, USA

Karl T. Weber
Division of Cardiovascular Diseases, University of Tennessee Health Science Center, Memphis, TN, USA

Lawrence S. Zisman
Ochsner Clinic Foundation, New Orleans, LA, USA

1

Intracellular Signaling and the Cardiac Renin Angiotensin System

George W. Booz and Kenneth M. Baker

Introduction

Angiotensin II (Ang II) has multiple actions in the heart that affect cardiac growth and performance (Booz and Baker, 1996, 1998; Bader, 2002). Most of these actions are attributed to interaction with the Ang II type 1 plasma membrane receptor (AT$_1$), a seven-transmembrane spanning, heterotrimeric G-protein coupled receptor that activates multiple signal transduction pathways (Berry et al., 2001). Humans express one form of AT$_1$, while rodents express two (AT$_{1A}$ and AT$_{1B}$) that are coded by separate genes, but are 95 percent homologous, exhibit the same ligand binding affinity, and are pharmacologically indistinguishable. In addition, nuclear Ang II-binding sites have been identified that are AT$_1$-like, but have different physiochemical properties, providing the basis for possible intracrine actions of Ang II (Booz et al., 1992; Tang et al., 1992). Evidence from clinical, animal, and cell culture studies support the idea that Ang II acts in an autocrine and paracrine manner in the heart, since the heart expresses all components of a renin angiotensin system (RAS) (Bader et al., 2001; Bader, 2002). The cardiac RAS is under control of tissue-specific regulatory influences that are activated by biomechanical stress, for example: increased levels of cardiac renin mRNA have been reported in patients sustaining a myocardial infarction (Endo-Mochizuki et al., 1995); cardiac renin and angiotensinogen

(Ao) are both upregulated in experimental animal models of infarction (Mascareno et al., 2001; Sun et al., 2001); a second renin transcript that may code for intracellular renin because it lacks the coding region of the secretory signal peptide, is upregulated in the left ventricle by myocardial infarction (Clausmeyer et al., 2000); and cardiac Ao gene expression is upregulated by experimental models of hypertension (Baker et al., 1990).

Regulation of cardiac remodeling by Ang II

There is evidence, both *in vitro* and *in vivo*, to support the role of Ang II as the primary modulator involved in the process of pathological cardiac remodeling that occurs as a result of pressure overload or ischemia (Booz and Baker, 1996, 1998; Kim and Iwao, 2000). The strongest evidence is provided by clinical and experimental studies that show efficacy of angiotensin-converting enzyme (ACE) inhibitors and AT_1 receptor antagonists (ARBs) in blocking cardiac hypertrophy and extracellular matrix (ECM) deposition (Booz and Baker, 1996). In addition, infusion of a subpressor dose of Ang II in rats induces cardiac hypertrophy via AT_1 (Dostal and Baker, 1992). The functional significance of a cardiac RAS is also supported by transgenic animal studies. Targeted overexpression of the Ao gene in cardiac myocytes resulted in increased cardiac Ang II concentration, and both right and left ventricular hypertrophy (Mazzolai et al., 1998, 2000). This was not accompanied by hypertension or increased circulating levels of Ang II. When AT_1 expression was targeted to cardiac ventricles in transgenic rats, the hypertrophic response to volume or pressure overload was increased compared to control animals, suggesting synergism between mechanical load and AT_1 activation in inducing cardiac hypertrophy (Hoffmann et al., 2001). However, in an AT_{1A} receptor knockout mouse, pressure overload-induced hypertrophy was not prevented, suggesting a contribution of AT_{1B} or, more likely, a compensatory mechanism activated upon AT_{1A} gene deletion during early embryogenesis (Harada et al., 1998a, b). In another study, AT_{1A} knockout mice showed diminished left ventricular remodeling and improved survival after myocardial infarction, suggesting that the effect of AT_{1A} knockout may depend upon the experimental pathology (Harada et al., 1999). Finally, hypertensive, transgenic mice that express Ao in liver and brain only (not the heart), exhibited significantly lower cardiac hypertrophy, as well as less perivascular and interstitial fibrosis (Bader, 2002).

The two cell types principally involved in cardiac remodeling are fibroblasts and myocytes, both of which express AT_1. Receptor levels on cardiac myocytes are substantially lower than on cardiac fibroblasts, but are increased by pressure overload and mechanical stretch (Booz and Baker, 1998). AP-1 and the cardiac-restricted transcription factor GATA4 are required for transcriptional activation of the AT_{1A} gene during hypertrophy (Herzig et al., 1997). AT_1-induced hypertrophy has been demonstrated in cultured cardiac myocytes, where Ang II also induces expression of early response genes, genes for growth factors (e.g., transforming growth factor-β (TGF-β), cardiotrophin-1), and fetal genes (skeletal α-actin and ANP), the latter being a feature of pathological cardiac hypertrophy. AT_1 activation induces upregulation of Ao by cardiac myocytes as well, and Ang II secreted from myocytes has a central role in stretch-induced hypertrophy, functioning in an autocrine manner (Sadoshima et al., 1993). AT_1 couples primarily to G_q in cardiac myocytes, but both G_q and G_i in cardiac fibroblasts (Schorb et al., 1994; Zou et al., 1998). In cardiac fibroblasts, AT_1 activation stimulates proliferation, migration, and synthesis of ECM proteins (Booz and Baker, 1995). AT_1 levels on cardiac fibroblasts are increased substantially after myocardial infarction, possibly from elevated levels of tumor necrosis factor-α (TNF-α) in the infarct zone (Peng et al., 2002). TNF-α (and interleukin (IL)-1β) was shown to upregulate AT_1 mRNA and protein in cardiac fibroblasts through activation of nuclear factor (NF)-κB (Cowling et al., 2002). In contrast, adrenomedullin downregulates AT_1 expression in cardiac fibroblasts possibly via an elevation in cAMP (Autelitano et al., 2003).

AT_1-mediated intracellular signaling

AT_1 activation in cardiac myocytes and fibroblasts induces phosphorylation of multiple proteins, including selective membrane transporters and channels, structural or contractile proteins, and proteins that control metabolism, protein synthesis, and gene expression (Booz and Baker, 1995, 1998; Berry et al., 2001). For the most part, these phosphorylation events are triggered by second messengers (Ca^{2+}, diacylglycerol (DAG), inositol phosphates, arachadonic acid, phosphatidic acid, reactive oxygen species (ROS)) that are generated by activation of phospholipases, phosphoinositide 3-kinase (PI3K), or NAD(P)H oxidase. Activation of phospholipase C-β (PLCβ) by AT_1 is direct via the G-protein α subunit; activation of PLCγ, phospholipase D (PLD), phospholipase A2 (PLA$_2$), PI3K and NAD(P)H oxidase is indirect, occurring via activation of PKC, nonreceptor tyrosine kinase, and/or small G-proteins (Griendling and Ushio-Fukai, 2000; Berry et al., 2001; Guo et al., 2001). In addition, AT_1 may activate phosphorylation cascades via transactivation of receptor tyrosine kinases (Guo et al., 2001).

Canonical signaling

Coupling to G_q/G_i and direct stimulation of PLCβ by the α-subunit is a well described intracellular signaling pathway, in which two second messengers, inositol 1,4,5-trisphosphate (IP_3) and diacylglycerol, are formed. IP_3 stimulates the release of Ca^{2+} from intracellular stores, and diacylglycerol activates protein kinase C (PKC). A key signaling intermediate that is activated by a rise in intracellular Ca^{2+} is the Ca^{2+}/calmodulin-dependent protein phosphatase, calcineurin. Accumulating evidence supports a role for calcineurin in cardiac hypertrophy resulting from various causes, including pressure overload (Frey and Olson, 2003), as well as Ang II stimulation. In cultured cardiac myocytes, Ang II was reported to increase calcineurin enzymatic activity, mRNA, and protein levels, and targeted inhibition of calcineurin attenuated Ang II-induced hypertrophy (Taigen et al., 2000). In hypertensive rats, a nonantihypertensive dose of an AT_1 antagonist attenuated both calcineurin activity and mRNA expression, as well as cardiac hypertrophy and fibrosis (Nagata et al., 2002).

In cardiac fibroblasts, AT_1 activates the three primary MAPK signaling cascades, ERK, JNK, and p38. Activation of the ERK and p38 MAPKs has been implicated in cardiac fibroblast proliferation, migration, and IL-6 expression (Booz et al., 1994; Sano et al., 2001; Stawowy et al., 2003). AT_1-mediated p38 MAPK activation was recently implicated in cyclooxygenase-2 expression and subsequent PGE(2) release, suggesting that Ang II may play a role in mediating an inflammatory response in the heart following myocardial infarction (Scheuren et al., 2002). Beyond being linked to c-jun gene transcription, the importance of AT_1-mediated JNK activation in cardiac fibroblasts has not been studied (Murasawa et al., 2000). Both ERK and JNK activation by AT_1 in cardiac fibroblasts are largely Ca^{2+}-dependent, proceeding through the intracellular Ca^{2+}-sensitive proline-rich tyrosine kinase, PYK2 and (at least for ERK) Src (Murasawa et al., 1998a, b; Zou et al., 1998; Wang et al., 1999; Murasawa et al., 2000), although for both MAPKs, a contribution from PKC activation has been noted (Booz et al., 1994; Murasawa et al., 2000). The mechanism of AT_1-mediated p38 MAPK activation in cardiac fibroblasts has not been well studied, although one report provided evidence that AT_1 may also activate the three primary MAPK cascades through NAD(P)H-mediated ROS generation (Sano et al., 2001).

AT_1 activates the major MAPK signaling cascades in cardiac myocytes as well: ERK via PKC (Zou et al., 1998), JNK via Ca^{2+} and PKC (Kudoh et al., 1997), and p38 via NAD(P)H oxidase and ROS generation (Wenzel et al., 2001). ERK activation by AT_1 has been implicated in pH_i recovery from acid load via Na^+–HCO_3^- cotransporter activation (Baetz et al., 2002), as well as induction of the fetal gene program (e.g., β-major histocompatibility complex (MHC) promoter activity and ANP expression (Aoki et al., 2000; Shih et al., 2001). Although the ERKs were implicated in AT_1-mediated 'activation' of translation elongation factor-2 in cardiac myocytes (Everett et al., 2001), the contribution of the ERKs to Ang II-induced protein synthesis appears to require other signaling cascades (such as PI3K and protein kinase B), and be dependent upon the age of the animal (Aoki et al., 2000; Ruf et al., 2002). Together with p38 MAPK activation, the ERKs have been implicated in AT_1-induced prostacyclin secretion from cardiac myocytes (Rebsamen et al., 2003). The p38 MAPK and JNK pathways, which play a role in Ang II-induced AP-1 binding activity, are responsible for increased TGF-β1 and endothelin-1 gene expression, respectively, in cardiac myocytes by AT_1 activation (Kudoh et al., 1997; Wenzel et al., 2001).

Novel signaling

Although AT_1 does not have intrinsic tyrosine kinase activity, the receptor couples to the activation of both nonreceptor (e.g., PYK2, Src and Jak family kinases, and FAK) and receptor (those for epidermal growth factor, platelet-derived growth factor, and insulin growth factor) tyrosine kinases (Berry et al., 2001; Guo et al., 2001). In some cases, the exact means by which AT_1 couples to the tyrosine kinase activation is not known, although with others activation has been shown to involve Ca^{2+} and/or PKC, in whole or in part. In addition, AT_1 has been shown to activate small G-proteins, including: Ras, which plays a role in Ang II-induced proliferation of cardiac fibroblasts (Murasawa et al., 1998b), and members of the Rho family, which have been implicated in Ang II-induced hypertrophy, fetal gene expression, and JNK activation of cardiac myocytes (Kudoh et al., 1997; Aikawa et al., 2000; Takemoto et al., 2001; Laufs et al., 2002).

Reactive oxygen species

Ang II induces the generation of ROS in cardiac myocytes, via AT_1-mediated activation of a membrane-bound NAD(P)H oxidase. Recently, ROS generation was implicated in Ang II-induced hypertrophy of cardiac myocytes via NF-κB activation, which involved the ROS-sensitive, mitogen-activated protein kinase, ASK1 and, presumably, p38 (Hirotani et al., 2002). ROS may also contribute to the pathophysiology of heart failure by exerting direct negative inotropic effects on the heart, and by initiating cardiac myocyte apoptosis. AT_1-mediated p38 MAPK activation due to ROS generation could underlie the reports of Ang II-induced cardiac myocyte apoptosis (Leri et al., 2000; Ravassa et al., 2000). Ang II was shown to induce apoptosis in cardiomyocytes from failing hearts by p38 MAPK activation linked to increased Fas ligand and decreased cyclin D_1 expression (Sharov et al., 2003). Additionally, AT_1-mediated ERK activation may enhance cardiac myocyte apoptosis by inactivating the cytoprotective transcription factor STAT3 (Booz et al., 2003).

Jak-STAT

As do cytokine receptors and receptor tyrosine kinases, AT_1 activates the tyrosine-phosphorylation based Jak-STAT signaling pathway. Jaks are nonreceptor tyrosine kinases, either constitutively associated with the cytoplasmic region of certain receptors, or recruited to a receptor upon ligand binding. Ligand-induced receptor oligomerization, brings about aggregation of associated Jaks, and subsequent activation via *trans*-autophosphorylation. Activated Jaks can recruit specific signal transducers and activators of transcription (STATs), by binding their SH2 domains, or by creating tyrosine-phosphorylated docking sites for STATs on the receptor or receptor-associated adapter protein. Recruited STATs are phosphorylated by Jaks, inducing their dimerization via intermolecular SH2-phosphotyrosine interactions. Dimerized STATs translocate to the nucleus, and induce expression of certain genes by binding target DNA sequences. AT_1 activates all three Jak family members expressed in the heart, Jak1, Jak2, and Tyk2 (Booz et al., 2002); however, only the mechanism behind AT_1-mediated Jak2 activation has been characterized, principally by studies on vascular smooth muscle cells. The cytoplasmic tail of AT_1 contains a YIPP motif (aa 319–322) important for activation and recruitment of Jak2 (Ali et al., 1997), which are temporally distinct events that do not require AT_1 Y319 phosphorylation (Ali et al., 2000). Association of Jak2 with AT_1

requires prior activation and SHP-2 acting as an adaptor protein (Marrero et al., 1998; Ali et al., 2000). Jak-receptor association is not necessary for AT_1-induced tyrosine phosphorylation of STATs; however, association is required for STAT recruitment to AT_1, and possibly, nuclear translocation (Ali et al., 2000; Sayeski et al., 2001). Conflicting reports suggest that AT_1 can couple to Jak2 activation by different means depending upon cell type or conditions. A conventional route involves PLC activation, with the subsequent rise in intracellular Ca^{2+} and activation of PKC serving to activate Jak2 through PYK2 (Frank et al., 2002). Others report that AT_1-induced Jak2 activation does not require Ca^{2+}, or even heterotrimeric G-protein activation, but proceeds through the generation of ROS by a mechanism involving the Rho family of small G-proteins (Doan et al., 2001; Pelletier et al., 2003).

There are seven members of the mammalian STAT family. In cardiac fibroblasts, AT_1 couples to STAT1 activation, the significance of which has not been established (Bhat et al., 1994). In cardiac myocytes, AT_1 has been shown to activate more STAT family members than any other stimulus (Booz et al., 2002). In addition, paracrine or autocrine release of Ang II has been implicated in activation of the Jak-STAT pathway in hearts by pressure overload or ischemia, and in cardiac myocytes by mechanical stretch. The principal STAT family members activated by AT_1 in cardiac myocytes are STATs 1 and 3, which have opposing roles: STAT1 has been implicated in apoptosis, while STAT3 is cytoprotective. Ang II-induced STAT1 activation is biphasic, with peaks at 15 and 120 min. Early STAT3 activation has either not been observed, or is modest and short-lived (Booz et al., 2003). More robust activation of STAT3 occurs after 2 hours and is caused by the upregulation of IL-6-related cytokines.

The STATs play an important role in Ao gene expression in cardiac myocytes. Ang II-induced Ao gene upregulation by AT_1-mediated STAT3 and STAT6 activation may constitute part of an autocrine, positive-feedback loop that contributes to cardiac hypertrophy *in vivo* (Booz et al., 2002). The STATs have also been implicated in enhanced Ao gene expression by cardiac myocytes induced by ischemia/reperfusion or cardiotrophin-1. The observation that two hypertrophic agonists, Ang II and cardiotrophin-1 induce each other's synthesis by cardiac myocytes suggests the possibility of synergism between the two in affecting cardiac hypertrophy *in vivo*.

Receptor transactivations/interactions

In cardiac fibroblasts, AT_1-induced ERK activation and mitogenic signaling (i.e., c-fos expression and DNA synthesis) are predominantly mediated by transactivation of the epidermal growth factor (EGF) receptor (Murasawa et al., 1998a; Wang et al., 2000; Seta and Sadoshima, 2003). Unlike AT_1, the EGF receptor continues to signal after it is internalized and, therefore, AT_1-mediated EGF receptor transactivation sets into motion the prolonged ERK activation necessary for inducing growth. Ang II induces tyrosine phosphorylation of the EGF receptor and its association with Shc and Grb2, leading to subsequent activation of the Ras-Raf-MEK-ERK1/2 cascade. The process of transactivation is specific for ERK signaling, and does not contribute to AT_1-mediated activation of Src, Jak2, or JNK (Murasawa et al., 1998a, Seta and Sadoshima, 2003). The mechanism of AT_1-mediated EGF receptor transactivation in cardiac fibroblasts is unclear, but does not involve autocrine release of EGF (Murasawa et al., 1998a). Evidence for and against involvement of Ca^{2+}/calmodulin has been reported (Murasawa et al., 1998a, b; Wang et al., 2000). Ca^{2+}-dependent EGF receptor transactivation proceeds through PYK2 in cooperation with Src-kinases. Other findings indicate that ROS may be involved in the transactivation process (Wang et al., 2000).

Seta and Sadoshima (2003) recently investigated the structural determinants of AT_1 involved in EGF receptor transactivation, and established the importance of Ang II-induced phosphorylation of Y319 within the conserved YIPP motif of the AT_1 carboxyl terminus. They demonstrated a transient association of AT_1 with the EGF receptor through SHP-2 acting as a scaffolding protein. The role of Y319 phosphorylation was specific for EGF receptor transactivation because Ang II-induced activation of other tyrosine kinases (Src and Jak2) was preserved in cells expressing AT_1-Y319F. The importance of AT_1-EGF receptor association to the mitogenic actions of Ang II was confirmed by experiments showing that overexpression of wild type AT_1 in cardiac fibroblasts enhanced Ang II-induced proliferation, while expression of AT_1-Y319F did not.

The low number of AT_1 on cultured ventricular myocytes makes it difficult to investigate the role of EGF receptor transactivation in Ang II-induced cardiomyocyte hypertrophy. However, using adenovirus to enhance AT_1 expression in neonatal rat ventricular myocytes, Thomas et al. (2002), recently demonstrated AT_1-mediated EGF receptor tyrosine phosphorylation, which was Ca^{2+}-independent but involved, in part, shedding of extracellular heparin-bound EGF. AT_1 overexpression enhanced Ang II-induced cardiac hypertrophy, and this response could be inhibited by an EGF receptor antagonist. In these studies, the increases in AT_1 levels were comparable to what might be observed *in vivo* in response to cardiac stress, supporting the possibility that EGF transactivation is involved in pathological hypertrophy of the heart.

Circumstantial evidence suggests that some sort of interaction of AT_1 with the Fas receptor contributes to Ang II-induced cardiomyocyte hypertrophy. Although the Fas/Fas ligand system is a potent activator of apoptosis in many cell types, at submaximal levels of Fas ligand, the Fas receptor has been linked to cardiac hypertrophy (Badorff et al., 2002). This response of Fas receptor activation proceeds through inactivation of glycogen synthase kinase 3β (GSK3β), a negative regulator of cardiomyocyte hypertrophy. Fas receptor activation was shown to induce hypertrophy of cultured cardiomyocytes and, in response to pressure overload, mice lacking a functional Fas receptor demonstrated rapid-onset left ventricular dilation and failure due to the absence of compensatory hypertrophy. Intriguingly, cardiomyocytes from these mice showed a significantly attenuated hypertrophic response to Ang II *in vitro* (Badorff et al., 2002).

AT_1 was recently reported to form functional heterodimers with two seven-transmembrane domain receptors, the bradykinin B_2 and the angiotensin II type 2 (AT_2) receptors, which generally activate responses that are antagonistic to the actions of AT_1. Dimerization of AT_1 with the B_2 receptor resulted in increased activation of $G\alpha_q$ and phospholipase C by Ang II, while the potency and efficacy of bradykinin in forming inositol phosphates was decreased (AbdAlla et al., 2000). In contrast, heterodimerization of AT_2 with AT_1 antagonized the function of AT_1 (AbdAlla et al., 2001). Surprisingly, AT_2-mediated inhibition was found to be independent of AT_2 activation and signaling, suggesting that AT_2 functions in part as an AT_1 antagonist.

Carboxyl terminal-dependent signaling

The cytoplasmic tail of AT_1 is important for receptor desensitization and internalization (Thomas, 1999; Guo et al., 2001). Because of a nuclear localization sequence, the carboxyl terminus of AT_1 may also target some internalized receptor to the nucleus (Lu et al., 1998). In addition to these functions, the tail plays an important role in intracellular signaling. Activation of PLCγ by AT_1 requires binding of the phospholipase to the YIPP motif that is phosphorylated upon agonist binding (Venema et al., 1998). Accumulating evidence indicates that the AT_1 tail may also couple to intracellular signaling events in a G-protein-independent manner by binding β-arrestins, which can then serve as scaffolds for the recruitment of signaling molecules (Tohgo et al., 2002). G-protein-independent, but tail-dependent, coupling of AT_1 to Src and ERK activation was recently reported (Seta et al., 2002). Whether heterotrimeric

G protein-dependent and -independent signaling by AT₁ have different roles to play in mediating the cellular response to Ang II will need to be determined.

Paracrine/autocrine actions of Ang II

Both ventricular cardiac myocytes and fibroblasts express all RAS components (Dostal et al., 2000). Production of Ao is under negative and positive feedback control of Ang II in cardiac fibroblasts and myocytes, respectively. Other stimuli that upregulate Ao gene expression by cardiac myocytes are cardiotrophin-1 (Fukuzawa et al., 2000), ischemia (Mascareno et al., 2001), mechanical stretch (Mascareno et al., 1998; Leri et al., 2000; Tamura et al., 2000), and pressure overload (Baker et al., 1990). Moreover, increased Ao production has been shown to contribute to cardiac myocyte hypertrophy in an autocrine manner in the case of cardiotrophin-1, mechanical stretch, and pressure overload. Ang II also stimulates cardiac myocyte hypertrophy in an autocrine manner due to enhanced endothelin-1 production (Ito et al., 1993), while Ang II-stimulated adrenomedullin production may serve to attenuate hypertrophy (Tsuruda et al., 2001).

We have documented that cardiac fibroblasts secrete a factor that upregulates Ao gene expression by cardiac myocytes, which could also lead to hypertrophy (Booz et al., 1999). Others have shown that Ang II stimulation of cardiac fibroblasts upregulates the production of hypertrophic factors for cardiac myocytes, including TGF-β1, endothelin-1, and the IL-6-related cytokines, LIF and cardiotrophin-1 (Gray et al., 1998; Sano et al., 2000). Like Ang II, endothelin-1 and cardiotrophin-1 have also been shown to stimulate cardiac fibroblast proliferation. Thus, local Ang II production in the heart more than likely contributes to pathological cardiac remodeling, by activating self-sustaining paracrine/autocrine loops involving both cardiac fibroblasts and myocytes.

Intracrine actions of Ang II

The most extensively studied and widely accepted mode of action of Ang II is through extracellular binding to the AT₁ plasma membrane receptor; however, the concept that Ang II acts intracellularly is gaining increasing support. Intracellular action does not require intracellular synthesis of Ang II, as presence inside the cell could also be due to uptake from the circulation by AT_1-mediated internalization. In addition to studies showing the presence of RAS components inside cells and increased concentrations of intracellular Ang II in diabetic and hypertensive patients (Frustaci et al., 2000), circumstantial evidence of intracellular Ang II action comes from studies showing the presence of intracellular Ang II binding sites (Booz et al., 1992; Tang et al., 1992). Direct evidence comes from recent observations that intracellular Ang II promotes growth in vascular smooth muscle cells and hepatocytes (Filipeanu et al., 2001). In cardiac myocytes, stimulation of voltage-operated Ca^{2+} channels and regulation of inward Ca^{2+} current by intracellular Ang II have also been reported (De Mello, 1998; Eto et al., 2002).

Our recent studies have shown that increased intracellular levels of Ang II in cardiac myocytes result in development of biventricular cardiac hypertrophy in the mouse. A plasmid construct that expressed Ang II peptide under control of the α-myosin heavy chain promoter, resulted in increased Ang II in cardiac ventricles and a 68 percent increase in the heart to body weight ratio over 96 hours. Intracellular Ang II increased cardiac mRNA levels of several genes, including c-jun, insulin-like growth factor-1, and TGF-β. Additionally, adenovirus-mediated delivery and expression of Ang II in cultured neonatal rat ventricular myocytes resulted in hypertrophic cell growth, as indexed by cell size and ^{3}H-leucine incorporation. The signaling mechanisms responsible for the growth effect of intracellular Ang II on cardiac myocytes are not known, nor has the physiological significance of intracellular Ang II been established. However, our working hypothesis is that the upregulation of cardiac myocyte Ao gene expression that occurs in response to hypertension or myocardial ischemia, amplifies and/or sustains cardiac myocyte growth, in part, through an intracellular Ang II-mediated process.

Summary

Cardiac hypertrophy is associated with an increased risk of morbidity and mortality, and thus determining the molecular mechanisms of cardiac myocyte hypertrophy should have significant impact on human health. The RAS has a major role in the development of cardiac hypertrophy, in response to pressure or volume overload, and ischemic damage. Although the 'traditional' RAS is systemic in nature, localized systems have now been well characterized in many organs and tissues and shown to have physiological and pathological relevance. We and others have presented evidence demonstrating the presence of an active RAS in cardiac tissue and have provided indirect evidence that the cardiac RAS is involved in pathological cardiac remodeling *in vivo*. Most of the effects of Ang II, the active octapeptide of the RAS, are mediated by the high affinity plasma membrane, G-protein-coupled receptor, AT_1. The signaling pathways that couple AT_1 to hypertrophy of cardiac myocytes, and proliferation and ECM deposition of cardiac fibroblasts have been extensively studied, and include both canonical, i.e., G-protein-associated, and novel mechanisms. Several studies have also suggested that Ang II acts intracellularly, possibly by activating ion channels, and gene transcription via direct binding to chromatin or an AT_1-like nuclear receptor. Our recent *in vivo* and *in vitro* studies demonstrating that intracellular Ang II induces hypertrophic growth of cardiac myocytes, suggests an additional mechanism by which Ang II controls physiological or pathological growth of the heart.

References

AbdAlla S, Lother H and Quitterer U (2000) AT_1-receptor heterodimers show enhanced G-protein activation and altered receptor sequestration. *Nature* **407**, 94–98.

AbdAlla S, Lother H, Abdel-tawab AM and Quitterer U (2001) The angiotensin II AT_2 receptor is an AT_1 receptor antagonist. *Journal of Biological Chemistry* **276**, 39721–39726.

Aikawa R, Komuro I, Nagai R and Yazaki Y (2000) Rho plays an important role in angiotensin II-induced hypertrophic responses in cardiac myocytes. *Molecular and Cellular Biochemistry* **212**, 177–182.

Ali MS, Sayeski PP, Dirksen LB, *et al.* (1997) Dependence on the motif YIPP for the physical association of Jak2 kinase with the intracellular carboxyl tail of the angiotensin II AT_1 receptor. *Journal of Biological Chemistry* **272**, 23382–23388.

Ali MS, Sayeski PP and Bernstein KE (2000) Jak2 acts as both a STAT1 kinase and as a molecular bridge linking STAT1 to the angiotensin II AT_1 receptor. *Journal of Biological Chemistry* **275**, 15586–15593.

Aoki H, Richmond M, Izumo S and Sadoshima J (2000) Specific role of the extracellular signal-regulated kinase pathway in angiotensin II-induced cardiac hypertrophy *in vitro*. *Biochemical Journal* **347**, 275–284.

Autelitano DJ, Ridings R, Pipolo L and Thomas WG (2003) Adrenomedullin inhibits angiotensin AT_{1A} receptor expression and function in cardiac fibroblasts. *Regulatory Peptides* **112**, 131–137.

Bader M (2002) Role of the local renin–angiotensin system in cardiac damage: a minireview focusing on transgenic animal models. *Journal of Molecular and Cellular Cardiology* **34**, 1455–1462.

Bader M, Peters J, Baltatu O, *et al.* (2001) Tissue renin–angiotensin systems: new insights from experimental animal models in hypertension research. *Journal of Molecular Medicine* **79**, 76–102.

Badorff C, Ruetten H, Mueller S, et al. (2002) Fas receptor signaling inhibits glycogen synthase kinase 3β and induces cardiac hypertrophy following pressure overload. *Journal of Clinical Investigation* **109**, 373–381.

Baetz D, Haworth RS, Avkiran M and Feuvray D (2002) The ERK pathway regulates $Na^+–HCO_3^-$ cotransport activity in adult rat cardiomyocytes. *American Journal of Physiology: Heart and Circulatory Physiology* **283**, H2102–H2109.

Baker KM, Chernin MI, Wixson SK and Aceto JF (1990) Renin-angiotensin system involvement in pressure-overload cardiac hypertrophy in rats. *American Journal of Physiology* **259**, H324–H332.

Berry C, Touyz R, Dominiczak AF, et al. (2001) Angiotensin receptors: signaling, vascular pathophysiology, and interactions with ceramide. *American Journal of Physiology: Heart and Circulatory Physiology* **281**, H2337–H2365.

Bhat GJ, Thekkumkara TJ, Thomas WG, et al. (1994) Angiotensin II stimulates *sis*-inducing factor-like DNA binding activity. Evidence that the AT_{1A} receptor activates transcription factor-Stat91 and/or a related protein. *Journal of Biological Chemistry* **269**, 31443–31449.

Booz GW and Baker KM (1995) Molecular signalling mechanisms controlling growth and function of cardiac fibroblasts. *Cardiovascular Research* **30**, 537–543.

Booz GW and Baker KM (1996) The role of the renin–angiotensin system in the pathophysiology of cardiac remodeling. *Blood Pressure* **5** (Suppl 2), 10–18.

Booz GW and Baker KM (1998) Actions of angiotensin II on isolated cardiac myocytes. *Heart Failure Reviews* **3**, 125–130.

Booz GW, Conrad KM, Hess AL, et al. (1992) Angiotensin-II-binding sites on hepatocyte nuclei. *Endocrinology* **130**, 3641–3649.

Booz GW, Dostal DE, Singer HA and Baker KM (1994) Involvement of protein kinase C and Ca^{2+} in angiotensin II-induced mitogenesis of cardiac fibroblasts. *American Journal of Physiology* **267**, C1308–C1318.

Booz GW, Dostal DE and Baker KM (1999) Paracrine actions of cardiac fibroblasts on cardiomyocytes: implications for the cardiac renin–angiotensin system. *American Journal of Cardiology* **83**, 44H–47H.

Booz GW, Day JN and Baker KM (2002) Interplay between the cardiac renin angiotensin system and Jak-STAT signaling: role in cardiac hypertrophy, ischemia/reperfusion dysfunction, and heart failure. *Journal of Molecular and Cellular Cardiology* **34**, 1443–1453.

Booz GW, Day JNE and Baker KM (2003) Angiotensin II effects on STAT3 phosphorylation in cardiomyocytes: evidence for Erk-dependent Tyr705 dephosphorylation. *Basic Research in Cardiology* **98**, 33–38.

Clausmeyer S, Reinecke A, Farrenkopf R, et al. (2000) Tissue-specific expression of a rat renin transcript lacking the coding sequence for the prefragment and its stimulation by myocardial infarction. *Endocrinology* **141**, 2963–2970.

Cowling RT, Gurantz D, Peng JF, et al. (2002) Transcription factor NF-κB is necessary for up-regulation of type 1 angiotensin II receptor mRNA in rat cardiac fibroblasts treated with tumor necrosis factor-α or interleukin-1β. *Journal of Biological Chemistry* **277**, 5719–5724.

De Mello WC (1998) Intracellular angiotensin II regulates the inward calcium current in cardiac myocytes. *Hypertension* **32**, 976–982.

Doan TN, Ali MS and Bernstein KE (2001) Tyrosine kinase activation by the angiotensin II receptor in the absence of calcium signaling. *Journal of Biological Chemistry* **276**, 20954–20958.

Dostal DE and Baker KM (1992) Angiotensin II stimulation of left ventricular hypertrophy in adult rat heart. Mediation by the AT$_1$ receptor. *American Journal of Hypertension* **5**, 276–280.

Dostal DE, Booz GW and Baker KM (2000) Regulation of angiotensinogen gene expression and protein in neonatal rat cardiac fibroblasts by glucocorticoid and β-adrenergic stimulation. *Basic Research in Cardiology* **95**, 485–491.

Endo-Mochizuki Y, Mochizuki N, Sawa H, et al. (1995) Expression of renin and angiotensin-converting enzyme in human hearts. *Heart and Vessels* **10**, 285–293.

Eto K, Ohya Y, Nakamura Y, et al. (2002) Intracellular angiotensin II stimulates voltage-operated Ca^{2+} channels in arterial myocytes. *Hypertension* **39**, 474–478.

Everett AD, Stoops TD, Nairn AC and Brautigan D (2001) Angiotensin II regulates phosphorylation of translation elongation factor-2 in cardiac myocytes. *American Journal of Physiology: Heart and Circulatory Physiology* **281**, H161–H167.

Filipeanu CM, Henning RH, de Zeeuw D and Nelemans A (2001) Intracellular Angiotensin II and cell growth of vascular smooth muscle cells. *British Journal of Pharmacology* **132**, 1590–1596.

Frank GD, Saito S, Motley ED, et al. (2002) Requirement of Ca^{2+} and PKCδ for Janus kinase 2 activation by angiotensin II: involvement of PYK2. *Molecular Endocrinology* **16**, 367–377.

Frey N and Olson EN (2003) Cardiac hypertrophy: the good, the bad, and the ugly. *Annual Review of Physiology* **65**, 45–79.

Frustaci A, Kajstura J, Chimenti C, et al. (2000) Myocardial cell death in human diabetes. *Circulation Research* **87**, 1123–1132.

Fukuzawa J, Booz GW, Hunt RA, et al. (2000) Cardiotrophin-1 increases angiotensinogen mRNA in rat cardiac myocytes through STAT3: an autocrine loop for hypertrophy. *Hypertension* **35**, 1191–1196.

Gray MO, Long CS, Kalinyak JE, et al. (1998) Angiotensin II stimulates cardiac myocyte hypertrophy via paracrine release of TGF-β1 and endothelin-1 from fibroblasts. *Cardiovascular Research* **40**, 352–363.

Griendling KK and Ushio-Fukai M (2000) Reactive oxygen species as mediators of angiotensin II signaling. *Regulatory Peptides* **91**, 21–27.

Guo DF, Sun YL, Hamet P and Inagami T (2001) The angiotensin II type 1 receptor and receptor-associated proteins. *Cell Research* **11**, 165–180.

Harada K, Komuro I, Shiojima I, et al. (1998a) Pressure overload induces cardiac hypertrophy in angiotensin II type 1A receptor knockout mice. *Circulation* **97**, 1952–1959.

Harada K, Komuro I, Zou Y, et al. (1998b) Acute pressure overload could induce hypertrophic responses in the heart of angiotensin II type 1a knockout mice. *Circulation Research* **82**, 779–785.

Harada K, Sugaya T, Murakami K, et al. (1999) Angiotensin II type 1A receptor knockout mice display less left ventricular remodeling and improved survival after myocardial infarction. *Circulation* **100**, 2093–2099.

Herzig TC, Jobe SM, Aoki H, et al. (1997) Angiotensin II type$_{1a}$ receptor gene expression in the heart: AP-1 and GATA-4 participate in the response to pressure overload. *Proceedings of the National Academy of Sciences of the United States of America* **94**, 7543–7548.

Hirotani S, Otsu K, Nishida K, et al. (2002) Involvement of nuclear factor-κB and apoptosis signal-regulating kinase 1 in G-protein-coupled receptor agonist-induced cardiomyocyte hypertrophy. *Circulation* **105**, 509–515.

Hoffmann S, Krause T, van Geel PP, et al. (2001) Overexpression of the human angiotensin II type 1 receptor in the rat heart augments load induced cardiac hypertrophy. *Journal of Molecular Medicine* **79**, 601–608.

Ito H, Hirata Y, Adachi S, et al. (1993) Endothelin-1 is an autocrine/paracrine factor in the mechanism of angiotensin II-induced hypertrophy in cultured rat cardiomyocytes. *Journal of Clinical Investigation* **92**, 398–403.

Kim S and Iwao H (2000) Molecular and cellular mechanisms of angiotensin II-mediated cardiovascular and renal diseases. *Pharmacological Reviews* **52**, 11–34.

Kudoh S, Komuro I, Mizuno T, et al. (1997) Angiotensin II stimulates c-Jun NH_2-terminal kinase in cultured cardiac myocytes of neonatal rats. *Circulation Research* **80**, 139–146.

Laufs U, Kilter H, Konkol C, et al. (2002) Impact of HMG CoA reductase inhibition on small GTPases in the heart. *Cardiovascular Research* **53**, 911–920.

Leri A, Fiordaliso F, Setoguchi M, et al. (2000) Inhibition of p53 function prevents renin–angiotensin system activation and stretch-mediated myocyte apoptosis. *American Journal of Pathology* **157**, 843–857.

Lu D, Yang H, Shaw G and Raizada MK (1998) Angiotensin II-induced nuclear targeting of the angiotensin type 1 (AT_1) receptor in brain neurons. *Endocrinology* **139**, 365–375.

Marrero MB, Venema VJ, Ju H, et al. (1998) Regulation of angiotensin II-induced Jak2 tyrosine phosphorylation: roles of SHP-1 and SHP-2. *American Journal of Physiology: Cell Physiology* **275**, C1216–C1223.

Mascareno E, Dhar M and Siddiqui MAQ (1998) Signal transduction and activator of transcription (STAT) protein-dependent activation of angiotensinogen promoter: a cellular signal for hypertrophy in cardiac muscle. *Proceedings of the National Academy of Sciences of the United States of America* **95**, 5590–5594.

Mascareno E, El-Shafei M, Maulik N, et al. (2001) Jak/STAT signaling is associated with cardiac dysfunction during ischemia and reperfusion. *Circulation* **104**, 325–329.

Mazzolai L, Nussberger J, Aubert JF, et al. (1998) Blood pressure-independent cardiac hypertrophy induced by locally activated renin–angiotensin system. *Hypertension* **31**, 1324–1330.

Mazzolai L, Pedrazzini T, Nicoud F, et al. (2000) Increased cardiac angiotensin II levels induce right and left ventricular hypertrophy in normotensive mice. *Hypertension* **35**, 985–991.

Murasawa S, Mori Y, Nozawa Y, et al. (1998a) Angiotensin II type 1 receptor-induced extracellular signal-regulated protein kinase activation is mediated by Ca^{2+}/calmodulin-dependent transactivation of epidermal growth factor receptor. *Circulation Research* **82**, 1338–1348.

Murasawa S, Mori Y, Nozawa Y, et al. (1998b) Role of calcium-sensitive tyrosine kinase Pyk2/CAKβ/RAFTK in angiotensin II induced Ras/ERK signaling. *Hypertension* **32**, 668–675.

Murasawa S, Matsubara H, Mori Y, et al. (2000) Angiotensin II initiates tyrosine kinase Pyk2-dependent signalings leading to activation of Rac1-mediated c-Jun NH_2-terminal kinase. *Journal of Biological Chemistry* **275**, 26856–26863.

Nagata K, Somura F, Obata K, et al. (2002) AT_1 receptor blockade reduces cardiac calcineurin activity in hypertensive rats. *Hypertension* **40**, 168–174.

Pelletier S, Duhamel F, Coulombe P, et al. (2003) Rho family GTPases are required for activation of Jak/STAT signaling by G protein-coupled receptors. *Molecular and Cellular Biology* **23**, 1316–1333.

Peng JF, Gurantz D, Tran V, et al. (2002) Tumor necrosis factor-α-induced AT₁ receptor upregulation enhances angiotensin II-mediated cardiac fibroblast responses that favor fibrosis. *Circulation Research* **91**, 1119–1126.

Ravassa S, Fortuno MA, Gonzalez A, et al. (2000) Mechanisms of increased susceptibility to angiotensin II-induced apoptosis in ventricular cardiomyocytes of spontaneously hypertensive rats. *Hypertension* **36**, 1065–1071.

Rebsamen MC, Capoccia R, Vallotton MB and Lang U (2003) Role of cyclooxygenase 2, p38 and p42/44 MAPK in the secretion of prostacyclin induced by epidermal growth factor, endothelin-1 and angiotensin II in rat ventricular cardiomyocytes. *Journal of Molecular and Cellular Cardiology* **35**, 81–89.

Ruf S, Piper HM and Schlüter KD (2002) Specific role for the extracellular signal-regulated kinase pathway in angiotensin II – but not phenylephrine-induced cardiac hypertrophy *in vitro*. *Pflügers Archiv* **443**, 483–490.

Sadoshima J, Xu Y, Slayter HS and Izumo S (1993) Autocrine release of angiotensin II mediates stretch-induced hypertrophy of cardiac myocytes *in vitro*. *Cell* **75**, 977–984.

Sano M, Fukuda K, Kodama H, et al. (2000) Interleukin-6 family of cytokines mediate angiotensin II-induced cardiac hypertrophy in rodent cardiomyocytes. *Journal of Biological Chemistry* **275**, 29717–29723.

Sano M, Fukuda K, Sato T, et al. (2001) ERK and p38 MAPK, but not NFκB, are critically involved in reactive oxygen species-mediated induction of IL-6 by angiotensin II in cardiac fibroblasts. *Circulation Research* **89**, 661–669.

Sayeski PP, Ali MS, Frank SJ and Bernstein KE (2001) The angiotensin II-dependent nuclear translocation of Stat1 is mediated by the Jak2 protein motif [231]YRFRR. *Journal of Biological Chemistry* **276**, 10556–10563.

Scheuren N, Jacobs M, Ertl G and Schorb W (2002) Cyclooxygenase-2 in myocardium stimulation by angiotensin-II in cultured cardiac fibroblasts and role at acute myocardial infarction. *Journal of Molecular and Cellular Cardiology* **34**, 29–37.

Schorb W, Peeler TC, Madigan NN, et al. (1994) Angiotensin II-induced protein tyrosine phosphorylation in neonatal rat cardiac fibroblasts. *Journal of Biological Chemistry* **269**, 19626–19632.

Seta K and Sadoshima J (2003) Phosphorylation of tyrosine 319 of the angiotensin II type 1 receptor mediates angiotensin II-induced *trans*-activation of the epidermal growth factor receptor. *Journal of Biological Chemistry* **278**, 9019–9026.

Seta K, Nanamori M, Modrall JG, et al. (2002) AT1 receptor mutant lacking heterotrimeric G protein coupling activates the Src-Ras-ERK pathway without nuclear translocation of ERKs. *Journal of Biological Chemistry* **277**, 9268–9277.

Sharov VG, Todor A, Suzuki G, et al. (2003) Hypoxia, angiotensin-II, and norepinephrine mediated apoptosis is stimulus specific in canine failed cardiomyocytes: a role for p38 MAPK, Fas-L and cyclin D_1. *European Journal of Heart Failure* **5**, 121–129.

Shih NL, Cheng TH, Loh SH, et al. (2001) Reactive oxygen species modulate angiotensin II-induced β-myosin heavy chain gene expression via Ras/Raf/extracellular signal-regulated kinase pathway in neonatal rat cardiomyocytes. *Biochemical and Biophysical Research Communications* **283**, 143–148.

Stawowy P, Goetze S, Margeta C, et al. (2003) LPS regulate ERK 1/2-dependent signaling in cardiac fibroblasts via PKC-mediated MKP-1 induction. *Biochemical and Biophysical Research Communications* **303**, 74–80.

REFERENCES

Sun Y, Zhang J, Zhang JQ and Weber KT (2001) Renin expression at sites of repair in the infarcted rat heart. *Journal of Molecular and Cellular Cardiology* **33**, 995–1003.

Taigen T, De Windt LJ, Lim HW and Molkentin JD (2000) Targeted inhibition of calcineurin prevents agonist-induced cardiomyocyte hypertrophy. *Proceedings of the National Academy of Sciences of the United States of America* **97**, 1196–1201.

Takemoto M, Node K, Nakagami H, *et al.* (2001) Statins as antioxidant therapy for preventing cardiac myocyte hypertrophy. *Journal of Clinical Investigation* **108**, 1429–1437.

Tamura K, Chen YE, Chen Q, *et al.* (2000) Expression of renin–angiotensin system and extracellular matrix genes in cardiovascular cells and its regulation through AT1 receptor. *Molecular and Cellular Biochemistry* **212**, 203–209.

Tang SS, Rogg H, Schumacher R and Dzau VJ (1992) Characterization of nuclear angiotensin-II-binding sites in rat liver and comparison with plasma membrane receptors. *Endocrinology* **131**, 374–380.

Thomas WG (1999) Regulation of angiotensin II type 1 (AT$_1$) receptor function. *Regulatory Peptides* **79**, 9–23.

Thomas WG, Brandenburger Y, Autelitano DJ, *et al.* (2002) Adenoviral-directed expression of the type 1A angiotensin receptor promotes cardiomyocyte hypertrophy via transactivation of the epidermal growth factor receptor. *Circulation Research* **90**, 135–142.

Tohgo A, Pierce KL, Choy EW, *et al.* (2002) β-Arrestin scaffolding of the ERK cascade enhances cytosolic ERK activity but inhibits ERK-mediated transcription following angiotensin AT1a receptor stimulation. *Journal of Biological Chemistry* **277**, 9429–9436.

Tsuruda T, Kato J, Kitamura K, *et al.* (2001) Roles of protein kinase C and Ca^{2+}-dependent signaling in angiotensin II-induced adrenomedullin production in rat cardiac myocytes. *Journal of Hypertension* **19**, 757–763.

Venema RC, Ju H, Venema VJ, *et al.* (1998) Angiotensin II-induced association of phospholipase Cγ1 with the G-protein-coupled AT$_1$ receptor. *Journal of Biological Chemistry* **273**, 7703–7708.

Wang D, Yu X and Brecher P (1999) Nitric oxide inhibits angiotensin II-induced activation of the calcium-sensitive tyrosine kinase proline-rich tyrosine kinase 2 without affecting epidermal growth factor receptor transactivation. *Journal of Biological Chemistry* **274**, 24342–24348.

Wang D, Yu X, Cohen RA and Brecher P (2000) Distinct effects of N-acetylcysteine and nitric oxide on angiotensin II-induced epidermal growth factor receptor phosphorylation and intracellular Ca^{2+} levels. *Journal of Biological Chemistry* **275**, 12223–12230.

Wenzel S, Taimor G, Piper HM and Schluter KD (2001) Redox-sensitive intermediates mediate angiotensin II-induced p38 MAP kinase activation, AP-1 binding activity, and TGF-β expression in adult ventricular cardiomyocytes. *FASEB Journal* **15**, 2291–2293.

Zou Y, Komuro I, Yamazaki T, Kudoh S, *et al.* (1998) Cell type-specific angiotensin II-evoked signal transduction pathways: critical roles of G$_{βγ}$ subunit, Src family, and Ras in cardiac fibroblasts. *Circulation Research* **82**, 337–345.

2

Cardiac Physiology and the Renin Angiotensin System: Lessons from Transgenic Animal Models

Alisdair Ryding and John J. Mullins

Introduction

The influence of the renin angiotensin system (RAS) on cardiac function and remodelling has long been appreciated. Not only does the RAS contribute to hypertension, it is also strongly implicated in cardiac hypertrophy, interstitial fibrosis, post-myocardial infarction remodelling, contractile dysfunction and vascular injury (De Mello and Danser, 2000; Ruiz-Ortega *et al.*, 2001).

In this chapter we review the application of transgenic techniques to understanding cardiac RAS physiology. In particular we address specific questions about the exact nature and mechanism of interaction between the RAS and the heart. Many of these questions can only be addressed satisfactorily by transgenic techniques. Firstly, does cardiac expression of RAS components exert effects on the heart? Does angiotensin II have direct hypertrophic effects on cardiomyocytes independently of its effect on blood pressure? Does the local RAS have effects on the heart distinct from the circulating RAS? Can prorenin exert biological functions independent of renin?

An overview of transgenesis

An exhaustive review of transgenic techniques is beyond the scope of this work, and the reader is referred to more detailed reviews (Lewandoski, 2001; Ryding et al., 2001).

Transgenic techniques allow the genetic manipulation of whole animals (usually mice) by introducing genetic changes in pluripotent cells, either fertilized eggs or mouse embryonic stem cells (ES cells). The strategy is either to introduce DNA encoding a specific gene (transgene) that will be overexpressed, or to disrupt ('knockout') a specific genetic locus within the genome. These two strategies are summarized in Figures 2.1 and 2.2, respectively.

Incorporation of specific promoters into a construct can direct transgene expression to a specific cell type, tissue, or developmental stage. For example the αMHC promoter is widely used to target transgene

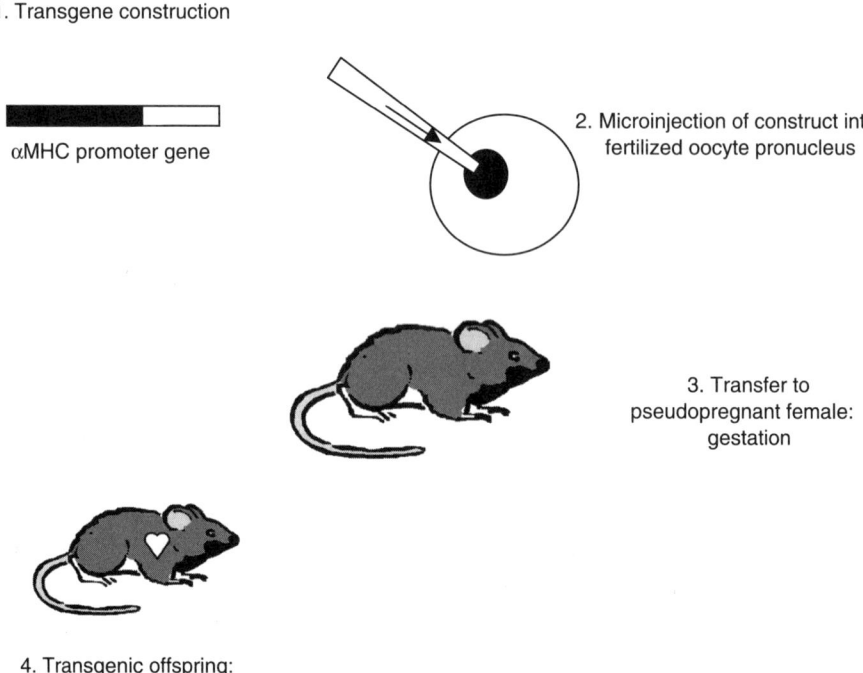

Figure 2.1 Generation of animals with cardiac-specific transgene expression. 1. Expression vector including gene of interest and cardiac specific promoter (e.g., αMHC) is constructed. 2. Vector is microinjected into the pronucleus of a fertilized oocyte. 3. Oocytes transferred to surrogate mother and allowed to reach gestation. 4. Transgenic offspring born, with cardiac specific transgene expression

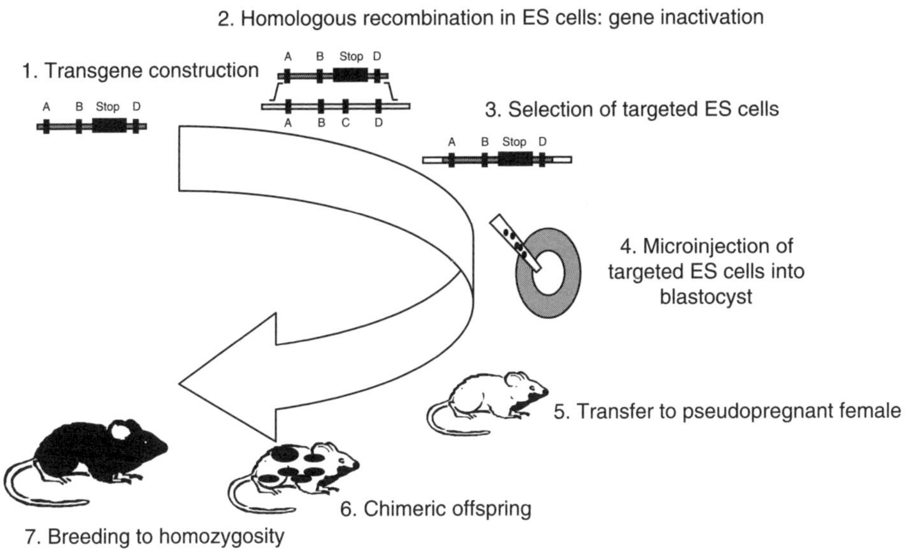

Figure 2.2 Generation of gene-targeted mice. 1. Gene-targeting vector is constructed. 2. Vector recombines with target gene in ES cells. 3. ES cells with the desired gene-targeting event are selected. 4. and 5. Targeted ES cells are microinjected into normal blastocysts and transferred to surrogate mother. 6. Chimeric offspring derived from blastocyst and ES cells are born. 7. Breeding from chimeras allows generation of heterozygotes, and eventually homozygotes for the gene deletion

expression to cardiomyocytes (Palermo *et al.*, 1996). Advanced knockout strategies take advantage of a bacterial phage enzyme (*Cre*) that mediates site-specific homologous recombination, allowing tissue-specific and even time-dependent disruption of targeted genes. Therefore, it is possible to produce animals that overexpress or completely lack a gene, and this can be controlled in time and place.

A further layer of sophistication is the addition of a marker molecule into the construct to allow identification of cells that express the transgene and, by implication, the wild-type gene. Such markers include fluorescent proteins (e.g., green fluorescent protein) or the chromogenic enzyme β-galactosidase. Genetically tagging cells in this way is a powerful method of determining the distribution and timing of gene expression.

Transgenic evidence of a cardiac-based RAS

Cardiac expression of most, if not all RAS components has been detected either in normal healthy hearts, or during disease processes such as cardiac hypertrophy or post-myocardial infarction remodelling (Danser et al., 1999). Such evidence has suggested the existence of a cardiac-based RAS. However, studying the cardiac RAS has been problematical because it is difficult to isolate the heart from the rest of the circulation.

A major strength of transgenic models is the feasibility of targeting transgene expression to specific tissues or cell types. Furthermore, selecting species-specific transgenes allows endogenous and transgene-derived products to be distinguished. Therefore transgenic models provide a useful tool for demonstrating the existence of the cardiac RAS, and for investigating its role.

Cardiac-specific overexpression of single components of the RAS demonstrates that this is sufficient to activate the RAS within the heart, with detrimental effects. Mice transgenic for mouse angiotensinogen under the cardiac-specific α-major histocompatibility complex (αMHC) promoter demonstrate activation of the cardiac RAS, causing cardiac hypertrophy without fibrosis (Mazzolai et al., 1998, 2000). This effect was independent of blood pressure in single-renin gene strains of mice, whilst two gene strains demonstrated an increase in blood pressure caused by systemic activation of the RAS. Similarly, cardiac-specific overexpression of mouse (Hein et al., 1997) or human (Paradis et al., 2000) AT_1 receptors in transgenic mice resulted in cardiac hypertrophy in the absence of hypertension, suggesting that the heart is exposed to Ang II constitutively. These studies provide compelling evidence that perturbations in the balance of the cardiac RAS have pathological consequences.

Further evidence can be drawn from studies of rats transgenic for mouse Ren-2d (TGR(mRen2)-27). These rats express Ren-2d from a variety of sites, including the adrenals, kidney, brain and heart, leading to accelerated hypertension and cardiac hypertrophy (Mullins et al., 1990; Zhao et al., 1993). Several studies have demonstrated increased cardiac Ang II, despite normal plasma levels, suggesting that cardiac Ren-2d expression specifically activates the cardiac RAS (Flesch et al., 1997; Zolk et al., 1998, 2002). Furthermore, studies have documented the efficacy of low-dose Ang II receptor blockade, angiotensin-converting enzyme (ACE) inhibition and intracardiac Ang II type I plasma membrane receptor (AT_1) antisense therapy in preventing cardiac hypertrophy, despite a minimal effect on blood pressure (Bohm et al., 1996; Ohta et al., 1996; Pachori et al., 2002). This indicates that cardiac hypertrophy is mediated by cardiac Ren-2d expression, as opposed to hypertension *per se*. However some recent studies suggest that hypertension is the predominant stimulus for hypertrophy (Bishop et al., 2000; Witte et al., 2001).

Transgenic evidence of cardiac renin uptake

Amongst the necessary components required for a complete RAS is the aspartyl protease, renin. Experiments in intact pigs (Danser et al., 1992, 1994), cardiomyocytes *in vitro* (van Kesteren et al., 1997; Saris et al., 2001, 2002) and heart preparations *ex vivo* (de Lannoy et al., 1997, 1998; Muller et al., 1998) have demonstrated that the heart probably imports renin from the circulating pool. However, such experiments have been limited in their ability to provide clear evidence that this phenomenon has physiological effects.

Transgenic experiments in mice and rats using heterologous renin transgenes provide *in vivo* evidence of cardiac renin accumulation, and cardiac RAS activation. Prescott et al. (2000) generated three transgenic mouse lines, one carrying a human angiotensinogen transgene under the control of the αMHC promoter, and the others expressing human renin, or prorenin from the liver via the transthyretin promoter (Prescott et al., 2000, 2002). By cross-breeding the lines they obtained mice transgenic for both angiotensinogen and renin, or angiotensinogen and prorenin. Because mouse renin is inactive towards human angiotensinogen, and vice versa, any change in cardiac RAS activation could be specifically attributed to the transgenes (Ganten et al., 1992). Compared to nontransgenic and single transgenic controls, mice carrying both angiotensinogen and renin transgenes demonstrated a marked increase in cardiac Ang I and II, suggesting that renin is taken up from the plasma, and contributes to the activity of the RAS within the heart (Prescott et al., 2000). Double transgenics with a human prorenin transgene demonstrated increased cardiac Ang I levels, but no increase in Ang II (Prescott et al., 2002). Unfortunately, the picture is complicated by the fact that mice transgenic for human renin alone developed hypertension, presumably via activation of mouse angiotensinogen within the liver, though cardiac angiotensin levels were not elevated. However, this does not detract from the basic conclusion that both renin and prorenin are imported by the heart and cause RAS activation at a local level. Immunoelectron microscopy demonstrated that human renin was localised to perivascular cells of uncertain identity.

Further evidence for uptake of renin by the heart is provided by analysis of transgenic rats overexpressing mouse Ren-2d. Although rat renin and mouse Ren-2d are highly conserved and both activate rat angiotensinogen, they are sufficiently different to be distinguishable immunologically, not least because Ren-2d is not glycosylated. Using a novel conditional rat model of hypertension, TGR (cyp1a1-Ren2) or inducible hypertensive rat

(IHR) (Kantachuvesiri et al., 2001) in which mouse Ren-2d is expressed in the liver, Peters et al. (2002) demonstrated clear evidence of elevated mouse Ren-2d internalized within cardiac tissues. Furthermore, since Ren-2d is nonglycosylated, uptake is unlikely to have been mediated by the mannose-6 phosphate receptor (M6PR) pathway (van Kesteren et al., 1997; Saris et al., 2001, 2002; van den Eijnden et al., 2001).

Another transgenic rat model, TGRhAT-rpR carries a rat prorenin cDNA transgene under the control of the human α_1-antitrypsin promoter. Male transgenic rats develop elevated levels of plasma prorenin, without increased plasma renin activity, leading to severe vascular damage and cardiac hypertrophy in the absence of hypertension (Veniant et al., 1996). A possible explanation for these observations is local uptake and activation of prorenin.

Although transgenic models have been useful in confirming the concept of cardiac renin uptake/activation of the cardiac RAS, they have not as yet contributed towards understanding the mechanism involved. Further work investigating the role of M6PR and the recently described renin receptor (Nguyen et al., 2002) by transgenic techniques is currently underway in a number of laboratories.

Prorenin activity

The great excess of prorenin over renin in the plasma has constantly intrigued scientists in this field, and several explanations have been postulated (Nielsen and Poulsen, 1988; Osmond et al., 1991; Laragh, 1992). Prorenin has traditionally been regarded as an inactive precursor of renin, the 43 amino acid prosegment serving to obstruct the active site. However, mutations of the prosegment or exposure to acid/cold conditions can lead to activation of prorenin by conformational changes (Derkx et al., 1992; Pitarresi et al., 1992; Mercure et al., 1995; Deinum et al., 1998). This suggests that prorenin may be active in vivo under appropriate conditions. However, short-term infusion studies of prorenin in monkeys (Lenz et al., 1990, 1991) and rats (Muller et al., 1999) have failed to demonstrate a significant effect on blood pressure or systemic/tissue levels of Ang II, suggesting that prorenin is truly inert.

Transgenic models have been used to address this question using mutant prorenin transgenes that cannot be processed to active renin. Human prorenin contains a protease recognition sequence (PMKRL) between amino acids 40 and 44. Mutation of the lysine in position 42 to alanine prevents cleavage by known proteases. Methot et al. (1999) designed an elegant experiment in which transgenic mice expressed human angiotensinogen, active renin, wild type or mutated human prorenin in the somatotrophs of the pituitary. Pituitary Ang I was elevated in animals transgenic for angiotensinogen and mutant prorenin, indicating that prorenin is enzymatically active *in vivo*.

We have developed rats transgenic for Ren-2d mutated at the prosegment cleavage site in a manner similar to that described above. These animals express mutant prorenin from the liver under the control of the α_1-antitrypsin promoter, resulting in high circulating prorenin levels. This resulted in severe hypertension and cardiac hypertrophy, as is seen in other Ren-2d-based transgenic rats (unpublished data). It is also notable that plasma levels of prorenin in TGR (cyp1a1-Ren2), TGRmren2-27 and TGR (hAT-rpR) greatly exceed those of active renin, which is barely elevated, if at all (Mullins *et al.*, 1990; Veniant *et al.*, 1996; Kantachuvesiri *et al.*, 2001). Therefore, there is substantial evidence that prorenin can exert biological effects similar to renin *in vivo* and that this may occur at extrarenal sites.

Role of the RAS in cardiac hypertrophy and fibrosis

Although it seems indisputable that Ang II causes cardiac hypertrophy, there is controversy as to whether this is a direct effect on cardiomyocytes, and if so, which receptor is responsible (Yamazaki and Yazaki, 1997). Transgenic experiments have shed light on this area, with surprising results. AT_{1a} receptor knockout mice appear to be fully susceptible to the hypertrophic effects of aortic/pulmonary banding (Hamawaki *et al.*, 1998; Harada *et al.*, 1998; Koide *et al.*, 1999), suggesting that Ang II is irrelevant to left ventricular hypertrophy (LVH). Indeed, transgenic mice overexpressing a fusion protein that liberates Ang II within cardiomyocytes, fail to develop cardiac hypertrophy in the absence of hypertension (van Kats *et al.*, 2001). However, mice deficient in AT_2 receptors resist hypertrophy induced by Ang II infusion or aortic banding (Senbonmatsu *et al.*, 2000; Ichihara *et al.*, 2001). This unexpected role for AT_2 receptors has not been universally confirmed (Akishita *et al.*, 2000; Schneider and Lorell, 2001). Indeed, cardiac overexpression of AT_2 receptor in mice does not lead to LVH in response to Ang II infusion (Masaki *et al.*, 1998; Sugino *et al.*, 2001), whilst it attenuates the development of perivascular fibrosis via kinin/NO-dependent mechanisms (Kurisu *et al.*, 2003).

Exactly why the AT_{1a} receptor appears to be superfluous when the overwhelming majority of pharmacological evidence points to its involvement is unclear. Interestingly, mice deficient in both $G\alpha q$ and $G\alpha_{11}$, the G-proteins for angiotensin, β-adrenergic and endothelin receptors, are protected from LVH (Wettschureck et al., 2001). This may support other evidence pointing to a co-operative autocrine/paracrine cascade involving Ang II, endothelin and TGF-β1 signaling between cardiomyocytes and noncardiomyocytes (Gray et al., 1998; Matsusaka et al., 1999; Sano et al., 2000; Schultz Jel et al., 2002). Therefore, the exact roles of AT_1R/AT_2R in LVH are complex and await further clarification.

Conclusions and questions

Transgenic models of RAS dysfunction have contributed greatly to our understanding of RAS and cardiac physiology, providing information that would otherwise have been impossible to obtain. There is now clear evidence from transgenic models that local activation of the RAS stimulates cardiac pathology independently of the circulating RAS. This appears to depend on cardiac uptake of renin and prorenin, although the mechanism responsible remains obscure. Prorenin itself has intrinsic enzymatic activity, and this may contribute to activation of the cardiac RAS. The effects of Ang II on the heart involve both cardiomyocyte and noncardiomyocyte interactions that are complex and poorly understood. Finally, detailed information about the level and cellular sites of RAS expression in the heart is lacking, and requires refinement.

References

Akishita M, Iwai M, Wu L, et al. (2000) Inhibitory effect of angiotensin II type 2 receptor on coronary arterial remodeling after aortic banding in mice. *Circulation* **102**(14), 1684–1689.

Bishop JE, Kiernan LA, Montogomery LE, et al. (2000) Raised blood pressure, not renin–angiotensin systems, causes cardiac fibrosis in TGRm(ren2)27 rats. *Cardiovascular Research* **47**(1), 57–67.

Bohm M, Lippoldt A, Wienen W, et al. (1996) Reduction of cardiac hypertrophy in TGR(mren2)27 by angiotensin II receptor blockade. *Molecular and Cellular Biochemistry* **163–164**, 217–221.

Danser AH, Koning MM, Admiraal PJ, et al. (1992) Production of angiotensins I and II at tissue sites in intact pigs. *American Journal of Physiology* **263**(2 Pt 2), H429–H437.

Danser AH, van Kats JP, Admiraal PJ, et al. (1994) Cardiac renin and angiotensins. Uptake from plasma versus in situ synthesis. *Hypertension* **24**(1), 37–48.

Danser AH, Saris JJ, Schuijt MP, et al. (1999) Is there a local renin–angiotensin system in the heart? *Cardiovascular Research* **44**(2), 252–265.

Deinum J, Derkx FH and Schalekamp MA (1998) Probing epitopes on human prorenin during its proteolytic and non-proteolytic activation. *Biochimica et Biophysica Acta* **1388**(2), 386–396.

De Mello WC and Danser AH (2000) Angiotensin II and the heart: on the intracrine renin–angiotensin system. *Hypertension* **35**(6), 1183–1188.

Derkx FH, Deinum J, Lipovski M, et al. (1992) Nonproteolytic 'activation' of prorenin by active site-directed renin inhibitors as demonstrated by renin-specific monoclonal antibody. *Journal of Biological Chemistry* **267**(32), 22837–22842.

van den Eijnden MM, Saris JJ, de Bruin RJ, et al. (2001) Prorenin accumulation and activation in human endothelial cells: importance of mannose 6-phosphate receptors. *Arteriosclerosis, Thrombosis and Vascular Biology* **21**(6), 911–916.

Flesch M, Schiffer F, Zolk O, et al. (1997) Contractile systolic and diastolic dysfunction in renin-induced hypertensive cardiomyopathy. *Hypertension* **30**(3), 383–391.

Ganten D, Wagner J, Zeh K, et al. (1992) Species specificity of renin kinetics in transgenic rats harboring the human renin and angiotensinogen genes. *Proceedings of the National Academy of Sciences of the United States of America* **89**(16), 7806–7810.

Gray MO, Long CS and Kalinyak JE (1998) Angiotensin II stimulates cardiac myocyte hypertrophy via paracrine release of TGF-beta I and endothelin-1 from fibroblasts. *Cardiovascular Research* **40**(2), 352–363.

Hamawaki M, Coffman TM, Lashus A, et al. (1998) Pressure-overload hypertrophy is unabated in mice devoid of AT1A receptors. *American Journal of Physiology* **274**(3 Pt 2), H868–H873.

Harada K, Komuro I, Zou Y, et al. (1998) Acute pressure overload could induce hypertrophic responses in the heart of angiotensin II type Ia knockout mice. *Circulation Research* **82**(7), 779–785.

Hein L, Stevens ME, Barsh GS, et al. (1997) Overexpression of angiotensin AT1 receptor transgene in the mouse myocardium produces a lethal phenotype associated with myocyte hyperplasia and heart block. *Proceedings of the National Academy of Sciences of the United States of America* **94**(12), 6391–6396.

Ichihara S, Senbonmatsu T, Price E, Jr, et al. (2001) Angiotensin II type 2 receptor is essential for left ventricular hypertrophy and cardiac fibrosis in chronic angiotensin II-induced hypertension. *Circulation* **104**(3), 346–351.

Kantachuvesiri S, Fleming S, Peters J, et al. (2001) Controlled hypertension, a transgenic toggle switch reveals differential mechanisms underlying vascular disease. *Journal of Biological Chemistry* **276**(39), 36727–36733.

van Kats JP, Methot D, Paradis P, et al. (2001) Use of a biological peptide pump to study chronic peptide hormone action in transgenic mice. Direct and indirect effects of angiotensin II on the heart. *Journal of Biological Chemistry* **276**(47), 44012–44017.

van Kesteren CAM, Danser AHJ, Derkx FF, et al. (1997) Mannose 6-phosphate receptor mediated internalization and activation of prorenin by cardiac cells. *Hypertension* **30**(6), 1389–1396.

Koide M, Carabello BA, Canrad CC, et al. (1999) Hypertrophic response to hemodynamic overload: role of load vs. renin–angiotensin system activation. *American Journal of Physiology* **276**(2 Pt 2), H350–H358.

Kurisu S, Ozono R, Oshima T, et al. (2003) Cardiac angiotensin II type 2 receptor activates the kinin/NO system and inhibits fibrosis. *Hypertension* **41**(1), 99–107.

de Lannoy LM, Danser AH, van Kats JP, et al. (1997) Renin–angiotensin system components in the interstitial fluid of the isolated perfused rat heart. Local production of angiotensin I. *Hypertension* **29**(6), 1240–1251.

de Lannoy LM, Danser AH, Bouhuizen AM, et al. (1998) Localization and production of angiotensin II in the isolated perfused rat heart. *Hypertension* **31**(5), 1111–1117.

Laragh JH (1992) Lewis K. Dahl Memorial Lecture. The renin system and four lines of hypertension research. Nephron heterogeneity, the calcium connection, the prorenin vasodilator limb, and plasma renin and heart attack. *Hypertension* **20**(3), 267–279.

Lenz T, Sealey JE, Lappe RW, et al. (1990) Infusion of recombinant human prorenin into rhesus monkeys. Effects on hemodynamics, renin–angiotensin–aldosterone axis and plasma testosterone. *American Journal of Hypertension* **3**(4), 257–261.

Lenz T, Sealey JE, Maack T, et al. (1991) Half-life, hemodynamic, renal, and hormonal effects of prorenin in cynomolgus monkeys. *American Journal of Physiology* **260**(4 Pt 2), R804–R810.

Lewandoski M (2001) Conditional control of gene expression in the mouse. *Nature Reviews Genetics* **2**(10), 743–755.

Masaki H, Kurihara T, Yamaki A, et al. (1998) Cardiac-specific overexpression of angiotensin II AT2 receptor causes attenuated response to AT1 receptor-mediated pressor and chronotropic effects. *Journal of Clinical Investigation* **101**(3), 527–535.

Matsusaka T, Katori H, Inagami T, et al. (1999) Communication between myocytes and fibroblasts in cardiac remodeling in angiotensin chimeric mice. *Journal of Clinical Investigation* **103**(10), 1451–1458.

Mazzolai L, Nussberger J, Aubert JF, et al. (1998) Blood pressure-independent cardiac hypertrophy induced by locally activated renin–angiotensin system. *Hypertension* **31**(6), 1324–1330.

Mazzolai L, Pedrazzini T, Nicoud F, et al. (2000) Increased cardiac angiotensin II levels induce right and left ventricular hypertrophy in normotensive mice. *Hypertension* **35**(4), 985–991.

Mercure C, Thibault G, Lussier-Cacan S, et al. (1995) Molecular analysis of human prorenin prosegment variants *in vitro* and *in vivo*. *Journal of Biological Chemistry* **270**(27), 16355–16359.

Methot D, Silversides DW and Reudelhuber TL (1999) *In vivo* enzymatic assay reveals catalytic activity of the human renin precursor in tissues. *Circulation Research* **84**(9), 1067–1072.

Muller DN, Fischli W, Clozel JP, et al. (1998) Local angiotensin II generation in the rat heart: role of renin uptake. *Circulation Research* **82**(1), 13–20.

Muller DN, Hilgers KF, Mathews S, et al. (1999) Effects of human prorenin in rats transgenic for human angiotensinogen. *Hypertension* **33**(1), 312–317.

Mullins JJ, Peters J and Ganten D (1990) Fulminant hypertension in transgenic rats harbouring the mouse ren-2 gene. *Nature* **344**(6266), 541A.

Nguyen G, Delarue F, Burckle C, et al. (2002) Pivotal role of the renin/prorenin receptor in angiotensin II production and cellular responses to renin. *Journal of Clinical Investigation* **109**(11), 1417–1427.

Nielsen AH and Poulsen K (1988) Is prorenin of physiological and clinical significance? *Journal of Hypertension* **6**(12), 949–958.

Ohta K, Kim S, Wanibuchi H, et al. (1996) Contribution of local renin–angiotensin system to cardiac hypertrophy, phenotypic modulation, and remodeling in TGR(mren2)27 transgenic rats. *Circulation* **94**(4), 785–791.

REFERENCES

Osmond DH, Sealey JE and McKenzie JK (1991) Activation and function of prorenin: different viewpoints. *Canadian Journal of Physiology and Pharmacology* **69**(9), 1308–1314.

Pachori AS, Numan MT, Ferrario CM, *et al.* (2002) Blood pressure-independent attenuation of cardiac hypertrophy by AT(1)RAS gene therapy. *Hypertension* **39**(5), 969–975.

Palermo J, Gulick J, Colbert M, *et al.* (1996) Transgenic remodeling of the contractile apparatus in the mammalian heart. *Circulation Research* **78**(3), 504–509.

Paradis P, Dali-Youcef N, Paradis FW, *et al.* (2000) Overexpression of angiotensin II type I receptor in cardiomyocytes induces cardiac hypertrophy and remodeling. *Proceedings of the National Academy of Sciences of the United States of America* **97**(2), 931–936.

Peters J, Farrenkopf R, Clausmeyer S, *et al.* (2002) Functional significance of prorenin internalization in the rat heart. *Circulation Research* **90**(10), 1135–1141.

Pitarresi TM, Rubattu S, Heinrickson R and Sealey JE (1992) Reversible cryo-activation of recombinant human prorenin. *Journal of Biological Chemistry* **267**(17), 11753–11759.

Prescott G, Silversides DW, Chiu SM and Reudelheuber TL (2000) Contribution of circulating renin to local synthesis of angiotensin peptides in the heart. *Physiological Genomics* **4**(1), 67–73.

Prescott G, Silversides DW and Reudelheuber TL (2002) Tissue activity of circulating prorenin. *American Journal of Hypertension* **15**(3), 280–285.

Ruiz-Ortega M, Lorenzo O, Ruperez M, *et al.* (2001) Role of the renin–angiotensin system in vascular diseases: expanding the field. *Hypertension* **38**(6), 1382–1387.

Ryding AD, Sharp MG and Mullins JJ (2001) Conditional transgenic technologies. *Journal of Endocrinology* **111**(1), 1–14.

Sano M, Fukuda K, Kodama H, *et al.* (2000) Interleukin-6 family of cytokines mediate angiotensin II-induced cardiac hypertrophy in rodent cardiomyocytes. *Journal of Biological Chemistry* **275**(38), 29717–29723.

Saris JJ, Derkx FH, Lamers JM, *et al.* (2001) Cardiomyocytes bind and activate native human prorenin: role of soluble mannose 6-phosphate receptors. *Hypertension* **37**, 710–715.

Saris JJ, van den Eijnden MM, Lamers JM, *et al.* (2002) Prorenin-induced myocyte proliferation: no role for intracellular angiotensin II. *Hypertension* **39**(2 Pt 2), 573–577.

Schneider MD and Lorell BH (2001) AT(2), judgment day: which angiotensin receptor is the culprit in cardiac hypertrophy? *Circulation* **104**(3), 247–248.

Schultz Jel J, Witt SA, Glascock BJ, *et al.* (2002) TGF-beta1 mediates the hypertrophic cardiomyocyte growth induced by angiotensin II. *Journal of Clinical Investigation* **109**(6), 787–796.

Senbonmatsu T, Ichihara S, Price E, Jr, *et al.* (2000) Evidence for angiotensin II type 2 receptor-mediated cardiac myocyte enlargement during *in vivo* pressure overload. *Journal of Clinical Investigation* **106**(3), R25–R29.

Sugino H, Ozono R, Kurisu S, *et al.* (2001) Apoptosis is not increased in myocardium overexpressing type 2 angiotensin II receptor in transgenic mice. *Hypertension* **37**(6), 1394–1398.

Veniant M, Menard J, Bruneval P, *et al.* (1996) Vascular damage without hypertension in transgenic rats expressing prorenin exclusively in the liver. *Journal of Clinical Investigation* **98**(9), 1966–1970.

Wettschureck N, Rutten H, Zywietz A, *et al.* (2001) Absence of pressure overload induced myocardial hypertrophy after conditional inactivation of Galphaq/Galpha11 in cardiomyocytes. *Nature Medicine* **7**(11), 1236–1240.

Witte K, Huser L, Knotter B, *et al.* (2001) Normalisation of blood pressure in hypertensive TGR(mren2)27 rats by amlodipine vs. enalapril: effects on cardiac hypertrophy and signal transduction pathways. *Naunyn Schmiedebergs Archiv für Pharmacologie* **363**(1), 101–109.

Yamazaki T and Yazaki Y (1997) Is there major involvement of the renin–angiotensin system in cardiac hypertrophy? *Circulation Research* **81**(5), 639–642.

Zhao Y, Bader M, Kreutz P, *et al.* (1993) Ontogenetic regulation of mouse ren-2^d renin gene in transgenic hypertensive rats, TGR(mren2)27. *American Journal of Physiology* **265**(5 Pt 1), E699–E707.

Zolk O, Flesch M, Nickenig G, *et al.* (1998) Alteration of intracellular Ca^{2+}-handling and receptor regulation in hypertensive cardiac hypertrophy: insights from ren2-transgenic rats. *Cardiovascular Research* **39**(1), 242–256.

Zolk O, Quattek J, Seeland U, *et al.* (2002) Activation of the cardiac endothelin system in left ventricular hypertrophy before onset of heart failure in TG(mren2)27 rats. *Cardiovascular Research* **53**(2), 363–371.

3

Prorenin Uptake in the Heart

A. H. Jan Danser

Introduction

The beneficial effects of angiotensin I-converting enzyme (ACE) inhibitors and angiotensin II (Ang II) type 1 (AT$_1$) receptor blockers in heart failure and following myocardial infarction are independent, at least in part, of the blood pressure lowering effect of these drugs (van Kats *et al.*, 1998; Yusuf *et al.*, 2000). It has therefore been suggested that Ang II is generated not only in the circulation, but also locally at cardiac tissue sites. Studies quantifying cardiac Ang II generation, using infusions of radiolabeled angiotensins to correct for uptake from plasma, have revealed that Ang II in the heart indeed largely, if not completely, originates from local synthesis at cardiac tissue sites, both under normal (van Kats *et al.*, 1998) and pathological (van Kats *et al.*, 2000) conditions (Figure 3.1). Originally it was thought that all components required to generate Ang II locally in the heart (i.e., renin, angiotensinogen and ACE) are also synthesized at cardiac tissue sites. However, recent studies have shown that this is not the case. In particular, there is no convincing evidence for renin synthesis in the heart:

- renin mRNA levels in the heart are low or undetectable (von Lutterotti *et al.*, 1994; Neri Serneri *et al.*, 2001);

- renin activity can no longer be demonstrated in cardiac tissue following a bilateral nephrectomy (Danser *et al.*, 1994; Katz *et al.*, 1997), nor does the isolated perfused rat Langendorff heart release or contain renin (Lindpaintner *et al.*, 1990; de Lannoy *et al.*, 1997);

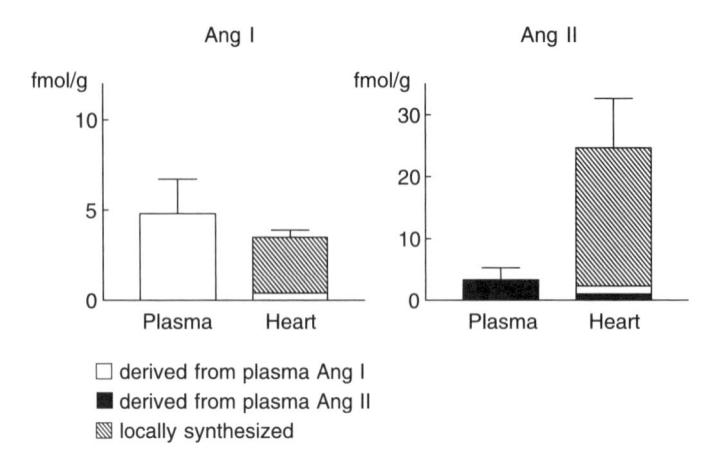

Figure 3.1 Origin of cardiac angiotensin (Ang) I and II in the pig. Modified from van Kats *et al.* (1998)

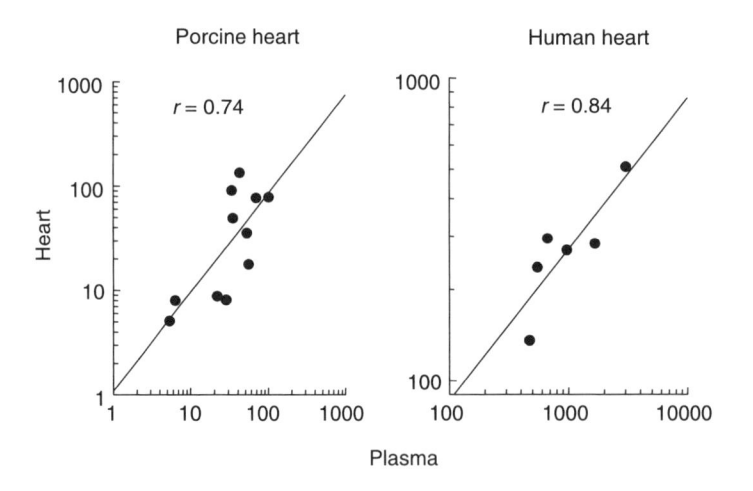

Figure 3.2 Correlation between plasma and cardiac renin in humans with end-stage cardiomyopathy (right) and healthy pigs (left). Data are from Danser *et al.* (1994, 1997)

- the cardiac tissue levels of renin closely correlate with the plasma levels of renin, both under normal and pathological conditions (Figure 3.2) (Danser *et al.*, 1994, 1997; Heller *et al.*, 1998; Hirsch *et al.*, 1999);

- cultured neonatal and adult rat cardiac myocytes and fibroblasts do not release renin or its inactive precursor, prorenin, into the medium (van Kesteren *et al.*, 1999; Katz *et al.*, 2001).

Taken together, therefore, it appears that the renin required for cardiac angiotensin generation is taken up from the circulation and, thus, is

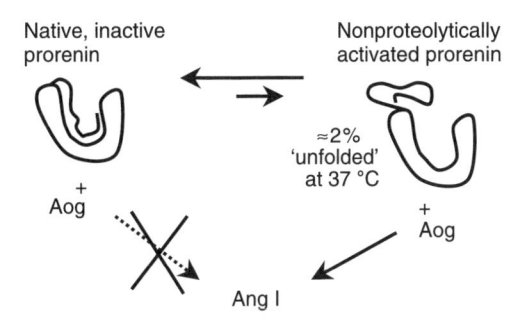

Figure 3.3 'Closed' (left) and 'open' (right) conformation of prorenin. Temporal nonproteolytic activation of prorenin, for instance at low pH, leads to exposure of the active site ('open' position) and display of enzymatic activity. At 37 °C, approximately 2 percent of prorenin is in the open conformation. Aog, angiotensinogen; Ang, angiotensin

kidney-derived. In addition, circulating prorenin may contribute to cardiac angiotensin generation, in particular because the prorenin levels in the circulation are almost ten times higher than those of renin (Danser et al., 1998a).

Prorenin uptake by tissues, if occurring, should be followed by local prorenin–renin conversion because prorenin displays either no or very limited enzymatic activity. The latter is due to temporal unfolding of the prosegment (so-called 'nonproteolytic activation') (Derkx et al., 1987), a situation which is enhanced by acid pH or low temperature (Figure 3.3). Therefore, to allow Ang I generation at tissue sites following prorenin uptake, either the prosegment should be cleaved by proteolytic enzymes, or prosegment unfolding should be enhanced (for instance because prorenin accumulates in intracellular, low pH-compartments).

How does the heart sequester circulating (pro)renin?

Cardiac renin levels (expressed per g wet weight) are too high to be explained based upon the amount of (renin- and prorenin-containing) blood plasma ($\approx$ 5 percent) in cardiac tissue, thereby confirming cardiac sequestration of circulating (pro)renin (Danser et al., 1994, 1997; Katz et al., 1997). Circulating renin and prorenin could either diffuse into the cardiac interstitial space and/or bind to cardiac (pro)renin receptors. Diffusion is supported by studies in a modified version of the isolated perfused rat Langendorff heart, allowing separate collection of coronary effluent and interstitial transudate. During perfusion of this heart preparation with renin, renin was found to diffuse slowly into the interstitial space, reaching steady-state levels that were equal to the renin levels in coronary effluent (de Lannoy *et al.*, 1997). Transport mechanisms other than diffusion could not be demonstrated for either renin or prorenin in a study investigating transcellular transport of renin angiotensin system components in human umbilical vein endothelial cells (van den Eijnden *et al.*, 2002). Furthermore, renin measurements in rat cardiac tissue are in full agreement with the concept that renin is present in cardiac interstitial fluid in concentrations that are as high as those in blood plasma (Katz *et al.*, 1997; Heller *et al.*, 1998; Hirsch *et al.*, 1999).

Studies in rat and porcine hearts subsequently showed that part of cardiac renin is membrane associated (Campbell and Valentijn, 1994; Danser *et al.*, 1994). Moreover, isolated perfused hearts of rats transgenic for human angiotensinogen release Ang I during renin infusion and this release continues after stopping the renin infusion (Müller *et al.*, 1998b). These data support the idea that circulating (pro)renin binds to a cardiac (pro)renin-binding protein/receptor, and that bound (pro)renin is catalytically active.

(Pro)renin receptors

Several groups have reported on the existence of (pro)renin-binding proteins and/or receptors (Figure 3.4). Such receptors may recognize the active site of renin (or the active site of prorenin, provided that the molecule is in the 'open' conformation), the prosegment (specific for prorenin), or any other part of the (pro)renin molecule. A fourth possibility would be binding to the carbohydrate portions which renin and prorenin contain. Both proteins display isoelectric heterogeneity (caused by differences in glycosylation and/or phosphorylation), and carbohydrate portions are known to be involved in their hepatic clearance (Kim *et al.*, 1988).

An intracellular renin-binding protein (RnBP) was first discovered in humans, rats and pigs (Takahashi *et al.*, 1983, 1992; Tada *et al.*, 1992). This RnBP, which reduces the Ang I-generating activity by more than 80 percent, was subsequently found to be equal to the enzyme N-acyl-D-glucosamine 2-epimerase (Maru *et al.*, 1996). The binding protein and renin do not colocalize in the rat kidney (Leckie *et al.*, 2000), and mice lacking the RnBP display normal blood pressure and renin activity (Schmitz *et al.*, 2000). Therefore, it is now generally assumed that renin and this RnBP are unrelated.

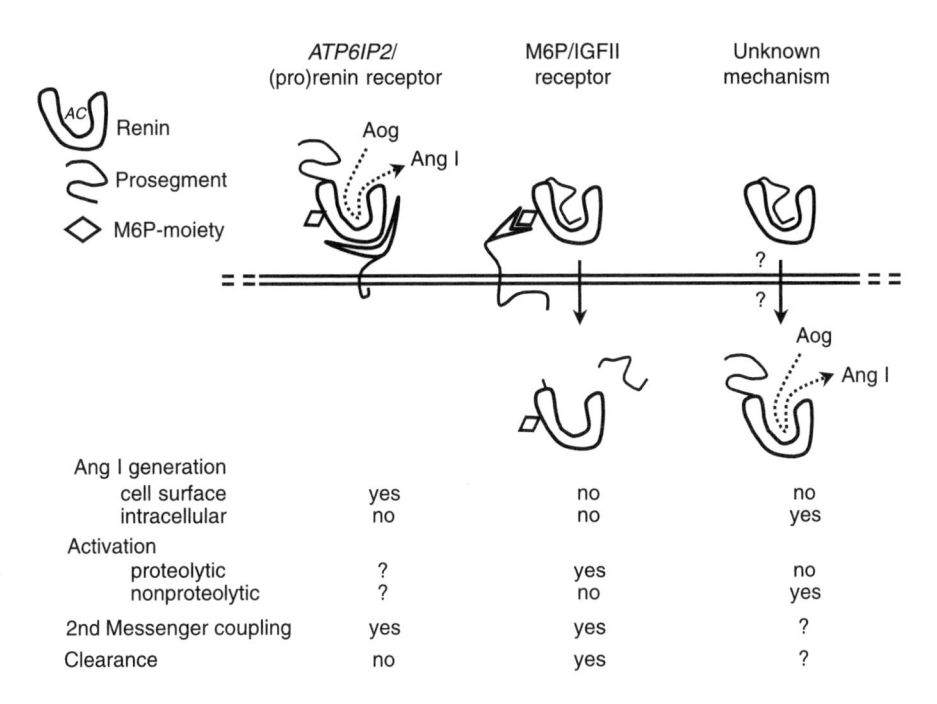

	ATP6IP2/ (pro)renin receptor	M6P/IGFII receptor	Unknown mechanism
Ang I generation			
cell surface	yes	no	no
intracellular	no	no	yes
Activation			
proteolytic	?	yes	no
nonproteolytic	?	no	yes
2nd Messenger coupling	yes	yes	?
Clearance	no	yes	?

Figure 3.4 Current status of prorenin receptors, prorenin internalization and prorenin-induced effects in the heart. The (pro)renin receptor cloned by Nguyen *et al.* (gene name *ATP6IP2*) facilitates cell surface angiotensin (Ang) generation from angiotensinogen (Aog) (Nguyen *et al.*, 2002), mannose 6-phosphate/insulin-like growth factor II (M6P/IGFII) receptor-induced internalization of M6P-containing prorenin results in prorenin clearance (Saris *et al.*, 2001), and an unknown mechanism allows nonglycosylated (i.e., nonM6P-containing) prorenin to internalize and to subsequently generate Ang I intracellularly (Peters *et al.*, 2002). AC, active center

Using chemical cross-linking, two vascular RnBPs were identified in membranes isolated from rat mesenteric arteries or cultured rat aortic smooth muscle cells (Campbell and Valentijn, 1994). Renin binding to these RnBPs was inhibited by a specific, active site-directed renin inhibitor, suggesting that the active site of the renin molecule is involved in the binding process. In contrast, Peters and colleagues using isolated adult rat cardiomyocytes and mouse *ren-2^d* (i.e., nonglycosylated) renin and prorenin, observed binding and internalization of prorenin only (Peters *et al.*, 2002). These data therefore suggest a role for the prosegment in the internalization process, although the underlying mechanism is not yet known. Importantly, internalized prorenin in this study displayed a 4–5-higher Ang I-generating activity than prorenin in the medium (3.3 percent vs. 0.7 percent of prorenin was in the 'open' conformation), suggesting partial activation of intracellular prorenin, for instance due to its presence in a low pH environment.

Nguyen and colleagues and Sealey and colleagues, using radio-labeled (pro)renin, demonstrated high-affinity renin-binding sites/receptors ($K_d \approx 1\,\text{nmol/l}$) in human mesangial cells and in membranes prepared from rat tissues, respectively (Nguyen et al., 1996; Sealey et al., 1996). These binding sites/receptors bound prorenin and renin equally well, which suggests that neither the prosegment nor the active site is involved in the binding process. The gene encoding the renin binding site in human mesangial cells has recently been cloned (Nguyen et al., 2002). It encodes for a 350-amino acid protein, part of which is identical to the previously reported 'M8-9 protein', a vacuolar proton–ATPase membrane associated sector associated protein (gene name *ATP6IP2*) (Ludwig et al., 1998). The receptor is predominantly present in vascular smooth muscle cells and glomerular mesangial cells. Interestingly, when bound to this receptor, renin displays increased catalytic activity as compared to soluble renin. It also induces cellular effects independent of angiotensin generation (e.g., mitogen-activated protein (MAP) kinase activation), thereby implying that renin acts as an endogenous agonist of this new receptor. Furthermore, prorenin displays full enzymatic activity when bound to this receptor, suggesting that prorenin binding either results in a conformational change ('nonproteolytic activation') or is accompanied by proteolytic removal of the prosegment. Binding of renin or prorenin to this receptor was not followed by internalization.

Finally, the mannose 6-phosphate (M6P)-moiety, which is present on the phosphomannosylated glycoforms of both renin and prorenin, determines (pro)renin binding and internalization by neonatal rat cardiac and human umbilical vein endothelial cells (van Kesteren et al., 1997; Admiraal et al., 1999; Saris et al., 2001; van den Eijnden et al., 2001). Moreover, following internalization, M6P-containing prorenin was proteolytically activated to renin.

Mannose 6-phosphate/insulin-like growth factor II receptors

M6P receptors function in the process of intracellular lysosomal enzyme sorting (Dahms et al., 1989; Ghosh et al., 2003). At present, two different M6P receptors have been identified: a large M6P receptor (molecular weight 300 kDa), which binds ligands independent of divalent cations (cation-independent M6P receptor), and a small M6P receptor (molecular weight 46 kDa), which requires divalent cations for optimal binding (cation-dependent M6P receptor) (Dahms et al., 1987). In 1987, it was discovered that the cation-independent M6P receptor and the insulin-like growth factor II receptor are the same protein (Morgan et al., 1987). Thus, the cation-independent M6P receptor is now also known as the M6P/IGFII receptor. This receptor binds IGFII, phosphomannosylated proteins (e.g., (pro)renin), and retinoic acid at distinct sites (Kornfeld, 1992; Kang et al., 1998). The M6P/IGFII receptor is involved in the activation of several M6P-containing precursor proteins, including procathepsin D and latent transforming growth factor-β (Helseth and Veis, 1984; Dennis and Rifkin, 1991; Danser et al., 1999). In view of the fact that, in cultured cells, we observed both M6P receptor-dependent binding and internalization of renin and prorenin, and intracellular prorenin activation, the M6P receptor involved in these processes is most likely the M6P/IGFII receptor. This conclusion is further supported by the high affinity binding ($K_d \approx 1$ nmol/l) of renin and prorenin to M6P receptors (Saris et al., 2001; van den Eijnden et al., 2001) since only M6P/IGFII receptors (and not cation-dependent M6P receptors) display such high affinity for phosphomannosylated proteins (Tong and Kornfeld, 1989).

The majority (90 percent) of the M6P/IGFII receptors is located in a late endosomal/prelysosomal compartment, with the rest being distributed over the plasma membrane, early endosomes, and the Golgi (Griffiths et al., 1990). Extracellular lysosomal enzymes which bind to the cell surface M6P/IGFII receptor are internalized via clathrin-coated pits. They dissociate from the receptor in acidified endosomal compartments and are subsequently delivered to lysosomes. The receptor is then reutilized; it can undergo many rounds of ligand delivery (Kornfeld and Mellman, 1989; Griffiths et al., 1990). Binding and internalization of IGFII to M6P/IGFII receptors results in the lysosomal degradation of this ligand (Oka et al., 1985). In addition, IGFII mediates growth-stimulatory responses via this receptor (Tally et al., 1987). Similarly, retinoic acid and phosphomannosylated proteins activate second messenger pathways in a G-protein-dependent manner through binding to M6P/IGFII receptors (Groskopf et al., 1997; Kang et al., 1999). Thus, M6P/IGFII receptors are not only involved in the binding and activation of M6P-containing proteins, but also respond to M6P-containing proteins in a G-protein-dependent manner.

M6P/IGFII receptor-mediated (pro)renin binding and prorenin activation

At 4 °C, cardiomyocytes, cardiac fibroblasts and endothelial cells bind recombinant human prorenin in a concentration-dependent manner

(Saris et al., 2001; van den Eijnden et al., 2001). Binding was significantly reduced by 10 mmol/l M6P. The difference between prorenin binding with and without M6P represents M6P/IGFII receptor-specific binding. The maximum number of cell surface M6P/IGFII receptors (B_{max}) was in the order of 650–4000/cell, and binding affinity was similar in all cells. The levels of cell-associated prorenin increased 10-fold when the incubations were performed at 37 °C. Moreover, at this temperature (but not at 4 °C) cell-associated prorenin was acid-resistant, thereby indicating that it is no longer present on the cell surface (i.e., has been internalized). Taken together, these data fully agree with the concept that M6P/IGFII receptors recycle continuously between the cell surface and the intracellular compartment. Recycling does not occur at 4 °C. Data obtained with renin were not different from those with prorenin (van Kesteren et al., 1997; Admiraal et al., 1999).

Intracellularly, prorenin was found to be activated to renin by proteolytic removal of the prosegment. Actual prosegment removal could be verified with monoclonal antibodies directed specifically against the carboxyterminal part of the prosegment (Saris et al., 2001; van den Eijnden et al., 2001).

Evidence for release of cell-activated prorenin or internalized renin into the medium could not be obtained (van den Eijnden et al., 2002), suggesting that renin may have intracellular actions. However, renin was also found to be degraded intracellularly ($t_{1/2} > 1$ h), and thus an alternative possibility is that M6P/IGFII receptor-mediated (pro)renin internalization represents (pro)renin clearance. Intracellular prorenin activation might then simply be the first step towards prorenin destruction.

Does prorenin mediate direct (Ang II-independent) effects?

There are at least three ways through which prorenin may induce cellular effects. First, prorenin binding *per se* (i.e., without subsequent Ang II generation), may yield an intracellular response. For instance, proliferin which, like prorenin, binds to M6P/IGFII receptors via its M6P group, induces endothelial cell chemotaxis via M6P/IGFII receptors in a G-protein- and mitogen-activated protein kinase-dependent manner (Groskopf et al., 1997). In addition, renin binding to the recently cloned (pro)renin receptor resulted in enhanced [^{3}H]-thymidine incorporation, plasminogen-activator inhibitor-1 release and MAP kinase activation without intermediate angiotensin generation (Nguyen et al., 1996, 2002). Second, prorenin may lead to intracellular Ang II generation following its intracellular activation. The underlying assumption for this hypothesis is that both angiotensinogen and ACE are present intracellularly. Intracellularly generated Ang II might activate intracellular AT_1 receptors, or, following its release from the cell, cell surface AT_1 receptors. Third, prorenin may result in extracellular Ang II generation, either because prorenin displays partial activity or because prorenin binding to the cell surface enhances its Ang I-generating capacity (Nguyen et al., 2002).

To investigate these possibilities, we measured [^{3}H]-thymidine incorporation by cardiomyocytes following their incubation with prorenin, angiotensinogen, prorenin plus angiotensinogen, or Ang II, in the absence and presence of M6P or eprosartan, to block M6P/IGFII receptors and AT_1 receptors, respectively (Saris et al., 2002).

The results show that prorenin combined with angiotensinogen, but not prorenin alone or angiotensinogen alone, enhanced [^{3}H]-thymidine incorporation. Remarkably, the effect of prorenin plus angiotensinogen on DNA synthesis was comparable to the effect of 100 nmol/l Ang II on [^{3}H]-thymidine incorporation, although the medium Ang II levels during combined prorenin plus angiotensinogen application were <1 nmol/l (Figure 3.5). Moreover, cellular Ang II was virtually undetectable during exposure to prorenin plus angiotensinogen, and only eprosartan, and not M6P, blocked the effects of both Ang II and prorenin plus

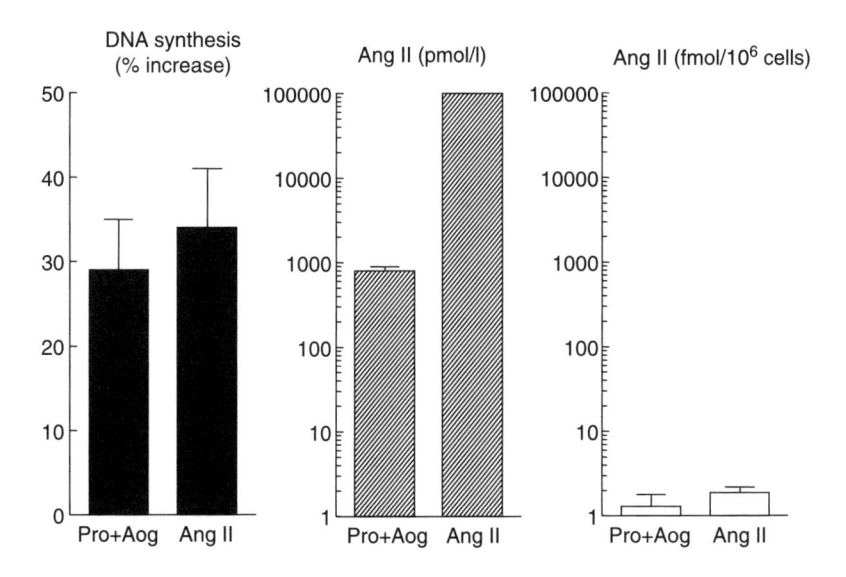

Figure 3.5 DNA synthesis rates (left panel) versus medium (middle panel) and cellular (right panel) angiotensin (Ang) II levels following incubation of neonatal rat cardiomyocytes with prorenin + angiotensinogen (Pro + Aog) or 100 nmol/l Ang II. Modified from Saris et al. (2002)

angiotensinogen. Since extracellularly applied AT_1 receptor antagonists do not internalize in significant amounts (Conchon et al., 1994), these data suggest that prorenin-induced myocyte proliferation depends on cell surface AT_1 receptor activation by extracellularly generated Ang II. M6P/IGFII receptors apparently do not contribute to this process, and thus the extracellular angiotensin generation occurs independently of these receptors. It may still occur on the cell surface, particularly in view of the low medium Ang II levels at which proliferation occurred during prorenin plus angiotensinogen exposure. Only cell-surface angiotensin generation will result in high Ang II levels in the microenvironment of AT_1 receptors. If this locally generated Ang II does not 'leak' into the medium, an explanation is provided for the comparable effects on myocyte proliferation of prorenin plus angiotensinogen versus Ang II despite a 100-fold difference in the Ang II levels in the medium.

Intracellular versus extracellular angiotensin generation

As discussed above, prorenin internalization and activation via M6P/IGFII receptors did not result in intracellular (i.e., cytoplasmic) Ang II generation in neonatal rat cardiomyocytes. The most likely explanation for the lack of intracellular Ang II generation is that angiotensinogen and/or ACE are not present in these cells. Neonatal rat cardiomyocytes synthesize ACE but not angiotensinogen (van Kesteren et al., 1999). Thus, to allow intracellular Ang II generation in these cardiomyocytes, angiotensinogen must first be sequestered from the extracellular fluid and then be translocated to the cytosol. Evidence for angiotensinogen internalization, however, could not be obtained (van den Eijnden et al., 2001). Moreover, ex-vivo measurements documented that angiotensinogen, unlike renin, does not bind to cardiac membranes (Campbell and Valentijn, 1994; Danser et al., 1994).

Thus, perhaps intracellular Ang II generation is possible only in cells that synthesize angiotensinogen themselves. This situation appears to exist in adult rat cardiomyocytes, since their incubation with mouse ren-2^d prorenin resulted in the intracellular appearance of both Ang I and II (Peters et al., 2002). Remarkably, such intracellular angiotensin generation did not occur following internalization of rat prorenin, leading the authors to suggest that the lack of glycosylation of mouse ren-2^d prorenin allows this prorenin to internalize via a different manner than rat prorenin.

An argument against intracellular Ang I generation is that all angiotensinogen-synthesizing cells normally release angiotensinogen into the medium, without storing it intracellularly (Eggena *et al.*, 1990; Klett *et al.*, 1993). This is due to the presence of an N-terminal signal sequence that directs angiotensinogen into the secretory pathway. Furthermore, a study in angiotensinogen-synthesizing rat hepatoma cells showed that intracellular Ang II generation occurred only following transfection of the cells with a mutated angiotensinogen cDNA that produces a nonsecreted form of angiotensinogen (i.e., angiotensinogen that lacks the N-terminal signal sequence) (Cook *et al.*, 2001). At present, there is no evidence for naturally occurring angiotensinogen variants lacking the signal peptide leading to secretion.

Taken together, the evidence that is currently available does not support the concept of intracellular Ang II generation under physiological conditions. This conclusion implies that the internalization of renin and prorenin, as well as the intracellular activation of prorenin via M6P/IGFII receptors, represents (pro)renin clearance rather than the initial step leading to intracellular angiotensin generation. Thus, M6P/IGFII receptors will affect local Ang II generation only indirectly (i.e., by decreasing the tissue levels of (pro)renin). In support of this concept, Ang I release from hearts of rats transgenic for human angiotensinogen doubled when perfusing the hearts with deglycosylated renin instead of wild type renin (Müller *et al.*, 1998a).

Angiotensin generation in the heart occurs on the cell surface of cardiac cells, and/or in the interstitial space if not intracellularly. Cell surface angiotensin generation is particularly supported by studies revealing that membrane-bound renin cleaves angiotensinogen much more efficiently than soluble renin (Nguyen *et al.*, 2002) and that Ang II-dependent effects occur at 100-fold lower extracellular Ang II levels during prorenin plus angiotensinogen application than during Ang II application (Saris *et al.*, 2002). The presence of ACE and/or renin in the microenvironment of AT receptors would allow maximum efficiency of local Ang II generation, i.e., immediate binding of Ang II to its receptors with minimal loss into the extracellular space. Indeed, when quantifying tissue angiotensin release using ^{125}I-Ang I infusions in humans and pigs, we were unable to demonstrate significant Ang II release from tissue sites (Danser *et al.*, 1992, 1998b; Admiraal *et al.*, 1993). Moreover, Ang II was barely detectable in interstitial fluid (Schuijt *et al.*, 1999).

Perspective

Cardiac angiotensin generation depends largely, if not completely, on circulating renin and/or prorenin. A range of studies has recently provided evidence for the presence of one or more (pro)renin receptors in the heart. Binding to such receptors most likely underlies the accumulation of circulating (pro)renin at cardiac tissue sites. Receptor binding not only results in prorenin activation and subsequent angiotensin generation, but it also leads to (pro)renin clearance. Taken together, these findings offer new and exciting insights into the mechanism of tissue angiotensin generation. Unravelling the contribution of each of the currently proposed (pro)renin receptors may lead to new ways to block the renin angiotensin system at the local level.

References

Admiraal PJJ, Danser AHJ, Jong MS, et al. (1993) Regional angiotensin II production in essential hypertension and renal artery stenosis. *Hypertension* **21**, 173–184.

Admiraal PJJ, van Kesteren CAM, Danser AHJ, et al. (1999) Uptake and proteolytic activation of prorenin by cultured human endothelial cells. *Journal of Hypertension* **17**, 621–629.

Campbell DJ and Valentijn AJ (1994) Identification of vascular renin-binding proteins by chemical cross-linking: inhibition of binding of renin by renin inhibitors. *Journal of Hypertension* **12**, 879–890.

Conchon S, Monnot C, Teutsch B, et al. (1994) Internalization of the rat AT1a and AT1b receptors: pharmacological and functional requirements. *FEBS Letters* **349**, 365–370.

Cook JL, Zhang Z and Re RN (2001) *In vitro* evidence for an intracellular site of angiotensin action. *Circulation Research* **89**, 1138–1146.

Dahms NM, Lobel P, Breitmeyer J, et al. (1987) 46 kd mannose 6-phosphate receptor: cloning, expression, and homology to the 215 kd mannose 6-phosphate receptor. *Cell* **50**, 181–192.

Dahms NM, Lobel P and Kornfeld S (1989) Mannose 6-phosphate receptors and lysosomal enzyme targeting. *Journal of Biological Chemistry* **264**, 12115–12118.

Danser AHJ, Koning MMG, Admiraal PJJ, et al. (1992) Production of angiotensins I and II at tissue sites in intact pigs. *American Journal of Physiology* **263**, H429–H437.

Danser AHJ, van Kats JP, Admiraal PJJ, et al. (1994) Cardiac renin and angiotensins. Uptake from plasma versus in situ synthesis. *Hypertension* **24**, 37–48.

Danser AHJ, van Kesteren CAM, Bax WA, et al. (1997) Prorenin, renin, angiotensinogen, and angiotensin-converting enzyme in normal and failing human hearts. Evidence for renin binding. *Circulation* **96**, 220–226.

Danser AHJ, Derkx FHM, Schalekamp MADH, et al. (1998a) Determinants of interindividual variation of renin and prorenin concentrations: evidence for a sexual dimorphism of (pro)renin levels in humans. *Journal of Hypertension* **16**, 853–862.

Danser AHJ, Admiraal PJJ, Derkx FHM and Schalekamp MADH (1998b) Angiotensin I-to-II conversion in the human renal vascular bed. *Journal of Hypertension* **16**, 2051–2056.

REFERENCES

Danser AHJ, Saris JJ, Schuijt MP and van Kats JP (1999) Is there a local renin–angiotensin system in the heart? *Cardiovascular Research* **44**, 252–265.

Dennis PA and Rifkin DB (1991) Cellular activation of latent transforming growth factor beta requires binding to the cation-independent mannose 6-phosphate/insulin-like growth factor type II receptor. *Proceedings of the National Academy of Sciences of the United States of America* **88**, 580–584.

Derkx FHM, Schalekamp MP and Schalekamp MADH (1987) Two-step prorenin–renin conversion. Isolation of an intermediary form of activated prorenin. *Journal of Biological Chemistry* **262**, 2472–2477.

Eggena P, Krall F, Eggena MP, et al. (1990) Production of angiotensinogen by cultured rat aortic smooth muscle cells. *Clinical and Experimental Hypertension A* **12**, 1175–1189.

van den Eijnden MMED, Saris JJ, de Bruin RJA, et al. (2001) Prorenin accumulation and activation in human endothelial cells. Importance of mannose 6-phosphate receptors. *Arteriosclerosis, Thrombosis and Vascular Biology* **21**, 911–916.

van den Eijnden MMED, de Bruin RJA, de Wit E, et al. (2002) Transendothelial transport of renin–angiotensin system components. *Journal of Hypertension* **20**, 2029–2037.

Ghosh P, Dahms NM and Kornfeld S (2003) Mannose 6-phosphate receptors: new twists in the tale. *Nature Reviews. Molecular and Cell Biology* **4**, 202–212.

Griffiths G, Matteoni R, Back R and Hoflack B (1990) Characterization of the cation-independent mannose 6-phosphate receptor-enriched prelysosomal compartment in NRK cells. *Journal of Cell Science* **95**, 441–461.

Groskopf JC, Syu LJ, Saltiel AR and Linzer DIH (1997) Proliferin induces endothelial cell chemotaxis through a G protein-coupled, mitogen-activated protein kinase-dependent pathway. *Endocrinology* **138**, 2835–2840.

Heller LJ, Opsahl JA, Wernsing SE, et al. (1998) Myocardial and plasma renin–angiotensinogen dynamics during pressure-induced cardiac hypertrophy. *American Journal of Physiology* **274**, R849–R856.

Helseth DL, Jr and Veis A (1984) Cathepsin D-mediated processing of procollagen: lysosomal enzyme involvement in secretory processing of procollagen. *Proceedings of the National Academy of Sciences of the United States of America* **81**, 3302–3306.

Hirsch AT, Opsahl JA, Lunzer MM and Katz SA (1999) Active renin and angiotensinogen in cardiac interstitial fluid after myocardial infarction. *American Journal of Physiology* **276**, H1818–H1826.

Kang JX, Li Y and Leaf A (1998) Mannose-6-phosphate/insulin-like growth factor-II receptor is a receptor for retinoic acid. *Proceedings of the National Academy of Sciences of the United States of America* **95**, 13671–13676.

Kang JX, Bell J, Beard RL and Chandraratna RAS (1999) Mannose 6-phosphate/insulin-like growth factor II receptor mediates the growth-inhibitory effects of retinoids. *Cell Growth and Differentiation* **10**, 591–600.

van Kats JP, Danser AHJ, van Meegen JR, et al. (1998) Angiotensin production by the heart: a quantitative study in pigs with the use of radiolabeled angiotensin infusions. *Circulation* **98**, 73–81.

van Kats JP, Duncker DJ, Haitsma DB, et al. (2000) Angiotensin-converting enzyme inhibition and angiotensin II type 1 receptor blockade prevent cardiac remodeling in pigs after myocardial infarction: role of tissue angiotensin II. *Circulation* **102**, 1556–1563.

Katz SA, Opsahl JA, Lunzer MM, *et al.* (1997) Effect of bilateral nephrectomy on active renin, angiotensinogen, and renin glycoforms in plasma and myocardium. *Hypertension* **30**, 259–266.

Katz SA, Opsahl JA and Forbis LM (2001) Myocardial enzymatic activity of renin and cathepsin D before and after bilateral nephrectomy. *Basic Research in Cardiology* **96**, 659–668.

van Kesteren CAM, Danser AHJ, Derkx FHM, *et al.* (1997) Mannose 6-phosphate receptor-mediated internalization and activation of prorenin by cardiac cells. *Hypertension* **30**, 1389–1396.

van Kesteren CAM, Saris JJ, Dekkers DHW, *et al.* (1999) Cultured neonatal rat cardiac myocytes and fibroblasts do not synthesize renin or angiotensinogen: evidence for stretch-induced cardiomyocyte hypertrophy independent of angiotensin II. *Cardiovascular Research* **43**, 148–156.

Kim S, Hiruma M, Ikemoto F and Yamamoto K (1988) Importance of glycosylation for hepatic clearance of renal renin. *American Journal of Physiology* **255**, E642–E651.

Klett C, Nobiling R, Gierschik P and Hackenthal E (1993) Angiotensin II stimulates the synthesis of angiotensinogen in hepatocytes by inhibiting adenylylcyclase activity and stabilizing angiotensinogen mRNA. *Journal of Biological Chemistry* **268**, 25095–25107.

Kornfeld S (1992) Structure and function of the mannose 6-phosphate/insulin like growth factor II receptors. *Annual Reviews in Biochemistry* **61**, 307–330.

Kornfeld S and Mellman I (1989) The biogenesis of lysosomes. *Annual Reviews in Cell Biology* **5**, 483–525.

de Lannoy LM, Danser AHJ, van Kats JP, *et al.* (1997) Renin–angiotensin system components in the interstitial fluid of the isolated perfused rat heart. Local production of angiotensin I. *Hypertension* **29**, 1240–1251.

Leckie BJ, Lacy PS and Lidder S (2000) The expression of renin-binding protein and renin in the kidneys of rats with two-kidney one-clip hypertension. *Journal of Hypertension* **18**, 935–943.

Lindpaintner K, Jin MW, Niedermaier N, *et al.* (1990) Cardiac angiotensinogen and its local activation in the isolated perfused beating heart. *Circulation Research* **67**, 564–573.

Ludwig J, Kerscher S, Brandt U, *et al.* (1998) Identification and characterization of a novel 9.2-kDa membrane sector-associated protein of vacuolar proton-ATPase from chromaffin granules. *Journal of Biological Chemistry* **273**, 10939–10947.

von Lutterotti N, Catanzaro DF, Sealey JE and Laragh JH (1994) Renin is not synthesized by cardiac and extrarenal vascular tissues. A review of experimental evidence. *Circulation* **89**, 458–470.

Maru I, Ohta Y, Murata K and Tsukada Y (1996) Molecular cloning and identification of N-acyl-D-glucosamine 2-epimerase from porcine kidney as a renin-binding protein. *Journal of Biological Chemistry* **271**, 16294–16299.

Morgan DO, Edman JC, Standring DN, *et al.* (1987) Insulin-like growth factor II receptor as a multifunctional binding protein. *Nature* **329**, 301–307.

Müller DN, Hilgers KF, Willnow T, *et al.* (1998a) Possible mechanisms of vascular renin uptake and metabolism: effects on local angiotensin formation. *Journal of Hypertension* **16** (Suppl 2), S3 (Abstract).

Müller DN, Fischli W, Clozel JP, *et al.* (1998b) Local angiotensin II generation in the rat heart: role of renin uptake. *Circulation Research* **82**, 13–20.

Neri Serneri GG, Boddi M, Poggesi L, et al. (2001) Activation of cardiac renin–angiotensin system in unstable angina. *Journal of the American College of Cardiologists* **38**, 49–55.

Nguyen G, Delarue F, Berrou J, et al. (1996) Specific receptor binding of renin on human mesangial cells in culture increases plasminogen activator inhibitor-1 antigen. *Kidney International* **50**, 1897–1903.

Nguyen G, Delarue F, Burcklé C, et al. (2002) Pivotal role of the renin/prorenin receptor in angiotensin II production and cellular responses to renin. *Journal of Clinical Investigation* **109**, 1417–1427.

Oka Y, Rozek LM and Czech MP (1985) Direct demonstration of rapid insulin-like growth factor II receptor internalization and recycling in rat adipocytes. Insulin stimulates 125I-insulin-like growth factor II degradation by modulating the IGF-II receptor recycling process. *Journal of Biological Chemistry* **260**, 9435–9442.

Peters J, Farrenkopf R, Clausmeyer S, et al. (2002) Functional significance of prorenin internalization in the rat heart. *Circulation Research* **90**, 1135–1141.

Saris JJ, Derkx FHM, de Bruin RJA, et al. (2001) High-affinity prorenin binding to cardiac man-6-P/IGF-II receptors precedes proteolytic activation to renin. *American Journal of Physiology* **280**, H1706–H1715.

Saris JJ, van den Eijnden MMED, Lamers JMJ, et al. (2002) Prorenin-induced myocyte proliferation: no role for intracellular angiotensin II. *Hypertension* **39**, 573–577.

Schmitz C, Gotthardt M, Hinderlich S, et al. (2000) Normal blood pressure and plasma renin activity in mice lacking the renin-binding protein, a cellular renin inhibitor. *Journal of Biological Chemistry* **275**, 15357–15362.

Schuijt MP, van Kats JP, de Zeeuw S, et al. (1999) Cardiac interstitial fluid levels of angiotensin I and II in the pig. *Journal of Hypertension* **17**, 1885–1891.

Sealey JE, Catanzaro DF, Lavin TN, et al. (1996) Specific prorenin/renin binding (ProBP). Identification and characterization of a novel membrane site. *American Journal of Hypertension* **9**, 491–502.

Tada M, Takahashi S, Miyano M and Miyake Y (1992) Tissue-specific regulation of renin-binding protein gene expression in rats. *Journal of Biochemistry* **112**, 175–182.

Takahashi S, Ohsawa T, Miura R and Miyake Y (1983) Purification of high molecular weight (HMW) renin from porcine kidney and direct evidence that the HMW renin is a complex of renin with renin binding protein (RnBP). *Journal of Biochemistry* **93**, 265–274.

Takahashi S, Inoue H and Miyake Y (1992) The human gene for renin-binding protein. *Journal of Biological Chemistry* **267**, 13007–13013.

Tally M, Li CH and Hall K (1987) IGF-2 stimulated growth mediated by the somatomedin type 2 receptor. *Biochemical and Biophysical Research Communications* **148**, 811–816.

Tong PY and Kornfeld S (1989) Ligand interactions of the cation-dependent mannose 6-phosphate receptor. Comparison with the cation-independent mannose 6-phosphate receptor. *Journal of Biological Chemistry* **264**, 7970–7975.

Yusuf S, Sleight P, Pogue J, et al. (2000) Effects of an angiotensin-converting-enzyme inhibitor, ramipril, on cardiovascular events in high-risk patients. The Heart Outcomes Prevention Evaluation Study Investigators. *New England Journal of Medicine* **342**, 145–153.

4

Role of Local Renin Angiotensin Systems in Cardiac Damage

Michael Bader

Introduction

The renin angiotensin system (RAS) recently celebrated its 100th anniversary. In 1898, renin was discovered by Tigerstedt and Bergman in rabbit kidney (Tigerstedt and Bergman, 1898). Renin turned out to be the rate limiting enzyme of a proteolytic cascade leading to the formation of angiotensin (Ang) I and Ang II. In this cascade renin splits the liver-derived renin substrate, angiotensinogen (AOGEN), in the plasma to form the decapeptide Ang I (Bader and Ganten, 2000). Ang I is then metabolized further into the octapeptide Ang II via the endothelium-bound angiotensin-converting enzyme (ACE). Ang II is one of the most potent vasopressor substances and releases aldosterone from the adrenal gland. The effects of the peptide are transmitted by two main G-protein-coupled receptors, AT_1 and AT_2, that were originally defined by the discovery of specific ligands and later confirmed by the cloning of two different genes (Murphy *et al.*, 1991; Sasaki *et al.*, 1991; Kambayashi *et al.*, 1993; Mukoyama *et al.*, 1993).

This was the classic view of the RAS. However, with additional research, it became clear that it is not the whole story. The local generation of angiotensin peptides in different tissues was detected mostly even by locally produced precursors and the concept of a tissue-based RAS emerged (Bader *et al.*, 2001). The most obvious example of such a tissue RAS was found in the brain, where AT_1 and AT_2 receptors have been located beyond the blood–brain barrier not accessible for circulating Ang II. However, Ang II can be generated in the brain from locally synthesized AOGEN and renin and activate these receptors playing an important role in vasopressin secretion, and in the control of the baroreflex and the sympathetic output (Bader and Ganten, 2002). Things are not so clear in the heart, where parts of the system are generated locally and others have to be imported from the circulation. However, the functional relevance of a local RAS in the heart in particular for pathophysiological processes of cardiac damage is beyond doubt.

In the heart, Ang I is generated by renin imported from the plasma (van Kesteren *et al.*, 1997; Müller *et al.*, 1998) which interacts with AOGEN partially also derived from the circulation but also locally produced (Campbell and Habener, 1986; Dzau *et al.*, 1987; Hellmann *et al.*, 1988; Lindpaintner *et al.*, 1990; Dostal *et al.*, 1992; Sawa *et al.*, 1992; Sadoshima *et al.*, 1993). Locally synthesized ACE (Zhou *et al.*, 1994; Katwa *et al.*, 1995) then converts Ang I to Ang II (Danser *et al.*, 1992; Neri Serneri *et al.*, 1996; de Lannoy *et al.*, 1998; Müller *et al.*, 1998). The peptide interacts with AT_1 and AT_2 receptors present on cardiac myocytes and fibroblasts (Rogers *et al.*, 1986; Saito *et al.*, 1987; Urata *et al.*, 1989; Rogg *et al.*, 1990, 1996; Sechi *et al.*, 1992; Crabos *et al.*, 1994; Lopez *et al.*, 1994; Matsubara *et al.*, 1994; Regitz-Zagrosek *et al.*, 1995; Booz and Baker, 1996; Haywood *et al.*, 1997; Ohkubo *et al.*, 1997; Wharton *et al.*, 1998). Additionally in the human heart, mast cells contain the enzyme chymase which also metabolizes Ang I to Ang II (Urata *et al.*, 1990, 1994). Circulating as well as locally generated Ang II induces vasoconstriction and exerts direct inotropic (Koch-Weser, 1964) and chronotropic actions on the heart. These effects are enhanced by a facilitation of noradrenaline release from sympathetic nerve endings. In addition, Ang II in the heart induces hypertrophy, inflammation and fibrosis by increasing endothelin, transforming growth factor (TGF)-β, oxidative stress, and cytokines.

An important development was the generation of transgenic and knockout technology in order to study the functionality of local RAS (Stec *et al.*, 1998; Bader *et al.*, 2000). Because polymorphisms in the gene for ACE were linked to the risk for cardiac diseases (Cambien *et al.*, 1992; Schunkert, 1997) and ACE inhibitors as well as AT_1 receptor antagonists were extremely effective drugs for the treatment of heart failure (CONSENSUS Trial Study Group, 1987; Pfeffer *et al.*, 1988, 1992; Sharpe *et al.*, 1988, 1991; SOLVD, 1992; Swedberg *et al.*, 1992; Pitt *et al.*, 1997, 2000; Yusuf *et al.*, 2000) numerous transgenic models have been generated to study the role of the RAS in cardiac damage. This chapter will summarize the pathophysiological functions of the cardiac RAS with a particular focus on the findings derived from transgenic animal models.

AT₁ and cardiac hypertrophy

Hypertrophy and fibrosis are the most important pathophysiological effects induced by Ang II in the heart. The growth-promoting actions of the peptide were originally discovered in adrenal cells and fibroblasts (Schelling *et al.*, 1991) where Ang II elicits DNA synthesis and proliferation. There is ample evidence that locally produced Ang II is also involved in the induction of cardiomyocyte growth and cardiac hypertrophy. ACE inhibitors and AT₁ antagonists prevent or decrease cardiac hypertrophy in humans (Nakashima *et al.*, 1984; Kaplan, 1985) and reduce or cause regression of left ventricular hypertrophy in experimental aortic banding (Kromer and Riegger, 1988), even at doses that do not reduce blood pressure (Linz *et al.*, 1989). Accordingly, other models of left ventricular hypertrophy like SHR, TGR(mREN2)27 (Mullins *et al.*, 1990), or isoproterenol-infused rats respond readily to these drugs with a reduction in left ventricular weight accompanied by a decreased myocardial fibrosis (Sen *et al.*, 1980; Brilla *et al.*, 1991; Nagano *et al.*, 1991, 1992; Pahor *et al.*, 1991; Böhm *et al.*, 1996). In some models, these changes were not correlated with blood pressure reduction or plasma Ang II levels, but instead with a reduction in cardiac Ang II concentrations (Nagano *et al.*, 1991, 1992; Böhm *et al.*, 1996).

The possible implication of the cardiac RAS has also been studied in the remodelling of the myocardium after myocardial infarction which for the most part is a hypertrophic process (Pfeffer, 1995). Some authors have reported transiently increased AOGEN mRNA in myocardial infarction and failure (Drexler *et al.*, 1989). In chronic heart failure induced by ligation of the left coronary artery in rats an enhancement of ACE mRNA was found, which correlated with the cardiac ACE activity, but not with ACE activity in other organs (Hirsch *et al.*, 1991).

To elicit cardiac hypertrophy, Ang II interacts with AT₁ receptors, which exerts its effects via several intracellular signalling pathways mediated by G proteins (Dostal, 2000; Eguchi and Inagami, 2000; Ruwhof and van der Laarse, 2000). Besides intracellular calcium surges and protein kinase C activation, small GTP-binding proteins like RAS and RhoA as well as tyrosine kinase cascades are activated including several members of the mitogen-activated protein (MAP) kinase family and the Jak/STAT pathway. Finally, transcription factors like AP₁ and the STATs are activated which initiate the expression of growth related genes. Moreover, the phosphorylation of the ribosomal protein S6 and thereby protein synthesis is increased.

Several cofactors have been implicated in the effects of Ang II on cardiomyocyte growth. Endothelin has been shown to be released by stretch and Ang II in the heart and in some models endothelin receptor antagonists block cardiac hypertrophy induced by Ang II (Ito et al., 1994; Arai et al., 1995; Yamazaki et al., 1996). The source of endothelin maybe the cardiac fibroblasts which also generate other growth factors when activated by Ang II such as TGF-β and fibroblast growth factor-2 (Kim et al., 1995; Gray et al., 1998; Pellieux et al., 2001). For these two factors a crucial involvement in Ang II-induced cardiac hypertrophy has been shown using specific knockout mouse models (Pellieux et al., 2001; Schultz et al., 2002).

Another possible mediator of Ang II-induced cardiac hypertrophy may be norepinephrine released by Ang II from sympathetic nerve endings in the heart. Norepinephrine was shown to trigger hypertrophy and in a positive feedback loop also RAS activation via α- and β-adrenergic receptors (Bogoyevitch et al., 1996; Yamazaki and Yazaki, 2000).

In addition, reactive oxygen species are generated by Ang II via the AT_1 receptor by the activation of NADPH oxidases in the heart. These free oxygen radicals are important for several signaling pathways including the transactivation of the epidermal growth factor (EGF) receptor by the AT_1 receptor (Griendling and Ushio-Fukai, 2000). It has been shown that in cardiac fibroblasts and vascular smooth muscle cells EGF-receptor transactivation is essential for the hypertrophic actions mediated by the AT_1 receptor (Eguchi and Inagami, 2000; Griendling and Ushio-Fukai, 2000). The relevance of reactive oxygen species was demonstrated using mice lacking a subunit of NADPH oxidase (Bendall et al., 2002). These animals were resistant against Ang II-induced cardiac hypertrophy.

Another important factor involved in cardiac hypertrophy is mechanical stretch of the cardiomyocytes. There is evidence that mechanical stretch induces Ang II generation and that this effect is crucial for the development of cardiac hypertrophy (Dostal, 2000). Stretch induces the release of Ang II in the myocardium as well as from cardiomyocytes in culture (Sadoshima et al., 1993; Leri et al., 1998). Ang II in turn increases the expression of RAS components such as AOGEN, ACE, AT_1, and AT_2 in a positive feedback loop (Kijima et al., 1996; Tamura et al., 1998; Malhotra et al., 1999). AOGEN and AT_1 are induced by p53 binding to the respective promoter regions after activation by the AT_1 receptor (Leri et al., 1998). AOGEN is additionally induced by the same receptor involving the Jak/STAT pathway of transcription factors, which was already mentioned above, to induce growth (Mascareno et al., 1998).

Transgenic animal models have been generated to solve the question whether mechanical stretch or whether the cardiac RAS alone are able to induce cardiac hypertrophy independently. Mice lacking AOGEN (own unpublished results) or AT_1 receptors (Hamawaki et al., 1998; Harada et al., 1998) develop cardiac hypertrophy after volume or pressure overload, respectively. Cardiomyocytes isolated from AOGEN knockout mice respond to mechanical stretch by activating MAP kinases as do control cells. However, in contrast to control cells this effect is not blocked by AT_1 antagonists (Nyui et al., 1997). These results indicate that there are redundant pathways of growth induction by stretch in cardiomyocytes circumventing the RAS. However, the default mechanisms involve Ang II and the AT_1 receptor.

Transgenic experiments designed to solve the opposite question, whether or not Ang II alone is able to induce cardiac hypertrophy without mechanical stretch gave controversial results. Transgenic rats overexpressing ACE predominantly in the heart have been produced (Tian et al., 1996). Despite very high cardiac levels of cardiac ACE activity, there were no morphological alterations unless the heart was pressure overloaded with aortic banding. This treatment resulted in a significantly higher hypertrophic response in the ACE-transgenic rats than in control animals. The results support the important role of Ang II in stretch-induced hypertrophy but deny an autonomous effect. In contrast, mice expressing AOGEN exclusively in the heart remained normotensive but nevertheless developed cardiac hypertrophy (Mazzolai et al., 1998). This finding indicates that the local formation of Ang II induces cardiac damage independent of blood pressure elevation. The importance of local angiotensin generation in end organs was confirmed in a hybrid mouse model carrying a rat AOGEN transgene on a knockout background (Kang et al., 2002). These animals developed hypertension due to the exclusive expression of AOGEN in liver and brain. However, since local AOGEN synthesis in kidney and heart was absent, cardiac hypertrophy and renal fibrosis was attenuated in these mice.

Transgenic animal models have been reported that overexpress AT_1-receptors in the heart by the use of the α-myosin-heavy chain promoter (Hein et al., 1997; Paradis et al., 2000; Hoffmann et al., 2001). However, the phenotypes of the transgenic animals generated were dramatically different. The mouse models exhibited a drastic cardiac hypertrophy and the animals died after several days (Hein et al., 1997) to weeks

(Paradis et al., 2000) of age. In sharp contrast, the rats appeared absolutely normal unless the heart was pressure-overloaded by aortic banding (Hoffmann et al., 2001). With this treatment, the AT_1 receptor transgenic rats also exhibited increased hypertrophy compared to controls, similar to the observations in the ACE transgenic rats. The difference may be related to a species-specific sensitivity of mouse and rat hearts for Ang II-related effects. However a transgenic mouse model was generated in which Ang II is produced exclusively in the heart and is independent of any other RAS component (van Kats et al., 2001). The investigators used a unique artificially engineered protein (Methot et al., 1997). The animals show dramatically enhanced Ang II levels in the heart but no cardiac hypertrophy. Thus, the issue whether or not Ang II alone can induce cardiac hypertrophy remains controversial. Mechanical stretch employs the local cardiac RAS for growth promotion, but can also use alternative pathways.

AT_1 and cardiac fibrosis

Concomitantly to hypertrophy, most stimuli also induce cardiac fibrosis namely the proliferation of cardiac fibroblasts and the excessive deposition of extracellular matrix in the cardiac interstitium (Booz and Baker, 1995). The resulting increase in stiffness causes ventricular dysfunction and finally heart failure mostly through diastolic dysfunction. Therefore, fibrosis is of major pathophysiological relevance. Ang II is directly involved in the development of cardiac fibrosis (Booz and Baker, 1995). Chronic Ang II infusion induces fibrosis and ACE inhibitors as well as AT_1 receptor antagonists can ameliorate fibrosis induced by pressure overload. Activation of the AT_1 receptor in fibroblasts again activates the MAP kinases and the Jak/STAT pathway which induce expression of angiotensinogen and fibrosis-related proteins such as collagens as well as cell proliferation (Booz and Baker, 1995; Murasawa et al., 2000).

A recent experiment employing chimeric mice that carry cardiac cells without AT_1 receptors surrounded by normal tissue has shown that the activation of fibroblasts by Ang II depends on the interaction of the peptide with neighbouring cardiomyocytes (Matsusaka et al., 1999). This observation indicates that cardiomyocytes release a paracrine factor after Ang II stimulation, possibly TGF-β, which is mitogenic for fibroblasts (Lee et al., 1995).

Endothelin may also play role in this conversation between cardiac myocytes and fibroblasts. It is released by cardiomyocytes after Ang II stimulation and activates collagen synthesis in fibroblasts (Guarda et al.,

1993; Rossi et al., 1999). This effect is direct but may be enhanced by stimulation of local TGF-β release (Belloni et al., 1996; Gandhi et al., 2000). Accordingly, two transgenic rat models with hypertension and marked end organ damage support the role of endothelin in Ang II-induced cardiac fibrosis. In transgenic rats, TGR(mREN2)27, carrying the mouse renin gene, *ren*-2 (Mullins et al., 1990), it was shown that cardiac fibrosis can be blunted by blockade with a combined ET_A/ET_B-endothelin receptor antagonist (Seccia et al., 2003). Furthermore, inhibition of the endothelin-converting enzyme in double transgenic rats expressing both, the human renin and angiotensinogen genes (Ganten et al., 1992), also attenuates the upregulated cardiac collagen synthesis (Müller et al., 2002). Another possible mediator of cardiac fibrosis in the double transgenic rat model is connective tissue growth factor, which may act via stimulation of TGF-β release (Finckenberg et al., 2003). The same rat model has also shed light on aldosterone as mediator of Ang II-induced fibrosis, since when these rats are treated with the mineralocorticoid receptor antagonist spironolactone, cardiac fibrosis is attenuated (Fiebeler et al., 2001). Aldosterone may facilitate Ang II signaling by upregulating AT_1 receptors (Sun and Weber, 1993; Robert et al., 1999) or the signaling of mediators of Ang II action such as EGF (Krug et al., 2002). Finally, reactive oxygen species seem to play a role in Ang II-induced cardiac fibrosis since mice lacking NADPH oxidase do not develop fibrosis (Bendall et al., 2002).

However, the issue of a crucial cardiomyocyte-derived mediator of the profibrotic actions of Ang II on fibroblasts such as endothelins and/or TGF-β remains controversial since growth-promoting actions of Ang II on pure cardiac fibroblasts in culture have been repeatedly demonstrated (Booz and Baker, 1995).

AT_2 in cardiac hypertrophy and fibrosis

Surprisingly, a recent study using AT_2-knockout mice has shown that this receptor is essential for cardiac hypertrophy induction by pressure overload (Senbonmatsu et al., 2000; Ichihara et al., 2001). This effect may be mediated by a reduced phosphorylation of the ribosomal protein S6. These results contradict earlier findings employing AT_2 antagonists, which showed antigrowth effects exerted by the AT_2 receptor (Booz and Baker, 1996). Furthermore, another strain of AT_2-deficient mice did not show any difference in hypertrophy development after pressure overload and vascular hypertrophy was even enhanced in these mice (Brede et al., 2001; Wu et al., 2002). Accordingly, a transgenic mouse overexpressing the AT_2 receptor in the heart was less susceptible to AT_1-mediated actions compared to controls (Masaki et al., 1998) and developed less fibrosis after Ang II infusion (Kurisu et al., 2003), whereas hypertrophy induction was equal (Sugino et al., 2001). Ang II-induced fibrosis is reduced in these animals by a mechanism involving the kallikrein kinin system (Kurisu et al., 2003), which has been shown to have antihypertrophic and antifibrotic actions in the heart by the use of tissue-kallikrein overexpressing transgenic rats (Silva et al., 2000).

After myocardial infarction, remodelling of the myocardium is part of the wound healing process implicating fibrosis and cardiomyocyte hypertrophy. In the AT_2 receptor overexpressing mice this remodelling is facilitated (Yang et al., 2002) and in AT_2-deficient animals it is blunted, development of heart failure is exacerbated (Adachi et al., 2003) and the heart may even rupture after infarction (Ichihara et al., 2002). Thus, the majority of data support an antihypertrophic and antifibrotic action of the AT_2 receptor but the issue still needs clarification (Inagami and Senbonmatsu, 2001).

Conclusion

Locally generated Ang II has numerous effects on the heart with significant pathophysiological impact. Cardiac hypertrophy is induced either by a direct action on cardiomyocytes in concert with mechanical stretch or by the release of mediators such as endothelin, TGF-β and reactive oxygen species from cardiac fibroblasts. This crosstalk between myocytes and fibroblasts in the heart is also of major importance for the Ang II-induced cardiac fibrosis which also implicates TGF-β and endothelin as well as aldosterone.

Cell type-specific transgenic and knockout animal models will help to clarify the pathophysiologically relevant communication between cardiac myocytes and fibroblasts and the relative importance of the two angiotensin receptors, AT_1 and AT_2 in these processes.

References

Adachi Y, Saito Y, Kishimoto I, et al. (2003) Angiotensin II type 2 receptor deficiency exacerbates heart failure and reduces survival after acute myocardial infarction in mice. *Circulation* **107**, 2406–2408.

Arai M, Yoguchi A, Iso T, et al. (1995) Endothelin-1 and its binding sites are upregulated in pressure overload cardiac hypertrophy. *American Journal of Physiology* **268**, H2084–H2091.

Bader M and Ganten D (2000) Regulation of renin. *Journal of Molecular Medicine* **78**, 130–139.

Bader M and Ganten D (2002) Editorial: it's renin in the brain. *Circulation Research* **90**, 8–10.

Bader M, Bohnemeier H, Zollmann FS, et al. (2000) Transgenic animals in cardiovascular disease research. *Experimental Physiology* **85**, 713–731.

Bader M, Peters J, Baltatu O, et al. (2001) Tissue renin–angiotensin systems: new insights from experimental animal models in hypertension research. *Journal of Molecular Medicine* **79**, 76–102.

Belloni AS, Rossi GP, Andreis PG, et al. (1996) Endothelin adrenocortical secretagogue effect is mediated by the B receptor in rats. *Hypertension* **27**, 1153–1159.

Bendall JK, Cave AC, Heymes C, et al. (2002) Pivotal role of a gp91(phox)-containing NADPH oxidase in angiotensin II-induced cardiac hypertrophy in mice. *Circulation* **105**, 293–296.

Bogoyevitch MA, Andersson MB, Gillespie-Brown J, et al. (1996) Adrenergic receptor stimulation of the mitogen-activated protein kinase cascade and cardiac hypertrophy. *Biochemical Journal* **314** (Pt 1), 115–121.

Böhm M, Lippoldt A, Wienen W, et al. (1996) Reduction of cardiac hypertrophy in TGR(mren2)27 by angiotensin II receptor blockade. *Molecular and Cellular Biochemistry* **163–164**, 217–221.

Booz GW and Baker KM (1995) Molecular signaling mechanisms controlling growth and function of cardiac fibroblasts. *Cardiovascular Research* **30**, 537–543.

Booz GW and Baker KM (1996) Role of type 1 and type 2 angiotensin receptors in angiotensin II-induced cardiomyocyte hypertrophy. *Hypertension* **28**, 635–640.

Brede M, Hadamek K, Meinel L, et al. (2001) Vascular hypertrophy and increased P70S6 kinase in mice lacking the angiotensin II AT(2) receptor. *Circulation* **104**, 2602–2607.

Brilla CG, Janicki JS and Weber KT (1991) Cardioprotective effects of lisinopril in rats with genetic hypertension and left ventricular hypertrophy. *Circulation* **83**, 1771–1779.

Cambien F, Poirier O, Lecerf L, et al. (1992) Deletion polymorphism in the gene for angiotensin-converting enzyme is a potent risk factor for myocardial infarction. *Nature* **359**, 641–644.

Campbell DJ and Habener JF (1986) Angiotensinogen gene is expressed and differentially regulated in multiple tissues of the rat. *Journal of Clinical Investigation* **78**, 31–39.

CONSENSUS Trial Study Group (1987) Effects of enalapril on mortality in severe congestive heart failure. Results of the Cooperative North Scandinavian Enalapril Survival Study (CONSENSUS). *New England Journal of Medicine* **316**, 1429–1435.

Crabos M, Roth M, Hahn AW and Erne P (1994) Characterization of angiotensin II receptors in cultured adult rat cardiac fibroblasts. Coupling to signaling systems and gene expression. *Journal of Clinical Investigation* **93**, 2372–2378.

Danser AH, Koning MM, Admiraal PJ, et al. (1992) Production of angiotensins I and II at tissue sites in intact pigs. *American Journal of Physiology* **263**, H429–H437.

Dostal DE (2000) The cardiac renin–angiotensin system: novel signaling mechanisms related to cardiac growth and function. *Regulatory Peptides* **91**, 1–11.

Dostal DE, Rothblum KN, Chernin MI, et al. (1992) Intracardiac detection of angiotensinogen and renin: a localized renin–angiotensin system in neonatal rat heart. *American Journal of Physiology* **263**, C838–C850.

Drexler H, Hänze J, Finckh M, et al. (1989) Atrial natriuretic peptide in a rat model of cardiac failure. *Circulation* **79**, 620–633.

Dzau VJ, Ellison KE, Brody T, et al. (1987) A comparative study of the distributions of renin and angiotensinogen messenger ribonucleic acids in rat and mouse tissues. *Endocrinology* **120**, 2334–2338.

Eguchi S and Inagami T (2000) Signal transduction of angiotensin II type 1 receptor through receptor tyrosine kinase. *Regulatory Peptides* **91**, 13–20.

Fiebeler A, Schmidt F, Müller DN, et al. (2001) Mineralocorticoid receptor affects AP_1 and nuclear factor-kappab activation in angiotensin II-induced cardiac injury. *Hypertension* **37**, 787–793.

Finckenberg P, Inkinen K, Ahonen J, et al. (2003) Angiotensin II induces connective tissue growth factor gene expression via calcineurin-dependent pathways. *American Journal of Pathology* **163**, 355–366.

Gandhi CR, Kuddus RH, Uemura T and Rao AS (2000) Endothelin stimulates transforming growth factor-beta1 and collagen synthesis in stellate cells from control but not cirrhotic rat liver. *European Journal of Pharmacology* **406**, 311–318.

Ganten D, Wagner J, Zeh K, et al. (1992) Species specificity of renin kinetics in transgenic rats harboring the human renin and angiotensinogen genes. *Proceedings of the National Academy of Science of the United States of America* **89**, 7806–7810.

Gray MO, Long CS, Kalinyak JE, et al. (1998) Angiotensin II stimulates cardiac myocyte hypertrophy via paracrine release of TGF-beta 1 and endothelin-1 from fibroblasts. *Cardiovascular Research* **40**, 352–363.

Griendling KK and Ushio-Fukai M (2000) Reactive oxygen species as mediators of angiotensin II signaling. *Regulatory Peptides* **91**, 21–27.

Guarda E, Katwa LC, Myers PR, et al. (1993) Effects of endothelins on collagen turnover in cardiac fibroblasts. *Cardiovascular Research* **27**, 2130–2134.

Hamawaki M, Coffman TM, Lashus A, et al. (1998) Pressure-overload hypertrophy is unabated in mice devoid of AT_{1A} receptors. *American Journal of Physiology* **274**, H868–H873.

Harada K, Komuro I, Zou Y, et al. (1998) Acute pressure overload could induce hypertrophic responses in the heart of angiotensin II type 1a knockout mice. *Circulation Research* **82**, 779–785.

Haywood GA, Gullestad L, Katsuya T, et al. (1997) AT_1 and AT_2 angiotensin receptor gene expression in human heart failure. *Circulation* **95**, 1201–1206.

Hein L, Stevens ME, Barsh GS, et al. (1997) Overexpression of angiotensin AT_1 receptor transgene in the mouse myocardium produces a lethal phenotype associated with myocyte hyperplasia and heart block. *Proceedings of the National Academy of Sciences of the United States of America* **94**, 6391–6396.

Hellmann W, Suzuki F, Ohkubo H, et al. (1988) Angiotensinogen gene expression in extrahepatic rat tissues: application of a solution hybridization assay. *Naunyn Schmiedeberg's Archives of Pharmacology* **338**, 327–331.

Hirsch AT, Talsness CE, Schunkert H, et al. (1991) Tissue-specific activation of cardiac angiotensin converting enzyme in experimental heart failure. *Circulation Research* **69**, 475–482.

Hoffmann S, Krause T, van Geel PP, et al. (2001) Overexpression of the human angiotensin II type 1 receptor in the rat heart augments load induced cardiac hypertrophy. *Journal of Molecular Medicine* **79**, 601–608.

Ichihara S, Senbonmatsu T, Price E, Jr, *et al.* (2001) Angiotensin II type 2 receptor is essential for left ventricular hypertrophy and cardiac fibrosis in chronic angiotensin II-induced hypertension. *Circulation* **104**, 346–351.

Ichihara S, Senbonmatsu T, Price E, Jr, *et al.* (2002) Targeted deletion of angiotensin II type 2 receptor caused cardiac rupture after acute myocardial infarction. *Circulation* **106**, 2244–2249.

Inagami T and Senbonmatsu T (2001) Dual effects of angiotensin II type 2 receptor on cardiovascular hypertrophy. *Trends in Cardiovascular Medicine* **11**, 324–328.

Ito H, Hiroe M, Hirata Y, *et al.* (1994) Endothelin ETA receptor antagonist blocks cardiac hypertrophy provoked by hemodynamic overload. *Circulation* **89**, 2198–2203.

Kambayashi Y, Bardhan S, Takahashi K, *et al.* (1993) Molecular cloning of a novel angiotensin II receptor isoform involved in phosphotyrosine phosphatase inhibition. *Journal of Biological Chemistry* **268**, 24543–24546.

Kang N, Walther T, Tian XL, *et al.* (2002) Reduced hypertension-induced end-organ damage in mice lacking cardiac and renal angiotensinogen synthesis. *Journal of Molecular Medicine* **80**, 359–366.

Kaplan NM (1985) New perspectives in the treatment of hypertension withy arterial disease. *Journal of Cardiovascular Pharmacology* **7**, S131–S134.

van Kats JP, Methot D, Paradis P, *et al.* (2001) Use of a biological peptide pump to study chronic peptide hormone action in transgenic mice. Direct and indirect effects of angiotensin II on the heart. *Journal of Biological Chemistry* **276**, 44012–44017.

Katwa LC, Ratajska A, Cleutjens JP, *et al.* (1995) Angiotensin converting enzyme and kininase-II-like activities in cultured valvular interstitial cells of the rat heart. *Cardiovascular Research* **29**, 57–64.

van Kesteren CA, Danser AH, Derkx FH, *et al.* (1997) Mannose 6-phosphate receptor-mediated internalization and activation of prorenin by cardiac cells. *Hypertension* **30**, 1389–1396.

Kijima K, Matsubara H, Murasawa S, *et al.* (1996) Mechanical stretch induces enhanced expression of angiotensin II receptor subtypes in neonatal rat cardiac myocytes. *Circulation Research* **79**, 887–897.

Kim NN, Villarreal FJ, Printz MP, *et al.* (1995) Trophic effects of angiotensin II on neonatal rat cardiac myocytes are mediated by cardiac fibroblasts. *American Journal of Physiology* **269**, E426–E437.

Koch-Weser J (1964) Myocardial actions of angiotensin. *Circulation Research* **14**, 337–344.

Kromer EP and Riegger GAJ (1988) Effects of longterm angiotensin converting enzyme inhibition on myocardial hypertrophy in experimental aortic stenosis in the rat. *American Journal of Cardiology* **62**, 161–163.

Krug AW, Schuster C, Gassner B, *et al.* (2002) Human epidermal growth factor receptor-1 expression renders Chinese hamster ovary cells sensitive to alternative aldosterone signaling. *Journal of Biological Chemistry* **277**, 45892–45897.

Kurisu S, Ozono R, Oshima T, *et al.* (2003) Cardiac angiotensin II type 2 receptor activates the kinin/NO system and inhibits fibrosis. *Hypertension* **41**, 99–107.

de Lannoy LM, Danser AH, Bouhuizen AM, *et al.* (1998) Localization and production of angiotensin II in the isolated perfused rat heart. *Hypertension* **31**, 1111–1117.

Lee AA, Dillmann WH, McCulloch AD and Villarreal FJ (1995) Angiotensin II stimulates the autocrine production of transforming growth factor-beta 1 in adult rat cardiac fibroblasts. *Journal of Molecular and Cellular Cardiology* **27**, 2347–2357.

Leri A, Claudio PP, Li Q, et al. (1998) Stretch-mediated release of angiotensin II induces myocyte apoptosis by activating p53 that enhances the local renin–angiotensin system and decreases the Bcl-2-to-Bax protein ratio in the cell. *Journal of Clinical Investigation* **101**, 1326–1342.

Lindpaintner K, Jin M, Niedermeier N, et al. (1990) Cardiac angiotensinogen and its local activation in the isolated perfused beating heart. *Circulation Research* **67**, 564–573.

Linz W, Schölkens BA and Ganten D (1989) Converting enzyme inhibition specifically prevents the development and induces regression of cardiac hypertrophy in rats. *Clinical and Experimental Hypertension [A]* **11**, 1325–1350.

Lopez JJ, Lorell BH, Ingelfinger JR, et al. (1994) Distribution and function of cardiac angiotensin AT_1- and AT_2-receptor subtypes in hypertrophied rat hearts. *American Journal of Physiology* **267**, H844–H852.

Malhotra R, Sadoshima J, Brosius FC, III and Izumo S (1999) Mechanical stretch and angiotensin II differentially upregulate the renin–angiotensin system in cardiac myocytes *in vitro*. *Circulation Research* **85**, 137–146.

Masaki H, Kurihara H, Yamaki A, et al. (1998) Cardiac-specific overexpression of angiotensin II AT_2 receptor causes attenuated response to AT_1 receptor-mediated pressor and chronotropic effects. *Journal of Clinical Investigation* **101**, 527–535.

Mascareno E, Dhar M and Siddiqui MA (1998) Signal transduction and activator of transcription (STAT) protein-dependent activation of angiotensinogen promoter: a cellular signal for hypertrophy in cardiac muscle. *Proceedings of the National Academy of Sciences of the United States of America* **95**, 5590–5594.

Matsubara H, Kanasaki M, Murasawa S, et al. (1994) Differential gene expression and regulation of angiotensin II receptor subtypes in rat cardiac fibroblasts and cardiomyocytes in culture. *Journal of Clinical Investigation* **93**, 1592–1601.

Matsusaka T, Katori H, Inagami T, et al. (1999) Communication between myocytes and fibroblasts in cardiac remodeling in angiotensin chimeric mice. *Journal of Clinical Investigation* **103**, 1451–1458.

Mazzolai L, Nussberger J, Aubert JF, et al. (1998) Blood pressure-independent cardiac hypertrophy induced by locally activated renin–angiotensin system. *Hypertension* **31**, 1324–1330.

Methot D, Lapointe MC, Touyz RM, et al. (1997) Tissue targeting of angiotensin peptides. *Journal of Biological Chemistry* **272**, 12994–12999.

Mukoyama M, Nakajima M, Horiuchi M, et al. (1993) Expression cloning of type 2 angiotensin II receptor reveals a unique class of seven-transmembrane receptors. *Journal of Biological Chemistry* **268**, 24539–24542.

Müller DN, Fischli W, Clozel JP, et al. (1998) Local angiotensin II generation in the rat heart: role of renin uptake. *Circulation Research* **82**, 13–20.

Müller DN, Mullally A, Dechend R, et al. (2002) Endothelin-converting enzyme inhibition ameliorates angiotensin II-induced cardiac damage. *Hypertension* **40**, 840–846.

Mullins JJ, Peters J and Ganten D (1990) Fulminant hypertension in transgenic rats harbouring the mouse ren-2 gene. *Nature* **344**, 541–544.

Murasawa S, Matsubara H, Mori Y, et al. (2000) Angiotensin II initiates tyrosine kinase Pyk2-dependent signalings leading to activation of Rac1-

mediated c-Jun NH₂-terminal kinase. *Journal of Biological Chemistry* **275**, 26856–26863.

Murphy TJ, Alexander RW, Griendling KK, *et al.* (1991) Isolation of a cDNA encoding the vascular type-1 angiotensin II receptor. *Nature* **351**, 233–236.

Nagano M, Higaki J, Mikami H, *et al.* (1991) Converting enzyme inhibitors regressed cardiac hypertrophy and reduced tissue angiotensin II in spontaneously hypertensive rats. *Journal of Hypertension* **9**, 595–599.

Nagano M, Higaki J, Nakamura F, *et al.* (1992) Role of cardiac angiotensin II in isoproterenol-induced left ventricular hypertrophy. *Hypertension* **19**, 708–712.

Nakashima Y, Fouad FM and Tarazi RC (1984) Regression of left ventricular hypertrophy from systemic hypertension by enalapril. *American Journal of Cardiology* **53**, 1044–1049.

Neri Serneri GG, Boddi M, Coppo M, *et al.* (1996) Evidence for the existence of a functional cardiac renin–angiotensin system in humans. *Circulation* **94**, 1886–1893.

Nyui N, Tamura K, Mizuno K, *et al.* (1997) Stretch-induced MAP kinase activation in cardiomyocytes of angiotensinogen-deficient mice. *Biochemical and Biophysical Research Communications* **235**, 36–41.

Ohkubo N, Matsubara H, Nozawa Y, *et al.* (1997) Angiotensin type 2 receptors are reexpressed by cardiac fibroblasts from failing myopathic hamster hearts and inhibit cell growth and fibrillar collagen metabolism. *Circulation* **96**, 3954–3962.

Pahor M, Bernabei R, Sgadari A, *et al.* (1991) Enalapril prevents cardiac fibrosis and arrhythmias in hypertensive rats. *Hypertension* **18**, 148–157.

Paradis P, Dali-Youcef N, Paradis FW, *et al.* (2000) Overexpression of angiotensin II type I receptor in cardiomyocytes induces cardiac hypertrophy and remodeling. *Proceedings of the National Academy of Sciences of the United States of America* **97**, 931–936.

Pellieux C, Foletti A, Peduto G, *et al.* (2001) Dilated cardiomyopathy and impaired cardiac hypertrophic response to angiotensin II in mice lacking FGF-2. *Journal of Clinical Investigation* **108**, 1843–1851.

Pfeffer MA (1995) Left ventricular remodeling after acute myocardial infarction. *Annual Reviews in Medicine* **46**, 455–456.

Pfeffer MA, Lamas GA, Vaughan DE, *et al.* (1988) Effect of captopril on progressive ventricular dilatation after anterior myocardial infarction. *New England Journal of Medicine* **319**, 80–86.

Pfeffer MA, Braunwald E, Moyé LA, *et al.* (1992) Effect of captopril on mortality and morbidity in patients with left ventricular dysfunction after myocardial infarction. *New England Journal of Medicine* **327**, 669–677.

Pitt B, Segal R, Martinez FA, *et al.* (1997) Randomised trial of losartan versus captopril in patients over 65 with heart failure (Evaluation of Losartan in the Elderly Study, ELITE). *Lancet* **349**, 747–752.

Pitt B, Poole-Wilson PA, Segal R, *et al.* (2000) Effect of losartan compared with captopril on mortality in patients with symptomatic heart failure: randomised trial – the Losartan Heart Failure Survival Study ELITE II. *Lancet* **355**, 1582–1587.

Regitz-Zagrosek V, Friedel N, Heymann A, *et al.* (1995) Regulation, chamber localization, and subtype distribution of angiotensin II receptors in human hearts. *Circulation* **91**, 1461–1471.

Robert V, Heymes C, Silvestre JS, et al. (1999) Angiotensin AT$_1$ receptor subtype as a cardiac target of aldosterone: role in aldosterone-salt-induced fibrosis. *Hypertension* **33**, 981–986.

Rogers TB, Gaa ST and Allen IS (1986) Identification and characterization of functional angiotensin II receptors on cultured heart myocytes. *Journal of Pharmacology and Experimental Therapeutics* **236**, 438–444.

Rogg H, Schmid A and de Gasparo M (1990) Identification and characterization of angiotensin II receptor subtypes in rabbit ventricular myocardium. *Biochemical and Biophysical Research Communications* **173**, 416–422.

Rogg H, de Gasparo M, Graedel E, et al. (1996) Angiotensin II-receptor subtypes in human atria and evidence for alterations in patients with cardiac dysfunction. *European Heart Journal* **17**, 1112–1120.

Rossi GP, Sacchetto A, Cesari M and Pessina AC (1999) Interactions between endothelin-1 and the renin–angiotensin–aldosterone system. *Cardiovascular Research* **43**, 300–307.

Ruwhof C and van der Laarse A (2000) Mechanical stress-induced cardiac hypertrophy: mechanisms and signal transduction pathways. *Cardiovascular Research* **47**, 23–37.

Sadoshima J, Xu Y, Slayter HS and Izumo S (1993) Autocrine release of angiotensin II mediates stretch-induced hypertrophy of cardiac myocytes *in vitro*. *Cell* **75**, 977–984.

Saito K, Gutkind JS and Saavedra JM (1987) Angiotensin II binding sites in the conduction system of rat hearts. *American Journal of Physiology* **253**, H1618–H1622.

Sasaki K, Yamano Y, Bardhan S, et al. (1991) Cloning and expression of a complementary DNA encoding a bovine adrenal angiotensin II type-1 receptor. *Nature* **351**, 230–232.

Sawa H, Tokuchi F, Mochizuki N, et al. (1992) Expression of the angiotensinogen gene and localization of its protein in the human heart. *Circulation* **86**, 138–146.

Schelling P, Fischer H and Ganten D (1991) Angiotensin and cell growth: a link to cardiovascular hypertrophy? *Journal of Hypertension* **9**, 3–15.

Schultz JJ, Witt SA, Glascock BJ, et al. (2002) TGF-beta1 mediates the hypertrophic cardiomyocyte growth induced by angiotensin II. *Journal of Clinical Investigation* **109**, 787–796.

Schunkert H (1997) Polymorphism of the angiotensin-converting enzyme gene and cardiovascular disease. *Journal of Molecular Medicine* **75**, 867–875.

Seccia TM, Belloni AS, Kreutz R, et al. (2003) Cardiac fibrosis occurs early and involves endothelin and AT$_1$ receptors in hypertension due to endogenous angiotensin II. *Journal of the American College of Cardiology* **41**, 666–673.

Sechi LA, Griffin CA, Grady EF, et al. (1992) Characterization of angiotensin II receptor subtypes in rat heart. *Circulation Research* **71**, 1482–1489.

Sen S, Tarazi RC and Bumpus FM (1980) Effect of converting enzyme inhibitor (SQ 14225) on myocardial hypertrophy in spontaneously hypertensive rats. *Hypertension* **2**, 169–176.

Senbonmatsu T, Ichihara S, Price E, Jr, et al. (2000) Evidence for angiotensin II type 2 receptor-mediated cardiac myocyte enlargement during *in vivo* pressure overload. *Journal of Clinical Investigation* **106**, R25–R29.

Sharpe N, Murphy J, Smith H and Hannan S (1988) Treatment of patients with symptomless left ventricular dysfunction after myocardial infarction. *Lancet* **I**, 255–259.

Sharpe N, Smith H, Murphy J, et al. (1991) Early prevention of left ventricular dysfunction after myocardial infarction with angiotensin-converting-enzyme inhibition. Lancet **337**, 872–876.

Silva JA, Jr, Araujo RC, Baltatu O, et al. (2000) Reduced cardiac hypertrophy and altered blood pressure control in transgenic rats with the human tissue kallikrein gene. FASEB Journal **14**, 1858–1860.

SOLVD (1992) Effects of enalapril on mortality and the development of heart failure in asymptomatic patients with reduced left ventricular ejection fractions. New England Journal of Medicine **327**, 685–691.

Stec DE, Davisson RL and Sigmund CD (1998) Transgenesis and gene targeting in the mouse. Tools for studying genetic determinants of hypertension. Trends in Cardiovascular Medicine **8**, 256–264.

Sugino H, Ozono R, Kurisu S, et al. (2001) Apoptosis is not increased in myocardium overexpressing type 2 angiotensin II receptor in transgenic mice. Hypertension **37**, 1394–1398.

Sun Y and Weber KT (1993) Angiotensin II and aldosterone receptor binding in rat heart and kidney: response to chronic angiotensin II or aldosterone administration. Journal of Laboratory and Clinical Medicine **122**, 404–411.

Swedberg K, Held P, Kjekshus J, et al. (1992) Effects of early administration of enalapril on mortality in patients with acute myocardial infarction. New England Journal of Medicine **327**, 678–684.

Tamura K, Umemura S, Nyui N, et al. (1998) Activation of angiotensinogen gene in cardiac myocytes by angiotensin II and mechanical stretch. American Journal of Physiology **44**, R1–R9.

Tian X-L, Costerousse O, Urata H, et al. (1996) A new transgenic rat model overexpressing human angiotensin-converting enzyme in the heart. Hypertension **28**, 520 (Abstract).

Tigerstedt R and Bergman PG (1898) Niere und Kreislauf. Archiv für Physiologie **8**, 223–271.

Urata H, Healy B, Stewart RW, et al. (1989) Angiotensin II receptors in normal and failing human hearts. Journal of Clinical and Endocrinological Metabolism **69**, 54–66.

Urata H, Kinoshita A, Misono KS, et al. (1990) Identification of a highly specific chymase as the major angiotensin II-forming enzyme in the human heart. Journal of Biological Chemistry **265**, 22348–22357.

Urata H, Strobel F and Ganten D (1994) Widespread tissue distribution of human chymase. Journal of Hypertension Supplement **12**, S17–S22.

Wharton J, Morgan K, Rutherford RA, et al. (1998) Differential distribution of angiotensin AT_2 receptors in the normal and failing human heart. Journal of Pharmacology and Experimental Therapeutics **284**, 323–336.

Wu L, Iwai M, Nakagami H, et al. (2002) Effect of angiotensin II type 1 receptor blockade on cardiac remodeling in angiotensin II type 2 receptor null mice. Arteriosclerosis, Thrombosis and Vascular Biology **22**, 49–54.

Yamazaki T and Yazaki Y (2000) Molecular basis of cardiac hypertrophy. Zeitschrift für Kardiologie **89**, 1–6.

Yamazaki T, Komuro I, Kudoh S, et al. (1996) Endothelin-1 is involved in mechanical stress-induced cardiomyocyte hypertrophy. Journal of Biological Chemistry **271**, 3221–3228.

Yang Z, Bove CM, French BA, et al. (2002) Angiotensin II type 2 receptor overexpression preserves left ventricular function after myocardial infarction. Circulation **106**, 106–111.

Yusuf S, Sleight P, Pogue J, *et al.* (2000) Effects of an angiotensin-converting-enzyme inhibitor, ramipril, on cardiovascular events in high-risk patients. The Heart Outcomes Prevention Evaluation Study Investigators. *New England Journal of Medicine* **342**, 145–153.

Zhou J, Allen AM, Yamada H, *et al.* (1994) Localization and properties of angiotensin-converting enzyme and angiotensin receptors in the heart. In *The Cardiac Renin–Angiotensin System*, Lindpaintner K and Ganten D (eds), Futura Publishing Co., Inc., Armonk, New York, pp. 63–88.

5

Cardiac Renin: *De Novo* Synthesis and Uptake

Jörg Peters

Introduction

It has long been proposed that a local renin angiotensin system (RAS) exists within the heart. Such a system could specifically regulate cardiac functions without affecting unnecessarily extracardiac tissues, blood pressure and electrolyte balance. The cardiac system could operate either independently from the circulating system or modulate (i.e., amplify or inhibit) the effects of the latter on the heart. A basic necessity for cardiac functions to be modulated according to local conditions by a local RAS is the separate regulation of the system. Such a separate regulation could principally take place on the level of expression and signal transduction of receptors of the system, availability of substrates or availability and activity of angiotensin-generating or -degrading enzymes.

A crucial step for the activity of the RAS is the generation of angiotensin I (Ang I) from angiotensinogen by the aspartyl protease renin. Therefore, the function of the system depends on the temporal and spatial presence of this enzyme. Cardiac-specific regulation of renin activity is, as will be discussed below, the result of both, differential regulation of renin transcript levels with consecutively *de novo* synthesis, as well as of local activation, uptake, concentration and clearance of circulating renin.

Renin Angiotensin System and the Heart Edited by Walmor De Mello
© 2004 by John Wiley & Sons Ltd. ISBN 0 470 86292 0

Presence of renin in the heart

Most studies on cardiac renin have been performed in the rat. There is no doubt that renin protein is present within the neonatal and adult rat heart (Dostal *et al.*, 1992; Danser *et al.*, 1994). Here renin is found in myocytes as well as in fibroblasts. By means of subcellular fractionation techniques we found the majority of renin in the adult rat heart to be located intracellularly and not just present within the extracellular space. Renin was found within fractions of low density, comigrating with lysosomes and vesicular fractions of low density. However, some renin also comigrated with mitochondria (Peters *et al.*, 2002). A considerable amount of renin was also found attached to the membranes of cardiac cells (Danser *et al.*, 1994). Whereas in nontreated rats cardiac levels of renin are very low, immunohistochemical studies revealed a marked increase of renin protein concentration after infarction of the left ventricle. Here renin was specifically localized in cells around the infarcted area (Passier *et al.*, 1996; Sun *et al.*, 2001), which were shown to represent predominantly macrophages and cardiac fibroblasts. Furthermore, a dissociation was observed between circulating and cardiac renin. Within the first week after myocardial infarction both plasma and cardiac renin activities increased. However, plasma renin declined again at week 3 and returned to normal by week 4, whereas renin activity in the heart rose progressively including week 4 (Sun *et al.*, 2001).

Uptake of renin into the heart

There is a large body of evidence that renin is taken up from the circulation into cardiac cells. Several studies support the hypothesis that renin is internalized by mannose-6-phosphate receptor-mediated endocytosis (Danser *et al.*, 1994; van Kesteren *et al.*, 1997; Saris *et al.*, 2001). For this pathway the glycosylation of renin as well as the mannose-6-phosphorylation is required (see also Chapter 3). We recently demonstrated another additional pathway of internalization. That pathway is independent of the mannose-6-phosphate receptor and transports predominantly prorenin, even if nonglycosylated, or probably because it is not mannose-6-phosphorylated. To confirm the uptake of unglycosylated prorenin we incubated isolated adult cardiomyocytes with *in vitro* translated radiolabeled or recombinant renin constructs and analyzed their intracellular renin content. The results show that unglycosylated prorenin of rat or mouse were internalized more efficiently than the corresponding unglycosylated active renins and equally efficient than glycosylated prorenin or renin. Furthermore, although unglycosylated prorenin was similarly well taken up into the cells than glycosylated prorenin, the functional consequences of uptake were apparently different. Uptake of nonglycosylated (mouse ren-2 gene-derived) prorenin was associated with an increase of intracellular angiotensin levels, uptake of glycosylated prorenin was not (Peters et al., 2002). Because uptake of angiotensins from the medium was excluded in control experiments incubating the cells with excess amounts of angiotensins, our data indicate intracellular generation of angiotensins after uptake of unglycosylated (mouse ren-2) prorenin.

These data suggest that glycosylated and nonglycosylated prorenin may be taken up by different pathways and, consequently may be transported into different intracellular compartments. Alternatively, ren-2 derived prorenin may be activated better than rat prorenin within the cells under certain conditions.

The functional significance of mannose-6-phosphate receptor mediated internalization could be a clearence of prorenin and therefore a reduction of the activity of the extracellular RAS. Such a mechanism has been discussed by van den Eijnden and Colleagues (2001) for endothelial cells. However, lysosomal targeting of renin not necessarily implies its lysosomal degradation. For instance, in the kidney, renin is targeted to the lysosomal pathway, with the result that the lysosomes modify to become secretory storage granules, which release renin into the extracellular space in a regulated manner. The suggestion that renin storage granules of the kidney are modified lysosomes is based on the following observations. First, renal renin granules contain lysosomal enzymes, such as acid phosphatase, cathepsins and β-glucosidase, although at lower levels than classic lysosomes. Second, the granules have phagocytotic properties (Hackenthal et al., 1990). Third, renin belongs itself to the family of lysosomal enzymes, having but shifted the optimal condition for its enzymatic activity to a more basic pH. Finally, the sorting of lysosomal enzymes to lysosomes is commonly known to be mediated by a mannose-6-phosphate receptor, recognizing mannose-6-phosphate residues at glycoside side chains of the proteins. In accordance with this, unglycosylated renin is not stored in the kidney in rats and mice at all (Hackenthal et al., 1992; Clark et al., 1997). Furthermore, mice expressing exclusively unglycosylated renin do not even develop renal renin storage granules (Clark et al., 1997). Correspondingly, we cannot exclude that in the heart uptake of glycosylated renin into lysosomes under certain conditions and cell type dependently may result in generation of storage granules ready for re-secretion.

In contrast to the uptake of renin via mannose-6-phosphate receptors, mannose-6-phosphate receptor independent uptake of renin appears to result in increased generation of angiotensins (Peters *et al.*, 2002). However, it remains to be shown that the presence or absence of mannose-6-phosphate residues alone is the critical factor. We still do not know, for instance, whether or not glycosylated (pro)renin without mannose-6-phosphate residues is transported similarly to nonglycosylated prorenin. The former is present in the circulation in many species, the latter probably only in mice.

It has been observed that prorenin elicits prohypertrophic and proliferative responses in neonatal cardiomyocytes via angiotensin generation independently of the mannose-6-phosphate receptor (Saris *et al.*, 2002). Recent *in vivo* experiments with transgenic rats indicate that this also holds true for the adult heart. In ren-2 transgenic rats, TGR(mren2)27, the development of hypertension and cardiac hypertrophy correlates well with elevated circulating prorenin levels, under several conditions, but not with active renin (Mullins *et al.*, 1990; Peters *et al.*, 1993; Djavidani *et al.*, 1995). Because it has been shown that prorenin cannot be converted to active renin in plasma, it must have been taken up into tissues, such as the heart, and cleaved to active renin or converted locally to a more active conformation. However, because in TGR(mren2)27 the ren-2 gene was found to be expressed in the heart, the functional significance of prorenin uptake *in vivo* could not be concluded with this model. Therefore we investigated another, more specific transgenic model, the cyp1a1-ren-2 transgenic rats (Kantachuvesiri *et al.*, 2001). These rats express the ren-2 gene under control of the cyp1a1 promotor inducibly and predominantly in the liver. After induction with 3-indol-carabinol plasma ren-2-derived prorenin levels and the intracardiac content of renin was markedly increased, and the rats develop hypertension as well as cardiac damage (Kantachuvesiri *et al.*, 2001; Peters *et al.*, 2002). High amounts of unglycosylated ren-2-derived renin were then found within the light vesicular fractions of the cardiac cells even in the absence of intracardiac ren-2 expression, as was to be expected, given the existence of a mannose-6-phosphate-independent pathway of internalization into cardiomyocytes.

Cardiac expression of renin

Results on the expression of renin within the heart have been controversial. Although in some studies the presence of renin mRNA was demonstrated (Lou *et al.*, 1991; Dostal *et al.*, 1992; Zhang *et al.*, 1995; Passier *et al.*,

1996; Flesch *et al.*, 1997); others failed to detect any renin transcript under nonstimulated conditions (Ekker *et al.*, 1989; Iwai *et al.*, 1992; Lou *et al.*, 1993; Zhao *et al.*, 1993). Several studies reported a marked increase in renin expression after myocardial infarction (Passier *et al.*, 1996; Sun *et al.*, 2001), in models of cardiac hypertrophy (Zhang *et al.*, 1995) and after stretch of cardiomyocytes (Boer *et al.*, 1994; Malhotra *et al.*, 1999).

The discrepancies regarding cardiac renin expression can be explained by several factors. First, there may be species-specific differences; second, the expression profile is age dependent (embryonal, neonatal, adult); third, the expression depends on a specific pathophysiological contex (ischemia, stretch), and, finally, there are different renin transcripts derived from the same gene that are differentially expressed. Those transcripts not only explain some of the discrepancies, but also provide a molecular basis for the existence of different renin angiotensin systems in the heart with completely different mode of actions (see below).

Discovery of a second transcript of the rat renin gene

When analyzing intracellular location of renin within the adrenal cortex, we were much surprised to find renin immunostaining not only within secretory vesicles, but also within mitochondria, where it resides in electron-dense intramitochondrial inclusion bodies (Peters *et al.*, 1996). To confirm these findings, intracellular organelles were separated by means of subcellular fractionation techniques and renin concentrations within the fractions were measured. We obtained two peaks of renin activity, one of which comigrated with the vesicular–lysosomal fraction, as indicated by the enrichment of the marker enzyme acid phosphatase and the other with the mitochondrial fraction, as indicated by the enrichment of the marker enzyme malate dehydrogenase. This fraction was then again analyzed by electron microscopy and was shown to contain exclusively mitochondria, some of which still contained renin, while renin vesicles were absent.

The question then arose of how renin is able to enter the mitochondria at all, since, as a secretory glycoprotein, it will be sorted to the endoplasmatic reticulum (ER) and packed into vesicles. Sorting to the ER is accomplished by means of a cotranslational transport mediated by the signal sequence residing in the prefragment of preprorenin. An import into mitochondria on the other hand would require cytoplasmatically localized renin protein, which therefore needs to be translated at free ribosomes.

A detailed analysis of the renin transcripts in the rat adrenal gland by 5′-RACE (rapid amplification of cDNA ends) indeed revealed the existence of an additional transcript lacking exon 1, which contains the coding sequence of the signal for the cotranslational transport to the ER. Instead, exon 2 is preceded by an alternative exon 1A, a domain of about 80 nucleotides originating in intron 1. The intervening sequence of intron 1 separating exon 1A from exon 2 is a region of about 830 nucleotides upstream of exon 2. The 3′ end of exon 1A and the following sequences of intron 1 agree well with the consensus sequences defining an exon/intron border. Upstream of exon 2, the splice acceptor site also agrees with the consensus sequences, as expected, as this site is used in the preprorenin transcript as well (Clausmeyer et al., 1999). Exon 1A, however, does not contain an in frame ATG translation start for renin. The reading frame of the alternative transcript starts in exon 2 and would code for a truncated prorenin. Because this mRNA lacks the prefragment, the encoded protein cannot be targeted to the secretory pathway and is therefore assumed to remain intracellular. These findings are supported by Lee-Kirsch, who also described the existence of the alternative renin transcript (Lee-Kirsch et al., 1999).

Furthermore, alternative transcripts of the renin gene were then identified for human renin, using mice transgenic for P1 phage artificial chromosomes containing the human renin gene (Sinn and Sigmund, 2000). A kidney-specific isoform uses the classic renin promotor and contains exon 1. A brain-specific isoform includes a so far unknown exon 1B, which originates from a transcription initiation upstream of the classic promotor. A third isoform has been found to be specific for the lung, containing an exon 1C, which is located immediately upstream of exon 2. To date, however, nothing is known about the corresponding proteins.

The question of how renin enters the mitochondria was investigated by *in vitro* import experiments, analyzing the transport of a series of amino-terminal deletion variants of renin into isolated mitochondria (Clausmeyer et al., 1999). A truncated prorenin, lacking 36 amino acids at the N-terminus, which comprise the complete secretory signal sequence of preprorenin and part of the profragment of prorenin, was found to be imported efficiently. This truncated prorenin exactly corresponds to the protein derived from exon 1A renin, using the first in frame ATG, which, in the absence of exon 1, is located in exon 2 of the renin gene. The import is dependent on an intact membrane potential and ATP synthesis, because inhibitors of ATP generation and electron transport completely prevented the import. In contrast, neither preprorenin nor a deletion mutant lacking 50 N-terminal amino acids nor active renin were imported at all. The region between amino acids 36 and 50 of the preprorenin thus is apparently indispensable for import. This region differs from known mitochondrial target sequences in that it contains some negatively charged amino acids in the vicinity of three arginine residues. Interestingly, however, some other mitochondrial proteins expressed in the adrenal cortex, such as Cyp11b1, Cyp11b2 and P450scc also include such negatively charged amino acids (von Heijne et al., 1989). We did not observe a proteolytic processing of the imported renin, however, which is usually found for nuclear encoded mitochondrial proteins. This would argue for the existence of an internal targeting sequence.

Differential expression of preprorenin and exon 1A renin transcripts

The detection of an alternative transcript of the renin gene suggested a possible role of intracellular renin within the adrenal gland, but also in other extrarenal tissues, that are known to express renin. Therefore, the expression of renin in rat tissues was analyzed by a nested reverse transcriptase–polymerase chain reaction of high sensitivity, differentiating between the full-length transcript coding for preprorenin and the alternative transcript coding for exon 1A renin. The alternative transcript was detected in various tissues, mostly in addition to the known full-length mRNA. Interestingly, in the heart exon 1A renin proved to be the only transcript of the renin gene being expressed (Clausmeyer et al., 2000). Even under conditions known to stimulate renin expression in the heart, such as cardiac hypertrophy (Zhang et al., 1995) or myocardial infarction (Passier et al., 1996), we found exclusively the exon 1A renin transcript. Moreover, the exon 1A renin transcript is markedly upregulated after myocardial infarction (Clausmeyer et al., 2000; Peters et al., 2002). These findings support the hypothesis of a possible role of intracellular generation of angiotensins in the heart in the remodeling or repair processes observed after myocardial infarction (Dostal et al., 1999; Lijnen and Petrov, 1999; Zimmermann et al., 1999; De Mello and Danser, 2000).

The differential regulation of preprorenin and exon 1A renin expression in the heart may explain the apparent discrepancies present in the literature regarding the expression of renin in the heart. Previous studies could not be aware of the existence of two different renin transcripts and therefore the methods applied were not designed to distinguish between them. Presumably, in former studies demonstrating renin expression in the adult rat heart, exon 1A renin was detected and not the transcript coding for preprorenin.

Possible functions of exon 1A renin

The functional consequences of exon 1A renin expression and intracellular renin sorting to mitochondria are not clear at present. Adrenal mitochondria are the site of aldosterone production. Several steroidogenic enzymes, such as aldosterone synthase, are located at their inner membrane. In the heart, expression of aldosterone synthase as well as aldosterone biosynthesis has been demonstrated as well (see also this book). Moreover, aldosterone production and aldosterone synthase expression increases after myocardial infarction (Silvestre et al., 1999), as is exon 1A expression. As a first indication for a function of exon 1A renin we observed a marked increase of exon 1A renin expression in the adrenal cortex after bilateral nephrectomy. This was associated with an increase of the number of mitochondria containing renin as well as with an increase of aldosterone production (Peters et al., 1996, 1999). Alternatively, given the expression and upregulation at sites of repair, exon 1A renin may be involved in apoptosis, particularly if exon 1A renin is imported into mitochondria. It still remains to be investigated, however, whether or not exon 1A-derived renin, like in adrenal cells, is imported into mitochondria of cardiac cells.

Significance of renin uptake and expression: concluding remarks

First, it is impossible to discriminate renin protein derived from exon 1A renin and preprorenin transcripts. The shorter one, exon 1A-derived renin, shares 100 percent identical sequence with preprorenin and the longer one, preprorenin-derived secretory prorenin certainly could well be shortened by protease cleavage to resemble exon 1A renin. Given the low expression of exon 1A renin transcripts in untreated rat hearts it is likely, that under physiological conditions most of cardiac renin protein represents secretory renin derived from the circulation. This view is further strengthened by the fact that bilateral nephrectomy not only eliminates circulating but also intracardiac renin with subsequently undetectable angiotensin levels in the heart (Danser et al., 1994). However, the effect of bilateral nephrectomy on exon 1A renin expression has not been investigated yet and thus, parallel absence of exon 1A renin cannot be ruled out in this context.

Under pathological conditions exon 1A renin may play a more important role than under physiological conditions. Upregulation of renin expression after myocardial infarction has been demonstrated. Renin expression was then particularly localized to sites of repair just around the infarcted area (Passier et al., 1996). Under these conditions, it is exon 1A renin, which is expressed and upregulated (Clausmeyer et al., 2000). Furthermore, if the circulating RAS is eliminated by bilateral nephrectomy prior to myocardial infarction, which stimulates cardiac exon 1A renin expression, angiotensin levels in the heart remain still detectable (Leenen et al., 1999). These data strongly indicate a role for exon 1A renin after infarction.

In conclusion, our understanding of the cardiac RAS becomes more and more sophisticated, although the situation does not become less complicated. We recognize that in the rat heart more than one local RAS exists. At least two means of internalization of renin have been defined. In addition, renin may be enriched at cardiac membranes. Furthermore, two different renin transcripts can be expressed. In each case, the consequences are unique. Uptake of renin via mannose-6-phosphate receptor may result in lysosomal degradation and represent a means to decrease generation of angiotensins in the extracellular space. Mannose-6-phosphate receptor-independent uptake of renin may increase cardiac angiotensin generation, as may enrichment of renin at cell membranes. Cardiac expression of preprorenin transcripts may still contribute to the tissue content of secretory renin in neonatal hearts, but this is unlikely in adult rat hearts. In the adult heart of the rat, particularly under pathological conditions, an alternative renin transcript is expressed, which remains intracellular and hence should exert primarily intracellular functions, if any. Furthermore, because a renin receptor has recently been discovered (Nguyen et al., 2002) and mitochondrial renin apparently exists (Clausmeyer et al., 1999), we need to keep in mind that renin may exert functions other than the generation of angiotensins. Careful dissection of the different fates of renin will still be needed to generate appropriate models for the modes of action of local RASs in the heart and other tissues.

References

Boer PH, Ruzicka M, Lear W, et al. (1994) Stretch mediated activation of cardiac renin gene. *American Journal of Physiology: Heart and Circulatory Physiology* **267**, H1630–H1636.

Clark AF, Sharp MGF, Morley SD, et al. (1997) Renin-1 is essential for normal renal juxtaglomerular cell granulation and macula densa morphology. *Journal of Biological Chemistry* **272**, 18185–18190.

Clausmeyer S, Stürzebecher R and Peters J (1999) An alternative transcript of the rat renin gene can result in truncated prorenin that is transported into adrenal mitochondria. *Circulation Research* **84**, 337–344.

Clausmeyer S, Reinecke A, Farrenkopf R, *et al.* (2000) Tissue-specific expression of a rat renin transcript lacking the coding sequence for the prefragment and its stimulation by myocardial infarction. *Endocrinology* **141**, 2963–2970.

Danser AHJ, Van Kats JP, Admiraal PJJ, *et al.* (1994) Cardiac renin and angiotensins. Uptake from plasma versus in situ synthesis. *Hypertension* **24**, 37–48.

Djavidani B, Sander M, Kreutz R, *et al.* (1995) Chronic dexamethasone treatment suppress hypertension development in the transgenic rat TGR(mren2)27. *Journal of Hypertension* **13**, 637–645.

Dostal DE and Baker KM (1999) The cardiac renin–angiotensin system. Conceptual or a regulator of cardiac function? *Circulation Research* **85**, 643–650.

Dostal DE, Rothblum KN, Chernin MI, *et al.* (1992) Intracardiac detection of angiotensinogen and renin: a localized renin–angiotensin system in neonatal rat heart. *American Journal of Physiology: Cell Physiology* **263**, C838–C850.

van den Eijnden MM, Saris JJ, de Bruin RJ, *et al.* (2001) Prorenin accumulation and activation in human endothelial cells: importance of mannose-6-phosphate receptors. *Arteriosclerosis, Thrombosis and Vascular Biology* **21**, 911–916.

Ekker M, Tronik D and Rougeon F (1989) Extra-renal transcription of the renin genes in multiple tissues of mice and rats. *Proceedings of the National Academy of Sciences of the United States of America* **86**, 5155–5158.

Flesch M, Schiffer F, Zolk O, *et al.* (1997) Contractile systolic and diastolic dysfunction in renin-induced hypertensive cardiomyopathy. *Hypertension* **30**, 383–391.

Hackenthal E, Paul M, Ganten D and Taugner R (1990) Morphology, physiology and molecular biology of renin secretion. *Physiological Reviews* **70**, 1067–1116.

Hackenthal E, Münter K and Fritsch S (1992) Kidney function and renin processing in transgenic rats, TGR(mren2)27. In *Genetic Hypertension*, Sassard J (ed), Colloque INSERM, Vol. 218, John Libbey Eurotext, Montrouge, London, Paris, pp. 349–351.

Von Heijne G, Steppuhn J and Herrmann RG (1989) Domain structure of mitochondrial and chloroplast targeting peptides. *European Journal of Biochemistry* **180**, 535–545.

Iwai N and Inagami T (1992) Quantitative analysis of renin gene expression in extrarenal tissues by polymerase chain reaction method. *Journal of Hypertension* **10**, 717–724.

Kantachuvesiri S, Fleming S, Peters J, *et al.* (2001) Controlled hypertension: a transgenic toggle switch reveals differential mechanisms underlying vascular disease. *Journal of Biological Chemistry* **276**, 36727–36733.

Van Kesteren CAM, Danser AH, Derkx FHM, *et al.* (1997) Mannose 6-phosphate receptor-mediated internalization and activation of prorenin by cardiac cells. *Hypertension* **30**, 1389–1396.

Lee-Kirsch MA, Gaudet F, Cardoso MC and Lindpaintner K (1999) Distinct renin isoforms generated by tissue-specific transcription initiation and alternative splicing. *Circulation Research* **84**, 240–246.

Leenen FHH, Skarda V, Yuan B and White R (1999) Changes in cardiac Ang II postmyocardial infarction in rats: effects of nephrectomy and ACE inhibitors. *American Journal of Physiology* **276**, H317–H325.

Lijnen P and Petrov V (1999) Renin–angiotensin system, hypertrophy and gene expression in cardiac myocytes. *Journal of Molecular and Cellular Cardiology* **31**, 949–970.

Lou Y, Smith DL, Robinson BC and Morris BJ (1991) Renin gene expression in various tissues determined by single-step polymerase chain reaction. *Clinical and Experimental Pharmacology and Physiology* **18**, 357–362.

Lou Y, Robinson BG and Morris BJ (1993) Renin messenger RNA, detected by polymerase chain reaction, can be switched on in rat atrium. *Journal of Hypertension* **11**, 237–243.

Malhotra R, Sadoshima J, Brosius FC and Izumo S (1999) Mechanical stretch and angiotensin II differentially upregulate the renin–angiotensin system in cardiac myocytes *in vitro*. *Circulation Research* **23**, 137–146.

De Mello W and Danser AHJ (2000) Angiotensin II and the heart. On the intracrine renin–angiotensin system. *Hypertension* **35**, 1183–1188.

Mullins JJ, Peters J and Ganten D (1990) Fulminant hypertension in transgenic rats harbouring the mouse ren-2 gene. *Nature* **344**, 541–544.

Nguyen G, Delarue F, Burckle C, *et al.* (2002) Pivotal role of the renin/prorenin receptor in angiotensin II production and cellular responses to renin. *Journal of Clinical Investigation* **109**(11), 1417–1427.

Passier RCJJ, Smits JFM, Verluyten MJA and Daemen MJAP (1996) Expression and localization of renin and angiotensinogen in rat heart after myocardial infarction. *American Journal of Physiology* **271**, H1040–H1048.

Peters J, Münter K, Bader M, *et al.* (1993) Increased adrenal renin in transgenic hypertensive rats, TGR(mren2)27, and its regulation by cAMP, angiotensin II, and calcium. *Journal of Clinical Investigation* **91**, 742–747.

Peters J, Kränzlin B, Schaeffer S, *et al.* (1996) Presence of renin within intramitochondrial dense bodies of the rat adrenal cortex. *American Journal of Physiology* **271**, E439–E450.

Peters J, Obermüller N, Woyth A, *et al.* (1999) Losartan and angiotensin II inhibit aldosterone production in anephric rats via different actions on the intraadrenal renin–angiotensin-system. *Endocrinology* **140**, 675–682.

Peters J, Farrenkopf R, Clausmeyer S, *et al.* (2002) Functional significance of prorenin internalisation in the rat heart. *Circulation Research* **90**, 1135–1141.

Saris JJ, Derkx FH, Lamers JM, *et al.* (2001) Cardiomyocytes bind and activate native human prorenin: role of soluble mannose-6-phosphate receptors. *Hypertension* **37**, 710–715.

Saris JJ, van den Eijnden MM, Lamers JM, *et al.* (2002) Prorenin-induced myocyte proliferation: no role for intracellular angiotensin II. *Hypertension* **39**, 573–577.

Silvestre JS, Heymes C, Oubenaissa A, *et al.* (1999) Activation of cardiac aldosterone production in rat myocardial infarction. *Circulation* **99**, 2694–2701.

Sinn PL and Sigmund CD (2000) Identification of three human renin mRNA isoforms from alternative tissue-specific transcriptional initiation. *Physiological Genomics* **3**, 25–31.

Sun Y, Zhang J, Zhang JQ and Weber KT (2001) Renin expression at sites of repair in the infarcted rat heart. *Journal of Molecular and Cellular Physiology* **33**, 995–1003.

Zhang X, Dostal DE, Reiss K, *et al.* (1995) Identification and activation of autocrine renin–angiotensin system in adult ventricular myocytes. *American Journal of Physiology* **269**, H1791–H1802.

Zhao Y, Bader M, Kreutz R, *et al.* (1993) Ontogenetic regulation of mouse ren-2^{d} renin gene in transgenic hypertensive rats, TGR(mren2)27. *American Journal of Physiology* **265**, E699–E707.

Zimmermann R, Kastens J, Linz W, *et al.* (1999) Effect of long-term ACE inhibition on myocardial tissue in hypertensive stroke-prone rats. *Journal of Molecular and Cellular Cardiology* **31**, 1447–1456.

6

The Cardiac Renin Receptors

Geneviève Nguyen, Céline Burckle
and Benjamin Tremey

Introduction

The renin angiotensin system (RAS) is a very complex regulatory system that plays a key role in controlling blood pressure and fluid and salt balance in mammals. Renin, a systemic aspartyl protease, is considered to have a unique function and an exclusive substrate: it cleaves angiotensinogen to generate angiotensin I (Ang I). Subsequently, the decapeptide Ang I is converted into the octapeptide Ang II by either angiotensin-converting enzyme (ACE) or chymase, a serine protease. To date, the classical dogma is that Ang II is the main, if not exclusive, effector of the RASs through binding to its receptors AT_1 and AT_2. This assumption is based on the belief that the RAS components preceding Ang II do not have functional receptors and that their generation only serves to produce Ang II. This was true until the demonstration (Nguyen et al., 1996) and the cloning of a functional receptor of (pro)renin (Nguyen et al., 2002).

It is well documented that the major source of (pro)renin in interstitial space, especially in cardiac tissue, is due to uptake of (pro)renin from the circulation (Danser et al., 1994; Müller et al., 1998). Furthermore, there are data indicating that tissue prorenin is active (Methot et al., 1999; Prescott et al., 2002) and that renin *per se* has cellular effects independent of Ang II generation (Nguyen et al., 1996, 2002). Renin uptake and increased activity on the cell surface (Nguyen et al., 2002) represents an essential component of the 'tissue renin angiotensin system' in which (pro)renin receptors play a major role. The tissue RAS is involved in several physiological and pathological processes such as: growth and remodeling (Tamura *et al.*, 2000); development (Guron and Friberg, 2000); inflammation and cardiac hypertrophy (Schieffer *et al.*, 2000); vascular hypertrophy and thrombosis (Brown and Vaughan, 2000); obesity (Engeli *et al.*, 2000).

Indeed, therapeutic and experimental data have clearly shown that antagonizing the RAS has beneficial impact on cardiovascular structure and function independently of the blood pressure lowering effect (Sleight *et al.*, 2001). Epidemiologic, experimental and therapeutical data also indicate that activation of the RAS has major role in increasing the risk of cardiovascular events. In particular, the Heart Outcome Prevention Evaluation (HOPE, 2000) study conclusively showed that administration of an ACE inhibitor reduces the risk of cardiovascular death, myocardial infarction and death in patients at risk for cardiovascular events but without heart failure and independently of their blood pressure lowering effect. Another very important finding of the HOPE study was the reduction of vascular events for patients with different types of underlying vascular disease and regardless of gender. These results strongly suggest that the RAS plays a more important role in the development and progression of atherosclerosis than expected. The results of HOPE and other clinical studies have stimulated the research in two directions. First, understanding how the modulation of the RAS may protect blood vessels and, second, elaborating clinical studies able to cover the large spectrum of potential effects resulting from interruption of the renin angiotensin cascade.

In line with the findings on the importance of a tissue RAS, several groups have been engaged in the search of a receptor of renin, and several binding proteins and receptors have been described so far.

The renin-binding proteins

Renin binding to membranes from different rat organs have been reported but no functional effects of renin binding were studied (Campbell and Valentijn, 1994; Sealey *et al.*, 1996). Renin also binds a 46-kDa protein called renin-binding rotein, RnBp, that was identified in rat, porcine and human tissues and was shown later to be identical to the *N*-acyl-D-glucosamine 2 epimerase (Maru *et al.*, 1996). Although RnBp was described as a renin inhibitor, mice lacking RnBp have normal blood pressure and plasma renin activity (Schmitz *et al.*, 2000), thus questionning the physiological role of RnBp on the control of plasma and renal renin activity.

More recently, the widely distributed mannose-6-phosphate (M6P) receptor has been shown to bind renin and prorenin on rat cardiac myocytes (van Kesteren *et al.*, 1997; Saris *et al.*, 2001a, b) and on human endothelial cells (Admiraal *et al.*, 1999; van den Eijnden *et al.*, 2001). Endothelial cells and cardiac myocytes exclusively bind glycosylated (pro)renin. The binding of prorenin is followed by internalization, activation by an unidentified protease, and degradation of renin. Co-incubation of prorenin and angiotensinogen on cardiac myocytes resulted in an increase of [^{3}H]thymidine incorporation and increased protein synthesis (Saris *et al.*, 2002). These effects were not attributed to the binding of prorenin to M6P receptor, but were due to the intrinsic activity of prorenin, responsible for the generation of Ang I and, subsequently, of Ang II on the cell surface. No intracellular Ang II could be detected. It is interesting to note that [^{3}H]thymidine incorporation provoked by 1 nM Ang II generated by co-incubation of prorenin plus angiotensinogen on cardiomyocytes, could only be reproduced by addition of a 100-fold higher concentration of exogenous Ang II (100 nM). This observation strongly suggests that formation of Ang II on a cell surface, at close vicinity of AT_1 receptors, is more efficient than in solution because it allows immediate binding to AT_1.

The role of M6P receptors on (pro)renin binding to cardiomyocytes and the absence of intracellular angiotensins generation is, however, still a matter of controversy. Rats transgenic for the mouse *ren-2^d* renin gene (coding for unglycosylated prorenin) are known to have extremely severe hypertension and cardiac damage (Mullins *et al.*, 1990). Using this model, with an inducible expression of *ren-2^d* renin gene restricted to the liver, Peters *et al.* have shown that increased synthesis of *ren-2^d* renin was associated with high circulating levels and increased concentration of *ren-2^d* renin within cardiac cells (Peters *et al.*, 2002). In addition, unglycosylated (pro)renin was demonstrated to be taken up *in vitro* by rat cardiomyocytes. The internalization of prorenin by mean of a yet unidentified binding protein was associated with an increased intrinsic activity of prorenin and with intracellular Ang I and Ang II generation. These results revive the controversy on the existence of an intracrine RAS and the mitogenic effect of intracellular Ang II (Sadoshima *et al.*, 1993; De Mello and Danser, 2000; Cook *et al.*, 2001). Whether intracellular accumulation of prorenin and angiotensin generation is directly linked to the cardiac cell hypertrophy and proliferation remains to be clearly established.

The reasons for these contradictory results of prorenin binding and effects on rat cardiomyocytes (binding of glycosylated prorenin via the M6P receptor vs. binding of nonglycosylated prorenin via an unidentified receptor, intracellular prorenin activation by proteolysis vs. increased intrinsic activity, no intracellular angiotensin generation vs. intracellular generation of Ang I and of Ang II) are still unclear. These discrepancies are unlikely due to the use of different rat strains. More likely, they could be attributed to the high expression of M6P receptors by neonatal cells that would mask the binding to another receptor. Nonetheless, two major facts have emerged from these studies: the importance of the cell surface-generation of Ang II to increase the efficiency of AT_1 receptor binding and activation, and the possibility for a functional role for prorenin. This functional role of prorenin is a very important issue because prorenin is the unique form of renin synthesised at tissue level.

The renin receptor

The cloning of a new renin receptor adds another degree to the complexity of (pro)renin binding and cellular effects. A functional receptor of renin was first identified on human mesangial cells in culture (Nguyen et al., 1996). Renin binding induced a hypertrophic effect and an increase of plasminogen activator inhibitor-1 synthesis. In contrast to the previously reported receptors, renin bound to the receptor was neither internalized nor degraded. This receptor which has been cloned (Nguyen et al., 2002) is a 350-amino-acid protein with a single transmembrane domain and no homology with any known membrane protein. The binding to this protein is specific for renin and prorenin. Receptor-bound renin displays a five-fold increase of the catalytic efficiency of angiotensinogen conversion to Ang I and induces an intracellular signal with phosphorylation of serine and tyrosine residues, associated to an activation of MAP kinases ERK1(p 44/2(p 42)). High levels of the receptor messenger RNA are detected in heart, brain and placenta, and lower levels in kidney, liver and pancreas. Immunofluorescence studies on normal frozen sections of human kidney and heart showed that the receptor is localized in the mesangium of glomeruli and in the subendothelium of coronary and kidney artery. Further, double staining with antismooth-muscle cell α-actin or with antirenin antibodies, and analysis by confocal microscopy showed that the receptor is associated to smooth-muscle cells and is colocalizes with renin.

The physiological implications of this receptor may be very important. First, it supports a functional role for prorenin. Indeed, the *in vivo* intrinsic activity of prorenin is confirmed by findings that prorenin also binds to the specific renin receptor and displays full activity.

The highest level of expression of the renin receptor mRNA was found in heart, brain, placenta and eye (Burcklé C and Nguyen G, personal observation). It is noteworthy that heart is a site of local generation of Ang II, brain, placenta and eye synthesize components of the RAS, and placenta and retina secrete high levels of prorenin (Deinum et al., 1996; Wagner et al., 1996). Prorenin intrinsic activity has been demonstrated in vivo (Methot et al., 1999; Prescott et al., 2002) and prorenin levels are increased in many physiological and pathological states such as pregnancy and in diabetic patients. In diabetic patients with proliferative retinopathy the vitreous fluid contains very high levels of prorenin and it has been reported that interruption of the RAS could prevent retinal neovascularization (Moravski et al., 2000). Could high prorenin levels play a pathological role through activation of the receptor and/or local, cell surface or intracellular generation of Ang II? This is an important issue.

Second, binding of (pro)renin activates the MAP kinases ERK1/2 pathway, known to be involved in cell hypertrophy and proliferation, independently of Ang II generation. Nullizygote mice for angiotensinogen, for ACE, for Ang II receptors, and for the renin gene display low blood pressure and severe renal vascular lesions associated with high or low plasma renin concentrations (Niimura et al., 1995; Esther et al., 1996; Tsuchida et al., 1998; Yanai et al., 2000). The vascular lesions have been attributed to the absence of Ang II during development but these data do not exclude a role of renin in the pathogenesis of vascular lesions. Moreover, rats expressing the prorenin transgene exclusively in the liver suffer severe nephroangiosclerosis, cardiac and aortic hypertrophy, and liver fibrosis, in the absence of hypertension (Véniant et al., 1996). This observation suggests that the effects observed in vitro on the activation of the ERK1/2 pathway, as well as the cellular hypertrophy and the increase of plasminogen activator inhibitor-1 synthesis (Nguyen et al., 1996) may be relevant in vivo.

Finally, this receptor may help to explain the local generation of Ang II, independently of the circulating RAS. The physiological plasma concentration of renin is in the picomolar range, but in tissues, especially in interstitial fluids, renin concentration may reach 10 nM. Based on the affinity of the receptor (approximately 0.5 nM) and on the concentration of renin in interstitial space it is possible that more than 50 percent of receptors are occupied. We have shown that receptor-bound renin activates angiotensinogen with kinetics different from those observed for renin in solution and, in particular, we showed a reduction in the K_m for angiotensinogen from 1 microM in solution to 0.15 microM with receptor-bound renin. This K_m is significantly below the normal plasma concentration of angiotensinogen, approximately 1 microM, suggesting that conversion of angiotensinogen by receptor-bound renin may be physiological in tissues where the concentration of angiotensinogen is lower than in plasma. The overall catalytic efficiency, k_{cat}/K_m of receptor-bound renin, increased about five times indicating that the cell-surface is an important site for angiotensinogen activation and Ang II generation (Nguyen et al., 2002).

In summary, the renin receptor is able to trigger intracellular signal by activating the ERK1/ERK2 pathway and it also acts as a co-factor by increasing the efficiency of angiotensinogen cleavage by receptor-bound renin, therefore facilitating Ang II generation and action on a cell surface.

Conclusion

The renin receptor appears to be an essential player in tissue RAS, by concentrating (pro)renin at cell surface and modulating the state of activation of vascular smooth-muscle cells either directly or indirectly by controlling the generation of Ang II at close vicinity of Ang II receptors. Moreover, the physiological concentration of circulating prorenin exceeds that of active renin, representing 50 to 70 percent of total renin, and this ratio even reaches 90 percent of total renin in diabetic patients. Therefore, blocking the binding of (pro)renin to the receptor and the cell-surface activation of angiotensinogen, may provide an efficient way to block renin concentration in tissue and to block renin angiotensin activation at its initial step.

The extremely high expression of the receptor in heart, brain, placenta and eye suggests that it may be physiologically important in these organs. Furthermore, in human heart, its exclusive localization on vascular smooth muscle cells of coronary arteries indicates that it may play an essential role in the modulation of smooth muscle cell tone and in the control of coronary artery function.

Finally, the existence of the renin receptor raises more questions than there are answers, but we are at the very beginning. This receptor may provide a new approach to a better understanding of the pathogenesis of cardiovascular diseases associated with (pro)renin angiotensin system activation in tissues. Indeed, activation of the tissue RAS is not only involved in cardiovascular diseases, hypertension, but also in other major diseases such as diabetes, obesity and fibrosis, in the pathogenesesis of atherosclerosis, inflammation and immune disease. For these reasons, blocking the RAS at its initial step of activation would have major impact far beyond the field of cardiovascular diseases. If the active site of renin is not involved in the binding, and this is supported by the increased catalytic activity of receptor-bound (pro)renin, then renin inhibitors may bind to receptor-bound (pro)renin, but they would not inhibit cell activation. Therefore, a bifunctional agent blocking renin activity and binding would represent the ideal pharmacological compound. If this receptor is physiologically relevant, (pro)renin receptor antagonists may provide a new therapeutic approach to block the renin angiotensin cascade at the initial step, inhibiting tissue generation of Ang II and cell activation by (pro)renin.

It is time now to study renin again, an aspartyl-protease with a unique substrate and a unique function (the cleavage of angiotensinogen) and, in the context of the renin receptor, to reconsider renin as a protease hormone.

References

Admiraal PJ, van Kesteren CA, Danser AH, et al. (1999) Uptake and proteolytic activation of prorenin by cultured human endothelial cells. *Journal of Hypertension* **17**, 621–629.

Brown NJ and Vaughan DE (2000) Prothrombotic effects of angiotensin. *Advances in Internal Medicine* **45**, 419–429.

Campbell DJ and Valentijn AJ (1994) Identification of vascular renin binding proteins by chemical cross-linking: inhibition of binding of renin by renin inhibitors. *Journal of Hypertension* **12**, 879–890.

Cook JL, Zhang Z and Re RN (2001) *In vitro* evidence for intracellular site of angiotensin action. *Circulation Research* **89**, 1138–1146.

Danser AJH, van Kats JP, Admiraal PJJ, et al. (1994) Cardiac renin and angiotensins: uptake from plasma versus in situ synthesis. *Hypertension* **24**, 37–48.

Deinum J, Derkx FHM, Danser AHJ and Schalekamp MADH (1990) Identification and quantification of renin and prorenin in the bovine eye. *Endocrinology* **126**, 1673–1682.

De Mello WC and Danser AHJ (2000) Angiotensin II and the hart. On the intracrine renin–angiotensin system. *Hypertension* **35**, 1183–1188.

Engeli S, Negret R and Sharma AM (2000) Physiology and pathophysiology of the adipose tissue renin–angiotensin system. *Hypertension* **35**, 1270–1277.

Esther C, Howard T, Marino E, et al. (1996) Mice lacking angiotensin converting enzyme have low blood pressure, renal pathology, and reduced male fertility. *Laboratory Investigation* **74**, 953–965.

Guron G and Friberg P (2000) An intact renin–angiotensin system is a prerequisite for renal development. *Journal of Hypertension* **181**, 23–137.

Maru I, Ohta Y, Murata K and Tsukada Y (1996) Molecular cloning and identification of N-acyl-D-glucosamine 2-epimerase from porcine kidney as renin-binding protein. *Journal of Biological Chemistry* **271**, 16294–16299.

Methot D, Silversides DW and Reudelhuber TL (1999) In vivo enzymatic assay reveals catalytic activity of the human renin precursor in tissues. *Circulation Research* **84**, 1067–1072.

Moravski CJ, Kelly DJ, Cooper ME, et al. (2000) Retinal neovascularization is prevented by blockade of the renin–angiotensin system. *Hypertension* **36**, 1099–1044.

Müller DN, Fischli W, Clozel J-P, et al. (1998) Local angiotensin II generation in the rat heart. Role of renin uptake. *Circulation Research* **82**, 13–20.

Mullins JJ, Peters J and Ganten D (1990) Fulminant hypertension in transgenic rats harbouring the mouse *ren*-2^d gene. *Nature* **344**, 541–544.

Nguyen G, Delarue F, Berrou J, et al. (1996) Specific receptor binding of renin on human mesangial cells in culture increases plasminogen activator inhibitor-1 antigen. *Kidney International* **50**, 1897–1903.

Nguyen G, Delarue F, Burckle C, et al. (2002) Pivotal role of the renin/prorenin receptor in angiotensin II production and cellular responses to renin. *Journal of Clinical Investigation* **109**, 1417–1427.

Niimura F, Labosky P, Kakuchi J, et al. (1995) Gene targeting in mice reveals a requirement for angiotensin in the development and maintenance of kidney morphology and growth factor regulation. *Journal of Clinical Investigation* **66**, 2947–2954.

Peters J, Farrenkopf R, Clausmeyer S, et al. (2002) Functional significance of prorenin internalization in the rat heart. *Circulation Research* **90**, 1135–1141.

Prescott G, Silverside DW and Reudelhuber TL (2002) Tissue activity of circulating prorenin. *American Journal of Hypertension* **13**, 280–285.

Sadoshima J, Xy Y, Slayter HS and Izumo S (1993) Autocrine release of angiotensin II mediates stretch-induced hypertrophy of cardiac myocytes *in vitro*. *Cell* **75**, 977–984.

Saris JJ, Derkx FHM, de Bruin RJA, et al. (2001) High-affinity protrenin binding to cardiac man-6-P/IGF-II receptors precedes proteolytic activation to renin. *American Journal of Physiology: Heart and Circulatory Physiology* **280**, H1706–H1715.

Saris JJ, Derkx FHM, Lamers JMJ, et al. (2001) Cardiomyocytes bind and activate native human prorenin. Role of soluble mannose-6-phoshate receptor. *Hypertension* **37** (part 2), 710–715.

Saris JJ, van den Eijnden MMED, Lamers JMJ, et al. (2002) Prorenin-induced myocyte proliferation. No role for intracellular angiotensin II. *Hypertension* **39** (part 2), 573–577.

Schieffer B, Schieffer E, Hilfiker-Kleiner D, et al. (2000) Expression of angiotensin II and interleukin 6 in human coronary atherosclerotic plaques. Potential implications for inflammation and plaque instability. *Circulation* **101**, 1372–1378.

Schmitz C, Gotthard M, Hinderlich S, et al. (2000) Normal blood pressure and plasma renin activity in mice lacking the renin-binding protein, a cellular renin inhibitor. *Journal of Biological Chemistry* **275**, 15357–15362.

Sealey JE, Catanzaro DF, Lavin TN, et al. (1996) Specific prorenin/renin binding (proBP). Identification and characterization of a novel membrane site. *American Journal of Hypertension* **9**, 491–502.

Sleight P, Yusuf S, Pogue J, et al. (2001) Blood-pressure reduction and cardiovascular risk in HOPE study. *Lancet* **358**, 2130–2131.

Tamura T, Said S, Harris J, et al. (2000) Reverse modeling of cardiac myocyte hypertrophy in hypertension and failure by targeting of the renin–angiotensin system. *Circulation* **102**, 253–259.

REFERENCES

The Heart Outcomes Prevention Evaluation Study Investigators (HOPE) (2000) Effects of an angiotensin-converting-enzyme inhibitor, ramipril, on cardiovascular events in high-risk patients. *New England Journal of Medicine* **342**, 145–153.

Tsuchida S, Matsusaka T, Chen X, *et al.* (1998) Murine double nullizygotes of the angiotensin type 1A and 1B receptors genes duplicate severe abnormal phenotypes of angiotensinogen nullizygotes. *Journal of Clinical Investigation* **101**, 755–760.

van den Eijnden MMED, Saris JJ, de Bruin RJA, *et al.* (2001) Prorenin accumulation and activation in human endothelial cells. Importance of the mannose-6-phosphate receptors. *Arteriosclerosis, Thrombosis and Vascular Biology* **21**, 911–916.

van Kesteren CAM, Danser AHJ, Derkx FH, *et al.* (1997) Mannose-6-phosphate receptor mediated internalization and activation of prorenin by cardiac cells. *Hypertension* **30**, 1389–1396.

Véniant M, Ménard J, Bruneval P, *et al.* (1996) Vascular damage without hypertension in transgenic rats expressing prorenin exclusively in the liver. *Journal of Clinical Investigation* **98**, 1966–1970.

Wagner J, Danser AHJ, Derkx FH, *et al.* (1996) Demonstration of renin mRNA, angiotensinogen mRNA, and angiotensin converting enzyme mRNA expression in the human eye: evidence for an intraocular renin–angiotensin system. *British Journal of Ophtalmology* **80**, 159–163.

Yanai K, Saito T, Kakimuna Y, Kon Y, *et al.* (2000) Renin-dependent cardiovascular functions and renin-independent blood–brain barrier function revealed by renin-deficient mice. *Journal of Biological Chemistry* **275**, 5–8.

7

Angiotensin II AT$_2$ Receptors and Cardiac Function

Jun Suzuki, Takanori Kanazawa, Masaru Iwai and **Masatsugu Horiuch**

Possible roles of AT$_2$ receptor stimulation associated with selective AT$_1$ receptor blockade

Cross-talk of signaling by AT$_1$ and AT$_2$ receptors

The peptide angiotensin (Ang) II exerts hemodynamic, and renal as well as cardiovascular structural effects. Multiple lines of evidence have suggested the existence of several Ang II receptor subtypes. The major cardiovascular actions of Ang II have been reported to be mediated by a seven-transmembrane-spanning, G-protein-coupled receptor (GPCR) that is termed the type 1 Ang II receptor or AT$_1$ receptor. In 1993, a second receptor subtype known as the Ang II type 2 (AT$_2$) receptor was cloned (Kambayashi *et al.*, 1993; Mukoyama *et al.*, 1993). While both the AT$_1$ and AT$_2$ receptors belong to the seven-transmembrane, GPCR family and share approximately 30 percent primary sequence homology, recent evidence has revealed that the functions of the AT$_1$ and AT$_2$ receptors are mutually antagonistic in various cells and tissues (Horiuchi *et al.*, 1999a; de Gasparo *et al.*, 2000; Gallinat *et al.*, 2000). Moreover, based on the restricted expression of the AT$_2$ receptor in fetal tissues as well as in disease states such as myocardial infarction and vascular injury, this receptor is thought to be involved in growth, development and/or differentiation.

Renin Angiotensin System and the Heart Edited by Walmor De Mello
© 2004 by John Wiley & Sons Ltd. ISBN 0 470 86292 0

The AT₂ receptor displays totally different signaling mechanisms from the AT₁ receptor. Indeed, AT₂ receptor stimulation leads to the activation of various phosphatases, while the AT₁ receptor activates a set of protein tyrosine kinases, which are involved in the induction of immediate early genes (Inagami et al., 1999; Horiuchi et al., 1999b). The overall cellular effect of AT₂ and AT₁ receptor costimulation is a premature termination of AT₁ receptor-elicited cell growth signals by the AT₂ receptor. The growth inhibitory effects of the AT₂ receptor are unique in that it is a seven-transmembrane, GPCR that counteracts the growth action of other receptors. The signaling mechanism of the AT₂ receptor has not been well defined compared with that of the AT₁ receptor. The growth inhibitory effects of the AT₂ receptor are reported to be at least partly mediated by activation of protein tyrosine phosphatases (PTPase), which results in the inactivation of AT₁ receptor- and/or growth factor-activated extracellular signal-regulated kinase (ERK). Several phosphatases that specifically couple to the AT₂ receptor have been identified. An immediate early gene product known as 3CH134 was identified recently as a phosphatase specific for MAP kinase and named MAP kinase phosphatase-1 (MKP-1). Interestingly, AT₂ receptor-mediated activation of MKP-1 in adult rat ventricular myocytes has been reported (Fischer et al., 1998). Consistent with this, our finding in PC12W cells that pretreatment with MKP-1 antisense oligonucleotide inhibited the proapoptotic effect of the AT₂ receptor suggests that MKP-1 is an AT₂ receptor-activated phosphatase (Yamada et al., 1996; Horiuchi et al., 1997). In addition to MKP-1, in N1E-115 neuroblastoma cells and in Chinese hamster ovary cells expressing recombinant human AT₂ receptor, Ang II rapidly stimulates the catalytic activity of SHP-1, a soluble PTPase that has been implicated in termination of signaling by cytokine and growth-factor receptors (Bedecs et al., 1997). In addition, serine/threonine phosphatase 2A (PP2A) activation and consequent ERK inactivation via the AT₂ receptor has been reported in neuronal cells cultured from neonatal rat hypothalamus and brainstem (Huang et al., 1996). Interestingly, MKP-1, SHP-1 and PP2A display different time courses of ERK inactivation, suggesting that they may regulate different steps of the ERK cascade. It would be an intriguing issue to find other target substrates, in addition to ERK, that are regulated by AT₂ receptor-activated phosphatases. We reported that stimulation of the AT₂ receptor in AT₂ receptor cDNA-transfected rat adult vascular smooth muscle cell (VSMC) inhibited AT₁ receptor-mediated tyrosine-phosphorylation of signal transducer and activator of transcription (STAT)1, STAT2 and STAT3 without influencing on Jak (Horiuchi et al., 1999c). This effect, together with the concurrent inhibition of serine-phosphorylation of STAT1 and STAT3 via the inactivation of ERK, attenuates STATs binding to a *sis*-inducing element in the *c-fos* promoter, resulting in decreased *c-fos* expression. In addition, AT_2 receptor activation seems to activate the bradykinin/NO system (Siragy *et al.*, 1999; Tsutsumi *et al.*, 1999).

Binding characteristics of AT_1 receptor blocker to AT_1 receptor

These results suggest that AT_2 receptor stimulation leads to the activation of a variety of phosphatases and NO, although the coupling mechanism still remains an enigma. Identification of specific phosphatases activated by the AT_2 receptor constitutes one of the future directions in AT_2 receptor research and may form the basis for the understanding of Ang II signaling events as well as for the development of new therapies for cardiovascular diseases.

It is of utmost importance to understand how the AT_1/AT_2 receptors interact with their ligands in terms of three-dimensional structure, in order to gain an insight into the mechanism of the receptors' physiological functions, such as receptor activation and coupling with G-proteins. Moreover, knowledge about the interactions between nonpeptide Ang II blockers and the Ang receptor will form the basis for understanding the pharmacological actions of Ang II receptor blockers. Elucidation of the three-dimensional structures of biological macromolecules by X-ray crystallography, nuclear magnetic resonance spectroscopy, or electron microscopy has contributed enormously to our understanding of their physiological functions and mechanisms as well as their structures. Although membrane proteins had not been amenable to structural determination for a long time, recent progress in X-ray crystallography has made it possible to resolve their structures at high resolution. Recently, the structure of bovine rhodopsin at 2.8 Å resolution was successfully determined (Palczewski *et al.*, 2000; Teller *et al.*, 2001), which is the first reported structure of a GPCR at the atomic resolution. Accordingly, we have built a three-dimensional structural model of the AT_1 and AT_2 receptors based on the high resolution X-ray structure of bovine rhodopsin (Figure 7.1(a) and (b). Ang II does not discriminate between these two receptors. AT_1 receptor blockers are new antihypertensive drugs and have already been used in the treatment of hypertension (Figure 7.1(c)). When the AT_1 receptor is blocked by an AT_1 receptor blocker, unbound Ang II acts preferentially on the AT_2 receptors. These results point to the pathophysiological importance of the

(a)

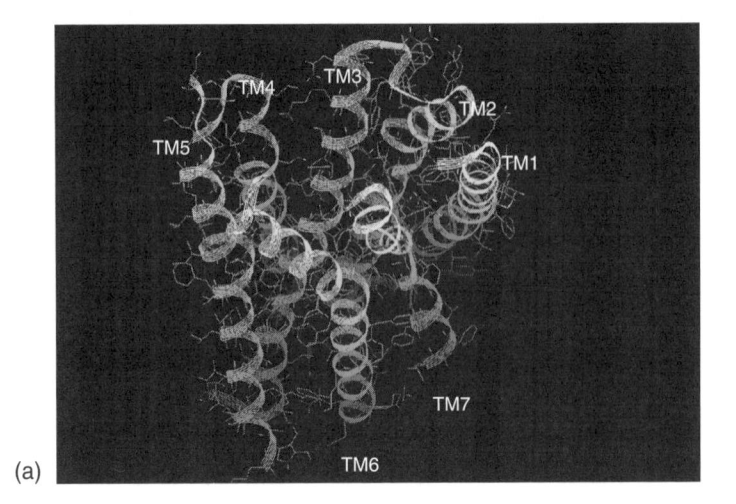

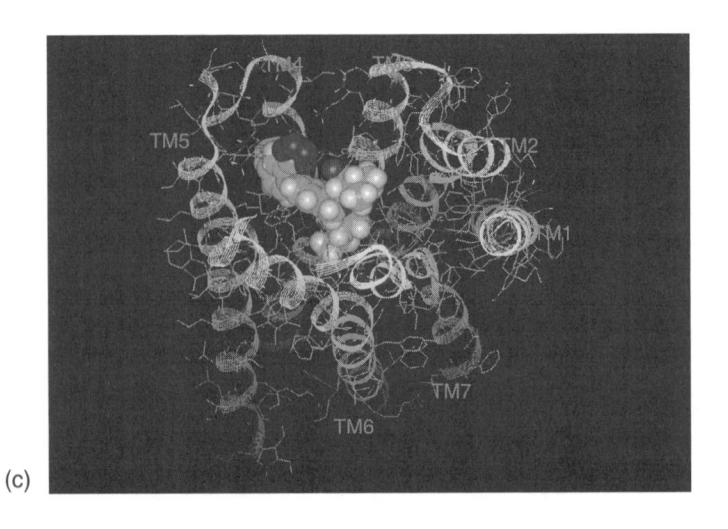

(b)

(c)

AT_2 receptor in the clinical use of AT_1 receptor blockers as well as ACE inhibitors. To fully understand the role(s) of Ang II in the cardiovascular system, additional work will be required to determine the nature of the interactions among the different signaling pathways regulated by AT_1 and AT_2 receptors and their roles in the pathogenesis of cardiovascular disease. In the following sections, we will review the roles of the AT_2 receptor in cardiac function.

Expression of AT_2 receptor in cardiac tissue

Although there are significant species differences in the distribution of Ang II receptor subtypes, both the AT_1 and AT_2 receptor are expressed in fetal and adult cardiac tissues. The AT_2 receptor is present at a high density in all fetal tissues but is much less abundant in adult tissues except for limited organs, including the brain, adrenal gland, uterus, and ovary (Unger *et al.*, 1998). The AT_2 receptor levels in cardiac myocytes and coronary vessels are significantly higher in neonatal than in young rats, but the AT_2 receptor could not be detected in neonatal fibroblasts or young rat aortic smooth muscle cells (Wang *et al.*, 1998). In sheep, cardiac AT_2 receptor mRNA expression is high during fetal development and decreases rapidly after birth, whereas AT_1 receptor gene expression is relatively unchanged during fetal and newborn life (Samyn *et al.*, 1998). These changes during development suggest that the AT_1 and AT_2 receptors exert different functions in the neonatal and adult heart. The AT_1 receptor predominates in the heart of most animal species including the rat (Shanmugam *et al.*, 1996) and hamster (Ohkubo *et al.*, 1997). In contrast, radioligand binding studies in humans revealed that the AT_2 receptor subtype predominates in the myocardium (Regitz-Zagrosec *et al.*, 1995; Tsutsumi *et al.*, 1998; Wharton *et al.*, 1998).

Figure 7.1 Three-dimensional structure of AT_1 receptor (a). The amino acid sequences of the transmembrane (TM) helices of the AT_1 receptor were aligned with those of bovine rhodopsin, and the three-dimensional structure of the AT_1 receptor was built based on the X-ray structure of bovine rhodopsin (PDB code: 1HZX) by homology modeling. Three-dimensional structure of AT_2 receptor (b). The structure was built in a manner similar to that used for the AT_1 receptor. AT_1 receptor blocker, valsartan, complexed with AT_1 receptor (c). Valsartan is docked in the AT_1 receptor, which is fully relaxed by energy minimization and subjected to 500 ps of molecular dynamics simulation. Valsartan has favorable vdW interactions with Val 108 of the AT_1 receptor. When the valine residue is replaced by a larger leucine residue as in the AT_2 receptor, the leucine residue will obviously be subjected to severe steric repulsion from valsartan, which will reduce binding affinity of valsartan to the AT_2 receptor. A color reproduction of this figure can be found in the color plate section

In an experimental model of myocardial infarction, the AT_2 receptor was increased in the infarcted area of myocardium 1 day after infarction, and AT_2 receptor expression was further upregulated 7 days after infarction in both the infarcted and noninfarcted areas (Nio et al., 1995). Recent studies demonstrated that approximately 40 percent of adult rat cardiomyocytes expressed the AT_1 receptor and approximately 10 percent expressed the AT_2 receptor (Busche et al., 2000). These proportions of receptor subtypes were unchanged 1 day after infarction, whereas the AT_2 receptor was expressed in 50 percent of cardiomyocytes 7 days after infarction. In the hypertrophied rat heart, the ratio of AT_2 to AT_1 receptor density is increased (Lopez et al., 1994). In the failing ventricle of the human heart, expression of the AT_1 receptor appears to decrease (Regitz-Zagrosec et al., 1995; Haywood et al., 1997; Tsutsumi et al., 1998; Wharton et al., 1998), whereas expression of the AT_2 receptor is unchanged (Regitz-Zagrosec et al., 1995; Wharton et al., 1998) or increased (Haywood et al., 1997; Tsutsumi et al., 1998). The density of AT_2 receptor binding sites is increased in endocardial, interstitial, and infarcted regions in the ventricle of patients with end-stage ischemic heart disease or dilated cardiomyopathy compared with the noninfarcted myocardium (Wharton et al., 1998). In chronic heart failure, the AT_2 receptor is upregulated in fibroblasts, associated with downregulation of the AT_1 receptor in atrial and left ventricular tissues (Tsutsumi et al., 1998). In our previous study, the AT_1 receptor was expressed in both cardiomyocytes and coronary artery, but the AT_2 receptor was mainly expressed in coronary artery (Akishita et al., 2000). Although the cell type-specific expression patterns of the AT_1 and AT_2 receptors are still undefined, these results suggest that the relative expression of the AT_1 and AT_2 receptors and their ratios may play an important pathophysiological role in cardiac remodeling.

Role of AT_2 receptor in cardiac structure and function

AT_2 receptor and cardiac growth

Several lines of *in vitro* and *in vivo* studies have demonstrated that the Ang II receptor is involved in cardiac growth (Table 7.1). Liu et al. (1998) showed, using cultured rat left ventricular myocytes isolated from normal and failing hearts after myocardial infarction, that Ang II stimulation induced myocyte hypertrophy. In both groups of myocytes, the AT_1 receptor blocker losartan completely inhibited cell growth and the increase in protein content per cell. Moreover, AT_1

Table 7.1 Pathophysiological roles of the AT_2 receptor in the heart

Effect	Reference
Coronary artery	
endothelial cell proliferation ↓	Stoll et al., 1995
thickness ↓	Akishita et al., 2000
Cardiac hypertrophy/apoptosis/fibrosis	
protein synthesis ↑/degeneration ↓	Booz et al., 1996
cardiac hypertrophy →	Liu et al., 1998; Makino et al., 1997
cardiac hypertrophy ↑	Senbonmatsu et al., 2000
cardiac apoptosis ↑	Goldenberg et al., 2001
cardiac apoptosis →	Sugino et al., 2001
cardiac fibrosis ↓	Okubo et al., 1997; Kurisu et al., 2003
cardiac fibrosis ↑	Senbonmatsu et al., 2000; Ichihara et al., 2002

receptor protein was increased in post-infarction myocytes. This result indicates that Ang II promotes myocyte growth through activation of the AT_1 receptor. Booz and Baker (1996) showed that the AT_2 receptor blocker PD123177 enhanced the stimulatory effect of Ang II on protein synthesis, and prevented Ang II-induced protein degradation in cultured neonatal rat ventricular myocytes. Thus, the authors concluded that the AT_2 receptor exerts an antagonistic action against AT_1 receptor-mediated growth. Using flaccid buffer-perfused adult hypertrophied rat heart, Bartunek et al. (1999) showed that inhibition of the cardiac AT_2 receptor amplified the immediate growth response of the left ventricle to Ang II, enhanced membrane translocation of protein kinase C and reduced left ventricular cGMP content. In coronary endothelial cells, the antiproliferative actions of the AT_2 receptor have been reported to offset the growth-promoting effects mediated by the AT_1 receptor (Stoll et al., 1995). We have also reported that in a mouse model of cardiac hypertrophy induced by aortic banding, the increase in heart/body weight ratio and cross-sectional area of cardiomyocytes were similar between wild-type and AT_2 receptor-deficient mice (Akishita et al., 2000). In contrast, the increase in coronary artery thickness was larger in AT_2 receptor-deficient mice than in wild-type mice. In this model, the AT_1 receptor blocker valsartan inhibited the heart/body weight ratio and cross-sectional area of cardiomyocytes to a similar extent in both wild type and AT_2 receptor-deficient mice (Wu et al., 2002). However, the inhibitory effect of valsartan on coronary artery thickness was significantly weaker in AT_2 receptor-deficient mice. These results suggest that the AT_1 receptor-mediated signal stimulates hypertrophy of cardiomyocytes, but remodeling of coronary arteries is regulated by both AT_1 and AT_2 receptors.

On the other hand, an increasing number of recent studies have revealed that the AT_2 receptor does not have an inhibitory effect on cardiac growth. Makino *et al.* (1997) and Liu *et al.* (1998) reported that administration of an AT_2 receptor antagonist did not affect left ventricular hypertrophy. Moreover, AT_2 receptor gene-deleted mice showed no ventricular hypertrophy in response to pressure overload by aortic constriction, although wild-type mice showed marked left ventricular hypertrophy (Senbonmatsu *et al.*, 2000).

AT_2 receptor and cardiac apoptosis

Apoptosis is well recognized to play a critical role in normal development and in pathological events in a wide variety of tissues, including the cardiovascular system. Indeed, apoptosis could be one of the alternative anti-growth mechanisms. It has been reported that the AT_2 receptor exerts proapoptotic effects on PC12W cells (Horiuchi *et al.*, 1997), R3T3 mouse fibroblasts (Tsuzuki *et al.*, 1996), AT_2-transfected adult rat VSMC (Yamada *et al.*, 1998) and fetal VSMC (Cui *et al.*, 2001). The intracellular signaling pathways leading to Ang II-mediated apoptosis are beginning to be defined. It is known that binding of Ang II to the AT_1 receptor activates ERK and serine/threonine kinase (Akt) (Haendeler *et al.*, 2000). Activation of ERK and Akt exerts antiapoptotic and pro-mitogenic effects (Franke *et al.*, 1997). AT_2 receptor stimulation activates phosphatases, which results in the inhibition of ERK and Akt activity and antagonizes the antiapoptotic effect of the AT_1 receptor (Horiuchi *et al.*, 1997; Horiuchi *et al.*, 1998; Takahashi *et al.*, 1999; Cui *et al.*, 2001). Moreover, AT_2 receptor stimulation increases ceramide production, an important mediator of apoptosis, in PC12W cells (Lehtonen *et al.*, 1999). Consistent with these *in vitro* studies, Suzuki *et al.* (2002) showed that the AT_2 receptor exerts antiproliferative effects and proapoptotic changes in VSMC by counteracting the AT_1 receptor in the process of neointimal formation after vascular injury. Thus, there are strong links between AT_2 receptor activity and the augmentation of apoptosis in a variety of tissues, including VSMC and fibroblasts. However, there is disparity regarding which receptor subtype is coupled with the mechanisms causing apoptosis in cardiac myocytes. Ang II induced irreversible double-strand cleavage of DNA in neonatal rat cardiomyocytes in culture (Cigola *et al.*, 1997). This phenomenon was mediated by an increase in intracellular free calcium and stimulation of calcium-dependent DNase I, through activation of the AT_1 receptor subtype. The ability of Ang II to initiate apoptosis in myocytes was completely inhibited by the AT₁ receptor blocker losartan. Diep *et al.* (2002) showed that Ang II infusion *in vivo* induced cardiomyocyte apoptosis associated with increased expression of bax and caspase 3 in rats. Ang II-infused rats treated with the AT₁ receptor blocker losartan exhibited normalized apoptosis, bax, and caspase 3 activity. Li *et al.* (2002) showed that lipopolysaccharide induces apoptosis *in vitro* and *in vivo* by activating the AT₁ receptor in adult rat cardiomyocytes. These results suggest that Ang II-induced apoptosis in rat cardiomyocytes is mediated through activation of the AT₁ receptor. In contrast, Goldenberg *et al.* (2001) showed that pretreatment with either the AT₁ receptor blocker irbesartan or AT₂ receptor blocker PD123319 prevented Ang II-induced apoptosis in neonatal rat cardiomyocytes, indicating that Ang II-induced apoptosis is mediated through activation of both the AT₁ and AT₂ receptor. However, Sugino *et al.* (2001) have recently shown that cardiomyocyte apoptosis is not increased by Ang II infusion in transgenic mice overexpressing the AT₂ receptor. These apparently conflicting results may provide evidence for heterogeneity of the effects of Ang II receptor stimulation in different tissues, cells, and/or different experimental conditions.

AT₂ receptor and cardiac fibrosis

Cardiac fibrosis is known to occur in pathological conditions such as the hypertrophied, infarcted, and failing heart. Excessive cardiac fibrosis contributes to ventricular dysfunction. Ang II stimulation of the AT₁ receptor induces fibroblast proliferation (Crabos *et al.*, 1994) and increased production of extracellular matrix proteins, fibronectin and collagen (Villarreal *et al.*, 1993). Varo *et al.* (2000) showed that the AT₁ receptor blocker losartan attenuated levels of tissue inhibitors of metalloproteinase-1 expression and stimulated collagenase activity in the left ventricle of adult SHR. These results indicate that Ang II stimulation of the AT₁ receptor facilitates cardiac fibrosis through increased collagen synthesis and inadequate collagen degradation. In cardiomyopathic hamsters, expression of the AT₂ receptor in the left ventricle was increased in the heart failure stage, and the AT₂ receptor was mainly localized in fibroblasts present in fibrous regions rather than in the myocardium (Ohkubo *et al.*, 1997). The AT₂ receptor blocker PD123319 increased the interstitial fibrosis by enhancing both Ang II-induced synthesis of fibrillar collagen and growth of cardiac fibroblasts, whereas the AT₁ receptor blocker TCV116 inhibited it. Akishita *et al.* (2000) showed that perivascular fibrosis in the hypertrophied heart induced by aortic banding was exaggerated in AT$_2$ receptor-deficient mice compared with wild-type control mice. In this model, the AT$_1$ receptor blocker valsartan inhibited perivascular fibrosis in both AT$_2$ receptor-deficient mice and wild-type control mice, whereas the inhibitory effect of valsartan was weaker in AT$_2$ receptor-deficient mice (Wu et al., 2002). Kurisu et al. (2003), using transgenic mice overexpressing the AT$_2$ receptor selectively in cardiomyocytes, showed that Ang II-induced perivascular fibrosis was significantly less in transgenic mice than in wild-type mice. The inhibition of perivascular fibrosis in transgenic mice was abolished by co-treatment with HOE140, a bradykinin B$_2$ receptor antagonist, or L-NAME, an inhibitor of NO synthase, suggesting that stimulation of the AT$_2$ receptor in cardiomyocytes attenuates perivascular fibrosis by a bradykinin/NO-dependent mechanism. In contrast, Senbonmatsu et al. (2000) showed that the left ventricular and interstitial fibrotic response to aortic banding was reduced in AT$_2$ receptor-deficient mice compared with wild-type control mice. Moreover, Ichihara et al. (2002) showed that excessive interstitial fibrosis and collagen accumulation after myocardial infarction were prevented in the infarcted and noninfarcted regions in AT$_2$ receptor-deficient mice, and that cardiac rupture after acute myocardial infarction occurred more frequently in AT$_2$ receptor-deficient mice than in wild-type control mice. Thus, the role of the AT$_2$ receptor in cardiac fibrosis is still an enigma.

AT$_2$ receptor and cardiac function

In human clinical trials, both angiotensin-converting enzyme inhibitors and AT$_1$ receptor blockers have been shown to improve cardiac function, attenuate remodeling, and prolong survival in patients with heart failure (Garg and Yusuf, 1995; Pitt et al., 2000; Cohn and Tognoni, 2001). Using a rat model of heart failure induced by myocardial infarction, Liu et al. (1997) showed that chronic treatment with the AT$_1$ receptor blocker L-158809 improved left ventricular function and attenuated left ventricular chamber remodeling, whereas the effect of the AT$_1$ receptor blocker was inhibited by the AT$_2$ receptor blocker PD123319. The authors speculated that blockade of the AT$_1$ receptor increases both rennin and angiotensin in heart failure, and this angiotensin stimulates the AT$_2$ receptor, which in turn has a therapeutic effect of the AT$_1$ receptor blocker. Xu et al. (2002) showed that the AT$_1$ receptor blocker valsartan increased the ejection fraction, cardiac output, and left ventricular diastolic dimension in wild-type control mice with heart failure

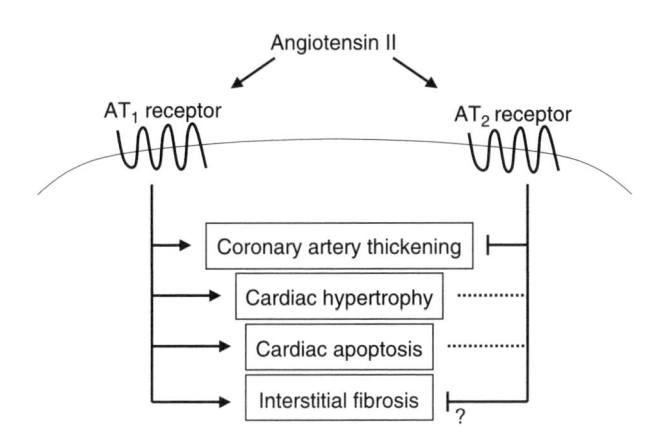

Figure 7.2 Effect of angiotensin II receptor subtypes on cardiac remodeling. The AT$_1$ receptor activation exerts coronary artery thickening, cardiac hypertrophy/apoptosis, and interstitial fibrosis. The AT$_2$ receptor stimulation has inhibitory effect on coronary artery thickening by counteracting against the AT$_1$ receptor. The roles of the AT$_2$ receptor in cardiac hypertrophy/apoptosis and interstitial fibrosis is still an enigma

induced by myocardial infarction, and that these effects of valsartan were significantly diminished in AT$_2$ receptor-deficient mice. Similar results were reported by Adachi et al. (2003) in the same mouse model of heart failure. They showed that cardiac function was significantly decreased in AT$_2$ receptor-deficient mice compared with wild-type control mice. Also, using transgenic mice overexpressing the AT$_2$ receptor, Yang et al. (2002) have shown that cardiac AT$_2$ receptor overexpression improves left ventricular systolic function at baseline and preserves function after myocardial infarction. Thus, the AT$_2$ receptor could exert cardioprotective effects (Figure 7.2).

References

Adachi Y, Saito Y, Kishimoto I, et al. (2003) Angiotensin II type 2 receptor deficiency exacerbates heart failure and reduces survival after acute myocardial infarction in mice. *Circulation* **107**, 2406–2408.

Akishita M, Iwai M, Wu L, et al. (2000) Inhibitory effect of angiotensin II type 2 receptor on coronary arterial remodeling after aortic banding in mice. *Circulation* **102**, 1684–1689.

Bartunek J, Weinberg EO, Tajima M, et al. (1999) Angiotensin II type 2 receptor blockade amplifies the early signals of cardiac growth response to angiotensin II in hypertrophied hearts. *Circulation* **99**, 22–25.

Bedecs K, Elbaz N, Sutren M, et al. (1997) Angiotensin II type 2 receptors mediate inhibition of mitogen-activated protein kinase cascade and functional activation of SHP-1 tyrosine phosphatase. *Biochemical Journal* **325** (Pt 2), 449–454.

Booz GW and Baker KM (1996) Role of type 1 and type 2 angiotensin receptors in angiotensin II-induced cardiomyocyte hypertrophy. *Hypertension* **28**, 635–640.

Busche S, Gallinat S, Bohle RM, et al. (2000) Expression of angiotensin AT(1) and AT(2) receptors in adult rat cardiomyocytes after myocardial infarction. A single-cell reverse transcriptase-polymerase chain reaction study. *American Journal of Pathology* **157**, 605–611.

Cigola E, Kajstura J, Li B, et al. (1997) Angiotensin II activates programmed myocyte cell death *in vitro*. *Experimental Cell Research* **231**, 363–371.

Cohn JN and Tognoni G (2001) A randomized trial of the angiotensin-receptor blocker valsartan in chronic heart failure. *New England Journal of Medicine* **345**, 1667–1675.

Crabos M, Roth M, Hahn AW and Erne P (1994) Characterization of angiotensin II receptors in cultured adult rat cardiac fibroblasts. Coupling to signaling systems and gene expression. *Journal of Clinical Investigation* **93**, 2372–2378.

Cui T, Nakagami H, Iwai M, et al. (2001) Pivotal role of tyrosine phosphatase SHP-1 in AT_2 receptor-mediated apoptosis in rat fetal vascular smooth muscle cell. *Cardiovascular Research* **49**, 863–871.

Diep QN, El Mabrouk M, Yue P and Schiffrin EL (2002) Effect of AT(1) receptor blockade on cardiac apoptosis in angiotensin II-induced hypertension. *American Journal of Physiology: Heart and Circulatory Physiology* **282**, H1635–H1641.

Fischer TA, Singh K, O'Hara DS, et al. (1998) Role of AT_1 and AT_2 receptors in regulation of MAPKs and MKP-1 by Ang II in adult cardiac myocytes. *American Journal of Physiology* **275**, H906–H916.

Franke TF, Kaplan DR and Cantley LC (1997) PI3K: downstream AKTion blocks apoptosis. *Cell* **88**, 435–437.

Gallinat S, Busche S, Raizada MK and Sumners C (2000) The angiotensin II type 2 receptor: an enigma with multiple variations. *American Journal of Physiology: Endocrinology and Metabolism* **278**, E357–E374.

Garg R and Yusuf S (1995) Overview of randomized trials of angiotensin-converting enzyme inhibitors on mortality and morbidity in patients with heart failure. Collaborative Group on ACE Inhibitor Trials. *JAMA* **273**, 1450–1456.

de Gasparo M, Catt KJ, Inagami T, et al. (2000) International union of pharmacology. XXIII. The angiotensin II receptors. *Pharmacology Reviews* **52**, 415–472.

Goldenberg I, Grossman E, Jacobson KA, et al. (2001) Angiotensin II-induced apoptosis in rat cardiomyocyte culture: a possible role of AT_1 and AT_2 receptors. *Journal of Hypertension* **19**, 1681–1689.

Haendeler J, Ishida M, Hunyady L and Berk BC (2000) The third cytoplasmic loop of the angiotensin II type 1 receptor exerts differential effects on extracellular signal-regulated kinase (ERK1/ERK2) and apoptosis via Ras- and Rap1-dependent pathways. *Circulation Research* **86**, 729–736.

Haywood GA, Gullestad L, Katsuya T, et al. (1997) AT_1 and AT_2 angiotensin receptor gene expression in human heart failure. *Circulation* **95**, 1201–1206.

Horiuchi M, Hayashida W, Kambe T, et al. (1997) Angiotensin type 2 receptor dephosphorylates Bcl-2 by activating mitogen-activated protein kinase phosphatase-1 and induces apoptosis. *Journal of Biological Chemistry* **272**, 19022–19026.

Horiuchi M, Akishita M and Dzau VJ (1998) Molecular and cellular mechanism of angiotensin II-mediated apoptosis. *Endocrinology Research* **24**, 307–314.

Horiuchi M, Akishita M and Dzau VJ (1999a) Recent progress in angiotensin II type 2 receptor research in the cardiovascular system. *Hypertension* **33**, 613–621.

Horiuchi M, Lehtonen JY and Daviet L (1999b) Signaling mechanism of the AT$_2$ angiotensin II receptor: crosstalk between AT$_1$ and AT$_2$ receptors in cell growth. *Trends in Endocrinology and Metabolism* **10**, 391–396.

Horiuchi M, Hayashida W, Akishita M, et al. (1999c) Stimulation of different subtypes of angiotensin II receptors, AT$_1$ and AT$_2$ receptors, regulates STAT activation by negative crosstalk. *Circulation Research* **84**, 876–882.

Huang XC, Richards EM and Sumners C (1996) Mitogen-activated protein kinases in rat brain neuronal cultures are activated by angiotensin II type 1 receptors and inhibited by angiotensin II type 2 receptors. *Journal of Biological Chemistry* **271**, 15635–15641.

Ichihara S, Senbonmatsu T, Price E, Jr, et al. (2002) Targeted deletion of angiotensin II type 2 receptor caused cardiac rupture after acute myocardial infarction. *Circulation* **106**, 2244–2249.

Inagami T, Eguchi S, Numaguchi K, et al. (1999) Cross-talk between angiotensin II receptors and the tyrosine kinases and phosphatases. *Journal of the American Society of Nephrology* **10** (Suppl 11), S57–S61.

Kambayashi Y, Bardhan S, Takahashi K, et al. (1993) Molecular cloning of a novel angiotensin II receptor isoform involved in phosphotyrosine phosphatase inhibition. *Journal of Biological Chemistry* **268**, 24543–24546.

Kurisu S, Ozono R, Oshima T, et al. (2003) Cardiac angiotensin II type 2 receptor activates the kinin/NO system and inhibits fibrosis. *Hypertension* **41**, 99–107.

Lehtonen JY, Horiuchi M, Daviet L, et al. (1999) Activation of the de novo biosynthesis of sphingolipids mediates angiotensin II type 2 receptor-induced apoptosis. *Journal of Biological Chemistry* **274**, 16901–16906.

Li HL, Suzuki J, Bayna E, et al. (2002) Lipopolysaccharide induces apoptosis in adult rat ventricular myocytes via cardiac AT(1) receptors. *American Journal of Physiology: Heart and Circulatory Physiology* **283**, H461–H467.

Liu Y, Leri A, Li B, et al. (1998) Angiotensin II stimulation in vitro induces hypertrophy of normal and postinfarcted ventricular myocytes. *Circulation Research* **82**, 1145–1159.

Liu YH, Yang XP, Sharov VG, et al. (1997) Effects of angiotensin-converting enzyme inhibitors and angiotensin II type 1 receptor antagonists in rats with heart failure. Role of kinins and angiotensin II type 2 receptors. *Journal of Clinical Investigation* **99**, 1926–1935.

Lopez JJ, Lorell BH, Ingelfinger JR, et al. (1994) Distribution and function of cardiac angiotensin AT$_1$- and AT$_2$-receptor subtypes in hypertrophied rat hearts. *American Journal of Physiology* **267**, H844–H852.

Makino N, Sugano M, Otsuka S and Hata T (1997) Molecular mechanism of angiotensin II type I and type II receptors in cardiac hypertrophy of spontaneously hypertensive rats. *Hypertension* **30**, 796–802.

Mukoyama M, Nakajima M, Horiuchi M, et al. (1993) Expression cloning of type 2 angiotensin II receptor reveals a unique class of seven-transmembrane receptors. *Journal of Biological Chemistry* **268**, 24539–24542.

Nio Y, Matsubara H, Murasawa S, et al. (1995) Regulation of gene transcription of angiotensin II receptor subtypes in myocardial infarction. *Journal of Clinical Investigation* **95**, 46–54.

Ohkubo N, Matsubara H, Nozawa Y, et al. (1997) Angiotensin type 2 receptors are reexpressed by cardiac fibroblasts from failing myopathic hamster hearts and inhibit cell growth and fibrillar collagen metabolism. *Circulation* **96**, 3954–3962.

Palczewski K, Kumasaka T, Hori T, et al. (2000) Crystal structure of rhodopsin: a G protein-coupled receptor. Science 289, 739–745.

Pitt B, Poole-Wilson PA, Segal R, et al. (2000) Effect of losartan compared with captopril on mortality in patients with symptomatic heart failure: randomised trial – the Losartan Heart Failure Survival Study ELITE II. Lancet 355, 1582–1587.

Regitz-Zagrosek V, Friedel N, Heymann A, et al. (1995) Regulation, chamber localization, and subtype distribution of angiotensin II receptors in human hearts. Circulation 91, 1461–1471.

Samyn ME, Petershack JA, Bedell KA, et al. (1998) Ontogeny and regulation of cardiac angiotensin types 1 and 2 receptors during fetal life in sheep. Pediatric Research 44, 323–329.

Senbonmatsu T, Ichihara S, Price E, Jr, et al. (2000) Evidence for angiotensin II type 2 receptor-mediated cardiac myocyte enlargement during in vivo pressure overload. Journal of Clinical Investigation 106, R1–R5.

Shanmugam S, Corvol P and Gasc JM (1996) Angiotensin II type 2 receptor mRNA expression in the developing cardiopulmonary system of the rat. Hypertension 28, 91–97.

Siragy HM, Inagami T, Ichiki T and Carey RM (1999) Sustained hypersensitivity to angiotensin II and its mechanism in mice lacking the subtype-2 (AT_2) angiotensin receptor. Proceedings of the National Academy of Sciences of the United States of America 96, 6506–6510.

Stoll M, Steckelings UM, Paul M, et al. (1995) The angiotensin AT_2-receptor mediates inhibition of cell proliferation in coronary endothelial cells. Journal of Clinical Investigation 95, 651–657.

Sugino H, Ozono R, Kurisu S, et al. (2001) Apoptosis is not increased in myocardium overexpressing type 2 angiotensin II receptor in transgenic mice. Hypertension 37, 1394–1398.

Suzuki J, Iwai M, Nakagami H, et al. (2002) Role of angiotensin II-regulated apoptosis through distinct AT_1 and AT_2 receptors in neointimal formation. Circulation 106, 847–853.

Takahashi T, Taniguchi T, Konishi H, et al. (1999) Activation of Akt/protein kinase B after stimulation with angiotensin II in vascular smooth muscle cells. American Journal of Physiology 276, H1927–H1934.

Teller DC, Okada T, Behnke CA, et al. (2001) Advances in determination of a high-resolution three-dimensional structure of rhodopsin, a model of G-protein-coupled receptors (GPCRs). Biochemistry 40, 7761–7772.

Tsutsumi Y, Matsubara H, Ohkubo N, et al. (1998) Angiotensin II type 2 receptor is upregulated in human heart with interstitial fibrosis, and cardiac fibroblasts are the major cell type for its expression. Circulation Research 83, 1035–1046.

Tsutsumi Y, Matsubara H, Masaki H, et al. (1999) Angiotensin II type 2 receptor overexpression activates the vascular kinin system and causes vasodilation. Journal of Clinical Investigation 104, 925–935.

Tsuzuki S, Eguchi S and Inagami T (1996) Inhibition of cell proliferation and activation of protein tyrosine phosphatase mediated by angiotensin II type 2 (AT_2) receptor in R3T3 cells. Biochemical and Biophysical Research Communications 228, 825–830.

Unger T, Culman J and Gohlke P (1998) Angiotensin II receptor blockade and end-organ protection: pharmacological rationale and evidence. Journal of Hypertension 16 (Suppl), S3–S9.

Varo N, Iraburu MJ, Varela M, et al. (2000) Chronic AT(1) blockade stimulates extracellular collagen type I degradation and reverses myocardial fibrosis in spontaneously hypertensive rats. *Hypertension* **35**, 1197–1202.

Villarreal FJ, Kim NN, Ungab GD, et al. (1993) Identification of functional angiotensin II receptors on rat cardiac fibroblasts. *Circulation* **88**, 2849–2861.

Wang ZQ, Moore AF, Ozono R, et al. (1998) Immunolocalization of subtype 2 angiotensin II (AT$_2$) receptor protein in rat heart. *Hypertension* **32**, 78–83.

Wharton J, Morgan K, Rutherford RA, et al. (1998) Differential distribution of angiotensin AT$_2$ receptors in the normal and failing human heart. *Journal of Pharmacology and Experimental Therapeutics* **284**, 323–336.

Wu L, Iwai M, Nakagami H, Chen R, et al. (2002) Effect of angiotensin II type 1 receptor blockade on cardiac remodeling in angiotensin II type 2 receptor null mice. *Arteriosclerosis, Thrombosis and Vascular Biology* **22**, 49–54.

Xu J, Carretero OA, Liu YH, et al. (2002) Role of AT$_2$ receptors in the cardioprotective effect of AT$_1$ antagonists in mice. *Hypertension* **40**, 244–250.

Yamada T, Horiuchi M and Dzau VJ (1996) Angiotensin II type 2 receptor mediates programmed cell death. *Proceedings of the National Academy of Sciences of the United States of America* **93**, 156–160.

Yamada T, Akishita M, Pollman MJ, et al. (1998) Angiotensin II type 2 receptor mediates vascular smooth muscle cell apoptosis and antagonizes angiotensin II type 1 receptor action: an *in vitro* gene transfer study. *Life Science* **63**, PL289–PL295.

Yang Z, Bove CM, French BA, et al. (2002) Angiotensin II type 2 receptor overexpression preserves left ventricular function after myocardial infarction. *Circulation* **106**, 106–111.

8

The Heart: A Target for the Renin Angiotensin System. Evidence of an Intracrine System

Walmor C. De Mello

Introduction

The finding that angiotensin II (Ang II) regulates heart contractility (Koch Weser, 1995), cell coupling and impulse propagation (De Mello, 1994, 1996, 1999; De Mello et al., 1997) and is responsible for remodeling and the induction of apoptosis (Harada et al., 1999; Horiuchi et al., 1999) certainly indicates that the heart is a target for the renin angiotensin system (RAS). The obvious question is how involved is the heart in the homeostatic role of the plasma RAS? Are the cardiac changes induced by the activation of the RAS part of the homeostatic response or an epiphenomenon independent of the classic role of this hormonal system? Is not the activation of the sympathetic nervous system enough to provide the cardiac response? These are important questions to be answered.

The relationship between the RAS and the heart goes beyond conventional ideas. The heart is not only influenced by the plasma RAS but has its own system.

The evidence that there is a local cardiac RAS, gained strength with the demonstration that renin, angiotensinogen, Ang I, Ang II and the angiotensin-converting enzyme (ACE) are present in the heart (Dzau, 1987; Jin et al., 1998). Moreover, the beneficial effects of ACE inhibitors in the treatment of congestive heart failure, myocardial ischemia and

Renin Angiotensin System and the Heart Edited by Walmor De Mello
© 2004 by John Wiley & Sons Ltd. ISBN 0 470 86292 0

myocardial hypertrophy (Ferrari, 1998; Nicholls *et al.*, 1998) at doses that does not change the arterial blood pressure, support this view.

However, there is a controversy concerning the synthesis of some of the RAS components inside the heart cell. The levels of cardiac renin are extremely low in nephrectomized animals (Katz *et al.*, 1997) suggesting that cardiac renin is dependent upon uptake from plasma at least in the normal heart (Campbell and Valentin, 1994; Danser *et al.*, 1994). Moreover, the source of angiotensinogen in the heart, for instance, is not known. Although angiotensinogen exists in the heart, no angiotensinogen is released from the perfused rat heart (de Lannoy *et al.*, 1997) and no angiotensinogen is present in the supernatant of serum deprived neonatal cardiac cells (van Kesteren *et al.*, 1999) what suggests that cardiac angiotensinogen is coming from the circulation. Similar observations have been published with respect to cardiac renin. Indeed, renin and renin mRNA levels in normal heart tissues are very low or even undetectable (de Lannoy *et al.*, 1997; van Kesteren *et al.*, 1999) suggesting that, under normal conditions, cardiac renin is coming from plasma through two possible pathways: (a) diffusion in the interstitial space; (b) binding to receptors (Passier *et al.*, 1996; Danser *et al.*, 1997; van Kesteren *et al.*, 1997; see also Chapter 6).

The contribution of plasma renin to cardiac renin was tested by using transgenic mice expressing human renin in the liver (TTRhren-A3) which were mated to mice expressing human angiotensinogen exclusively in the heart (MHChAgt-2). The results indicated low or undetectable angiotensin peptide in the heart of single transgenic animals while double transgenic mice showed a remarkable increase in cardiac levels of Ang I and Ang II, indicating that plasma renin is able to act on its substract within the heart (Prescott *et al.*, 2000).

However, this is not the whole history. It has been demonstrated that in some tissues a second renin gene transcription start site can be utilized leading to the synthesis of renin but lacking the secretory signal peptide. Initially found in the brain, the nonsecreted transcript was found also in the myocardium, particularly during myocardial infarction (Lee-Kirsch *et al.*, 1999; Clausmeyer *et al.*, 2000), when the cardiac RAS is activated. Indeed, the expression of exon 1A-renin mRNA in the left ventricle was found to be stimulated four-fold during myocardial ischemia, supporting the view of an intracellular function of renin (Clausmeyer *et al.*, 2000).

More recently, it has been shown that transgenic animal models used to investigate the role of the cardiac RAS, provide important information. Overexpression of the angiotensinogen gene in normal heart muscle cells of mice, for instance, caused an increase of Ang II concentration in the right and left ventricles and elicited hypertrophy of both ventricles without any change in arterial blood pressure (Mazzolai et al., 1998, 2000). These observations substantiate the notion of a cardiac RAS at the level of cardiac myocytes.

Classically, a hormonal action involves the release of the hormone, its interaction with specific receptors located at the surface cell membrane of the target cell with consequent activation of second messengers. The concept of an intracrine hormonal system implies that the hormone as well as the intracellular receptor and chemical machinery needed for the intracellular action of the hormone are available inside the cell (De Mello and Re, 2003).

This concept is particularly important under pathological conditions when an increased expression of renin and angiotensinogen genes seems to occur in cardiac muscle. Evidence has been presented, for instance, that stretch of myocardial fibers enhanced the expression of these genes (Tamura et al., 1998; Malhotra et al., 1999). On the other hand, it is known that ACE and Ang II, at cardiac sites, are increased after myocardial infarction and ventricular hypertrophy induced by pressure-overload (Yamada et al., 1991; Passier et al., 1995; van Katz et al., 1998). Cardiac Ang II generation increases the expression of renin, angiotensinogen, the Ang I/II plasma membrane receptors, AT_1 and AT_2, forming a positive feedback loop (Tamura et al., 1998). The left ventricular hypertrophy induced by aortic coarctation leads to an increase of renin and angiotensinogen mRNA in the left ventricle while the renin levels in plasma are only transiently elevated (Baker et al., 1990). The major question remains: what is the physiological or physiopathological meaning of a cardiac RAS and particularly of an intracellular system?

RAS and intercellular signaling

Although contraction is the most important function of the heart, one cannot forget that the heart is a complex electrochemical machine in which generation of electrical propagated responses is essential for the trigger of the contractile process. An increase in resistance of the gap junctions to electrical current flow can result in impairment of impulse propagation and cardiac arrhythmias (De Mello, 2001) (Figure 8.1). Moreover, suppression of cell communication reduces heart contractions by sequestering a large number of myocytes which are not able to participate in the contractile process (De Mello, 2002b).

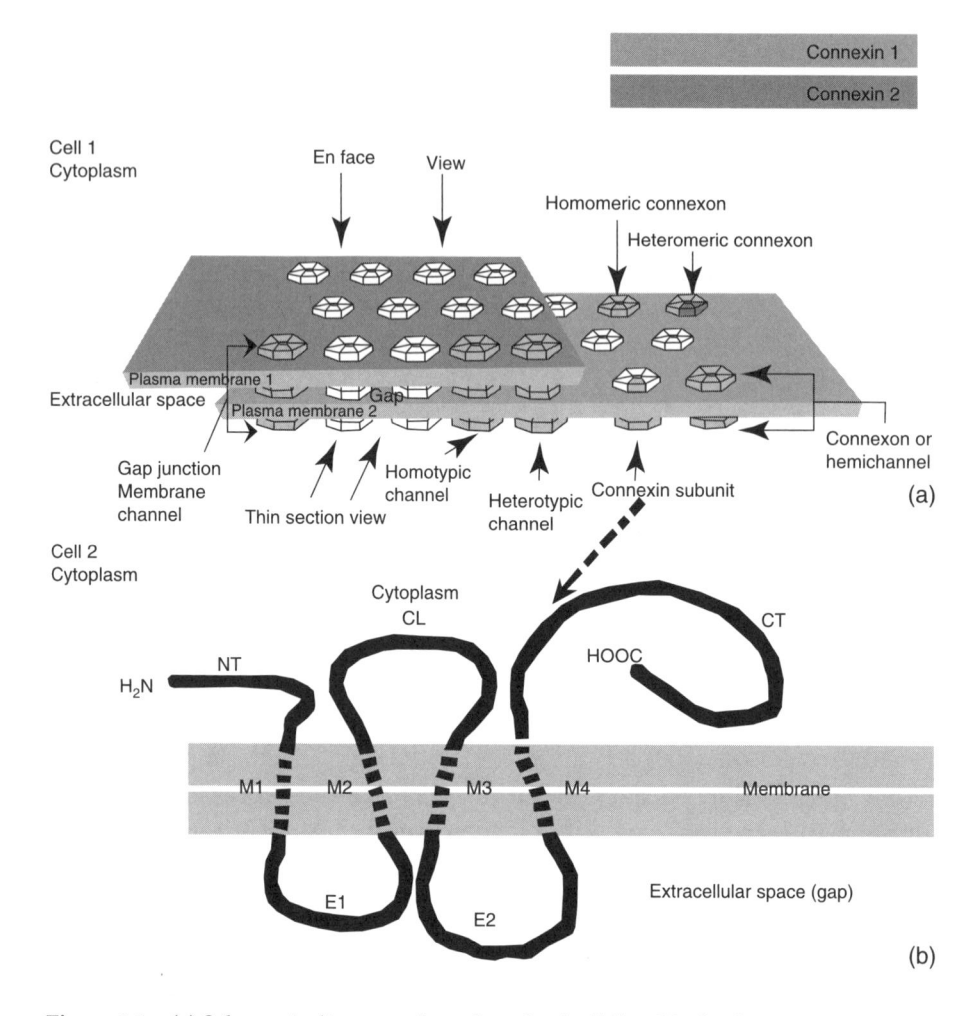

Figure 8.1 (a) Schematic diagram of gap junction building block of connexin molecule. The half-channel is a hexamer of connexin subunits. Two connexons dock in the intracellular space to form the membrane channel. (b) Topology diagram of the connexin primary sequence with three domains (cytoplasmic, membrane and extracellular domains). From Sosinsky, 2000 with permission from Academic press

Evidence is provided that intercellular communication is impaired in the failing heart (De Mello, 1999, 2002b). Indeed, the values of gap junction conductance (gj) measured in cell pairs isolated from the failing heart of cardiomyopathic hamsters, showed areas in which the gap junction conductance was extremely low (0.8–2.5 nS) and incompatible with impulse propagation (De Mello, 1996). Indeed, measurements of transmembrane action potentials performed on isolated ventricles of the failing heart, at an advanced stage of the disease, showed some areas of the ventricular wall in which the impulse propagation was normal, while in others, block of impulse conduction occurs. Histological studies revealed interstitial fibrosis, necrosis and calcifications in the failing heart (De Mello et al., 1997) that explain, at least in part, the anisotropy and the impairment of impulse propagation. Moreover, the distribution of connexin 43, which is the main gap junction protein in mammals, is altered (De Mello, 2002b) in the failing heart, which might explain, at least in part, the abnormalities of impulse propagation (see Figure 8.2).

The question whether the activation of the cardiac RAS is responsible for the changes of cell communication and impulse propagation in the

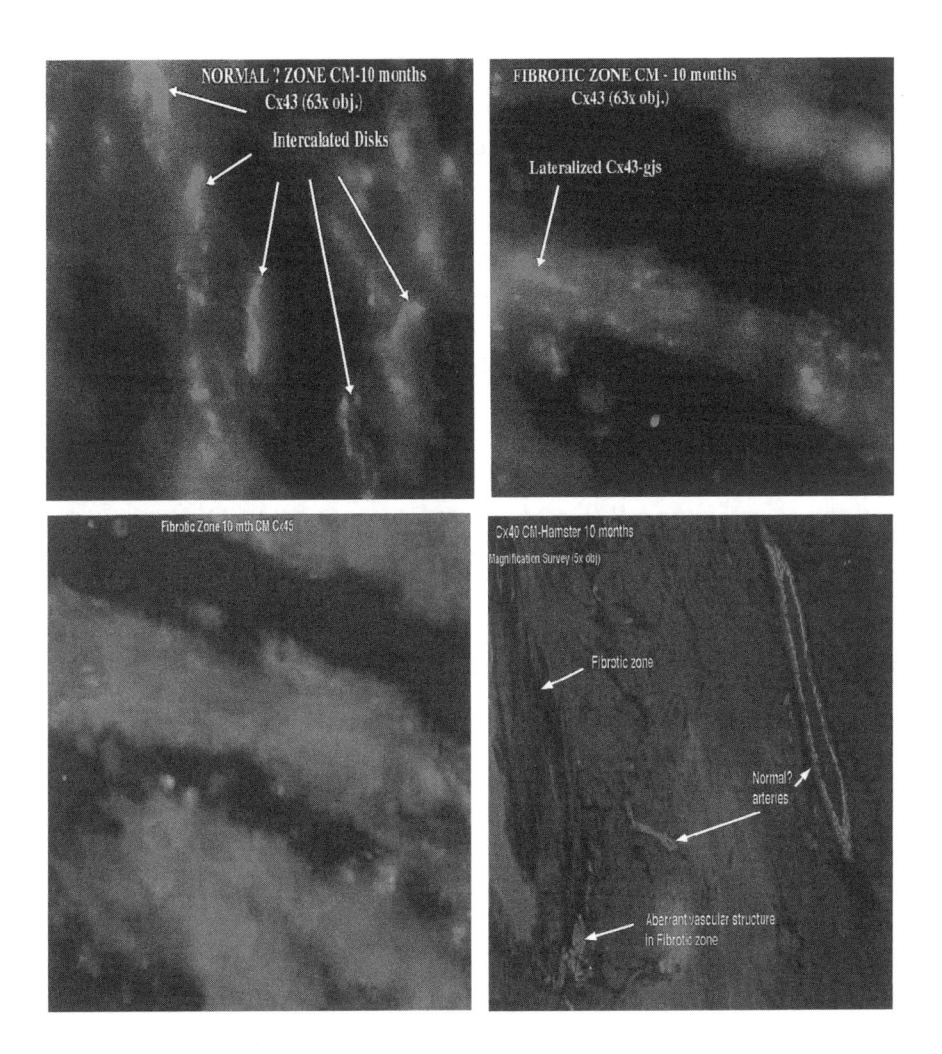

Figure 8.2 Left-normal distribution of connexin 43 in normal zone of the ventricle of cardiomyopathic hamster (TO-2) 10 months old. Right-abnormal distribution (lateral) of connexin 43 near damaged zone from the same preparation shown at left. From De Mello, 2002b, with permission from Kluwer Academic Publishers. A colour version of this figure can be found in the color plate section

failing heart is of seminal importance. It is known that activation of the plasma RAS during the process of heart failure, is largely responsible for the impairment of heart function and the remodeling of the ventricle (Dzau, 1987; Lindpaintner et al., 1990). Furthermore, the activation of a local RAS in the failing heart (for a review see De Mello and Danser, 2000), might be implicated in cell abnormalities seen during this condition.

The mechanism by which the cardiac RAS is activated is not well known. Some hemodynamic changes or glucocorticoid treatment seem to increase the angiotensinogen mRNA levels in the heart, (Lindpaintner et al., 1990). Only local factors seem to be involved because stretch of the right ventricle activates the system in this ventricle but not in the left ventricle (Lee et al., 1996).

Initial studies (De Mello, 1996) demonstrated that in cardiomyopathic hamsters at an advanced stage of the disease with overt heart failure, Ang II (10^{-8} M) added to the extracellular medium, caused cell uncoupling in cell pairs with very low values of junctional conductance (0.8–2.5 nS) and reduced gj by 53 ± 6.6 percent in cell pairs with higher gj values (7–35 nS) (De Mello, 1996). The effect of the peptide is not related to a fall in surface membrane resistance (1.4 GΩ) which remained unchanged during the experiments. The decline or suppression of cell coupling elicited by extracellular Ang II administration, requires the activation of protein kinase C (PKC) because PKC inhibitors abolished the effect of Ang II (De Mello and Altieri, 1992). The activation of this kinase leads to phosphorylation of gap junction proteins with consequent decline of cell coupling. The effect of PKC activation on cell communication, however, seems to vary with the different states of phosphorylation of connexin 43 before the activation of PKC (Imanaga et al., 2000).

It is known that tyrosine kinase represents a quite large family of molecules which play an important role on signal transduction and are involved on regulatory mechanisms such as growth and differentiation (Hunter, 1996). It has been shown that viral scr tyrosine protein kinase suppresses cell communication in fibroblasts (Atkinson et al., 1981). Ulterior studies showed that connexin 43 is a MAP kinase substrate *in vivo* and that phosphorylation of Ser 255, Ser 279 and Ser 282 initiates the downregulation of junctional communication (Zhou et al., 1999). The levels of tyrosine phosphorylated connexin 43 are increased in the heart of cardiomyopathic hamsters at an advanced stage of the disease (Toyofuku et al., 1999). These and other findings open the possibility that Ang II reduced the junctional conductance in the failing heart through tyrosine phosphorylation, an idea supported by the evidence that tyrosine phosphorylation is involved in Ang II-mediated signal transduction in different systems (Haendeler and Berk, 2000).

Ang II, cell coupling and growth; an important relationship?

Cell-to-cell communication occurs through hormones, cytokines and growth factors which are released into bloodstream or through local generation and responses to several ions and molecules such as growth factors, nitric oxide, calcium ions or cytokines.

The exchange of second messengers and other signal molecules which are involved in cell proliferation and function pass through gap junctions which make possible the electrical synchronization of cardiac myocytes (see De Mello, 2002b) and the metabolic co-operation between cells. Many growth factors like the epidermal growth factor (EGF), the platelet derived growth factor (PDGF), the basic fibroblast growth factor (bFGF) and the hepatic growth factor (HGF) inhibit gap junctional communication when applied to cultured cell (Trosko et al., 1990). The inhibition of cell coupling by EGF is quite rapid and is related to the phosphorylation of connexin 43 (Cx43) on serine residues by mitogen-activated protein kinase (MAPK) (Warn-Cramer et al., 1998).

Ang II is an important growth factor which elicit hypertrophy through the activation of AT_1 and consequently of several intracellular pathways including PKC, increases intracellular calcium and activates the MAP kinase family (Dostal, 2000).

Several cytoplasmic ions and regulatory molecules (inositol phosphate, cyclic AMP, etc.) that have an important role in growth pass through gap junctions. The relation between growth and cell coupling is well known. Cancer cells, for instance, are weakly coupled (see Trosko et al., 1990; Wilgenbus et al., 1992) and factors that increase connexin expression such as retinoids, inhibit neoplastic transformation in target tissues (Ruch, 1994). On the other hand, ACE inhibitors that increase cell coupling (De Mello and Altieri, 1992) decrease ventricular hypertrophy. These observations raise the possibility that growth, decrease of cell communication and Ang II are all connected.

Evidence for an intracellular RAS

The presence of a RAS inside the cardiomyocyte (intracrine system) has been supported experimentally (see De Mello, 1994, 1995, 1996;

De Mello and Danser, 2000; Cook et al., 2001; De Mello and Re, 2003). Similar results were described in vascular smooth muscle cells in which intracellular Ang II promotes growth (Filipenu et al., 2001; Eto et al., 2002). Indeed, when Ang I (10^{-9} M) is dialyzed inside myocytes isolated from the failing ventricle, the junctional conductance was greatly reduced (De Mello, 1996), an effect practically suppressed by enalaprilat given to the cytosol. This finding is indicative that the effect of intracellular Ang I was related to its convertion to Ang II because intracellular Ang II, by itself, reduced or abolished cell coupling (De Mello, 1996). Furthermore, the decline in cell communication caused by intracellular dialysis of Ang II in isolated cell pairs of the failing heart, was suppressed by intracellular administration of losartan (10^{-7} M) but not by the administration of the AT_1 blocker to the extracellular space. This finding indicates that the peptide is acting intracellularly and that an intracellular Ang II receptor similar to AT_1 is involved in the decline of cell coupling. Furthermore, quantifying tissue angiotensin release studies using ^{125}Ang I infusions (see Admiraal et al., 1993) did not show significant Ang II release from tissues. On the other hand, evidence is available that there is an intracellular Ang II receptor (Baker et al., 1984). Indeed, cytoplasmic Ang II receptors and a soluble angiotensin-binding cytosolic protein with a molecular weight of 75 kDa have been described in liver cells (Sen and Rajasekaran, 1991). Moreover, nuclear and chromatin Ang II receptors have been identified (Re et al., 1983). Immunochemical studies also indicated the presence of intracellular Ang II receptors in cardiomyocytes and fibroblasts (Fu et al., 1998). This finding, however, contrasts with previous studies of Kato et al. (1994) which demonstrated that the porcine soluble angiotensin-binding protein is a microsomal endopeptidase – a finding that does not support the idea of an intracellular Ang II receptor.

Concerning the ACE there is reliable evidence that the enzyme is synthesized at cardiac sites because ACE and ACE mRNA are detectable in the heart by autoradiography as well as in homogenate of cardiac muscle (Yamada et al., 1991; De Mello and Crespo, 1999; see also De Mello and Danser, 2000).

On the possible role of endogenous Ang II on heart cell communication

The internalization of prorenin and the formation of renin inside the cardiac myocyte lead to two possible consequences: formation of Ang II inside the cell with consequent intracellular action of the peptide

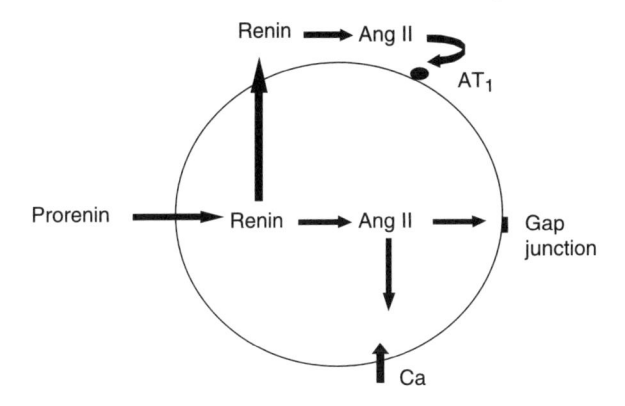

Figure 8.3 Diagram showing the possible role of prorenin uptake and generation of Ang II on gap junction communication and inwards calcium current

(see Figure 8.3) or release of renin to the extracellular medium and formation of Ang II outside the cell with activation of AT_1 (see also Chapters 3, 5 and 6).

It is thus conceivable that if Ang I is formed inside the cardiomyocyte, the administration of enalaprilat into the cytosol will suppress its conversion to Ang II. Considering that intracellular Ang II has a modulatory role on cell communication (De Mello, 1996), it is expected that intracellular enalaprilat increments the value of junctional conductance by inhibiting Ang II formation. This hypothesis is substantiated by the finding that intracellular administration of enalaprilat, *per se*, on cell pairs of cardiomyopathic hamsters at 4 months of age when the ACE activity is enhanced, drastically reduced the effect of intracellular Ang I on cell coupling. Moreover, no effect of the ACE inhibitor was found in cells of 2 month-old animals in which the ACE activity is not increased (Figure 8.4) (De Mello, 1996; De Mello and Crespo, 1999). This finding might indicate that the lack of action of the ACE inhibitor was due to absence of Ang I formation at early stages of the disease probably because no renin is available for the formation of the peptide.

The concept that endogenous levels of Ang II plays an important role on cell functions is supported by recent studies showing that the intracellular administration of losartan (10^{-8} M) on cell pairs of cardiomyopathic hamster's heart increased *gj* by 15.9 ± 3.1 percent (De Mello, 2003). The possibility that losartan is suppressing the action of intracellular Ang II from exogenous origin cannot be discounted. It is not known, for instance, if the internalization of Ang II–receptor complex is a source of intracellular Ang II. Because in our model of isolated cells

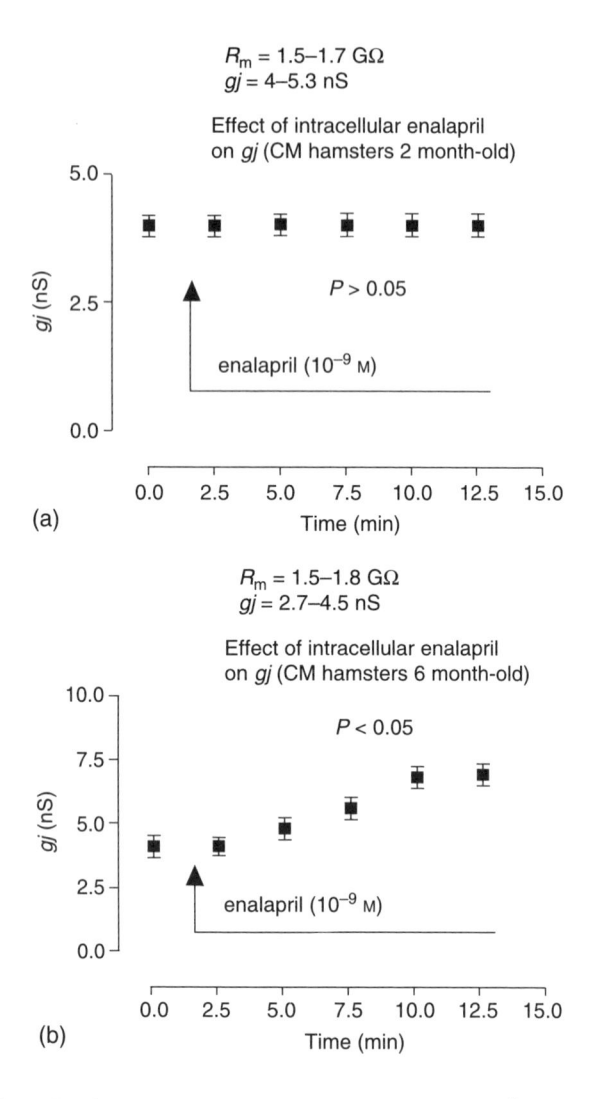

Figure 8.4 (a) Lack of action of intracellular enalaprilat (10^{-8} M) on junctional conductance (gj) of ventricular cells from 2 month-old cardiomyopathic hamsters in which the ACE activity is not above control levels. Values of gj were expressed in nS. Arrow indicates the moment enalaprilat was administered. Each point is the average of 35 cell pairs. Vertical lines at each point ± SE. (b) Increase of gj caused by intracellular enalaprilat (10^{-8} M) on gj of ventricular cells from 6 month-old cardiomyopathic hamsters with an appreciable increase of ACE activity (average of 33 cells). Arrow indicates the moment enalaprilat was administered intracellularly. Vertical lines each point ± SE. From De Mello, 2003, with permission from Elsevier

no extracellular Ang II is available, it is reasonable to conclude that the effect of intracellular losartan on cell coupling is related to solely to the suppression of the action of endogenous Ang II.

However, is the ACE located intracellularly or at the surface cell membrane? This is an important question because the uptake of renin by the heart might be followed by its release from the cardiomyocyte and consequent formation of Ang II at the level of the cell membrane. Previous observations indicated that in endothelial cells the enzyme is membrane bound with the active site projecting into the extracellular space (Soubrier et al., 1988) and that the majority of its molecule is bound to the plasma membrane by a C terminal transmembrane spanning region (Soubrier et al., 1988). If this is the case for cardiomyocytes, it is expected that Ang I, added to the cytosol, be unable to change cell coupling. However, experimental evidence is available that Ang I (10^{-8} M) dialyzed intracellularly reduced or abolished cell coupling, an effect suppressed by intracellular enalaprilat (De Mello, 1996). These observations indicate that ACE is available inside the cardiomyocytes.

Conceivably, the decline in cell-to-cell coupling caused by Ang II increases the intracellular resistance in cardiac muscle with consequent decrease of impulse propagation. We have carried on studies on the influence of the peptide on the electrical properties of intact rat ventricle and the results showed a decrease of conduction velocity from 59.5 ± 2.5 cm/s to 35 ± 3.6 cm/s (De Mello et al., 1993) while enalapril, an angiotensin converting enzyme inhibitor, reduced the intracellular resistance and increased cell coupling (De Mello, 1996) as well as the conduction velocity within 5 min (De Mello et al., 1993). The improvement of impulse propagation elicited by the drug, however, is in part related to the hyperpolarization induced by the drug through the activation of the Na–K pump (De Mello, 2002c).

The intracellular injection of Ang II (10^{-10} M) inside the cells of intact ventricular muscle of 4 month-old cardiomyopathic hamsters, elicited a decrease of resting potential of 7.5 ± 1.4 mV ($P < 0.05$) and an increase in duration of the action potential by 108 ± 1.3 percent at 50 percent repolarization and 33 ± 1.5 percent at 90 percent repolarization ($P < 0.05$). Some ventricular cells, however, seem insensitive to Ang II (De Mello, unpublished) but the reason for this insensitivity is not known.

Aldosterone modulates the effect of Ang II

It is well known that Ang II releases aldosterone from adrenal gland. The obvious question is how influencial is aldosterone on the effects of Ang II? Recent studies indicated that in rats treated with aldosterone for 48 h, Ang II added to the bath, increases the action potential duration and refractoriness contrary to the effect in the controls in which both parameters were reduced by the same dose of Ang II (De Mello, 2002a). The increment in action potential duration elicited by Ang II was suppressed by verapamil what may indicate that it is related to an increased inward calcium current. Interestingly, the effect of isoproterenol on cardiac excitability and action potential duration was not altered by aldosterone. This finding shows that the effect of Ang II on heart functions must be evaluated considering the presence or absence of aldosterone. Recently, it has been reported that not only aldosterone receptors are present in the heart (Bonvalet et al., 1995) but that the hormone is produced by the heart. Chronic treatment with Ang II as well as low sodium/high potassium diet, for instance, increased the production of aldosterone (Silvestre et al., 1999; Takeda et al., 2000) raising the possibility of a cross-talk between angiotensin II and aldosterone in the heart (see Chapter 11).

Effect of intracellular and extracellular Ang II on the inward calcium current

In cardiomyocytes of adult rats, in which Ang II has a negative inotropic action, the intracellular administration of the peptide reduced the inward calcium current, whereas in normal hamsters, in which the peptide elicit a positive inotropic action, the intracellular administration of Ang II increased the inward calcium current (De Mello, 1998). Similar result was found when Ang II was applied extracellularly. Stimulation of I_{Ca} by exogenous cAMP or inhibition of PKC did not alter the effect of intracellular Ang II on I_{Ca} but zaprinast, an inhibitor of cGMP phosphodiesterase, increased appreciably the effect of the peptide on I_{Ca} of rat cardiomyocytes. The mechanism by which intracellular Ang II increments I_{Ca} on normal hamster cardiomyocytes involves the activation of PKC (De Mello, 1998). Recently, it was found that intracellular dialysis of Ang II into myocytes of cardiomyopathic hamsters at 4 months of age, when the ACE activity is increased above control levels (De Mello and Crespo, 1999), increases the inward calcium current.

Changes in cardiac gene expression and activation of the local RAS might be implicated in ventricular remodeling. In isolated and perfused rat heart the increase of coronary perfusion pressure and consequent stretch increased the steady state c-fos mRNA expression 2.3-fold (Kang et al., 1996). Mechanical stretch also enhanced the expression of renin and angiotensinogen genes (Tamura et al., 1998; Malhotra et al., 1999). Figure 8.5 illustrates the possible relationship between ventricular dilatation, stretch, increased expression of renin and angiotensinogen

```
        Heart failure
            ⇩
Increase of end diastolic volume
            ⇩
  Stretch of ventricular fibers
            ⇩
Increased expression of renin and angiotensinogen genes
            ⇩
Increase of renin and Ang II in heart fibers
            ⇩
Increase of inward calcium current
            ⇩
Increase of heart contractility
```

Figure 8.5 Flow diagram of events involved in heart failure

genes, increase of intracellular Ang II and consequent increment of heart contractility.

Although intracellular Ang II can be beneficial for the failing heart through an increase of contractility, the changes in cell coupling and the remodeling induced by the peptide can generate re-entrant rhythms (De Mello, 2001) and impair the ventricular function. These and other observations indicate that prevention of a rise of intracellular renin and angiotensin levels can be an important aspect of therapeutics of heart failure and other pathological conditions which involves the activation of the cardiac renin angiotensin system.

Acknowledgments

I want to thank Mrs Maria Gonzalez for the technical work and the American Heart Association and NIH (HL-34148; GM 61838) for support.

References

Admiraal PJJ, Danser AHJ, Jong MS, *et al.* (1993) Regional angiotensin II production in essential hypertension and renal artery stenosis. *Hypertension* **21**, 173–184.

Atkinson MM, Menko AS, Johnson RG, *et al.* (1981) Rapid and reversible reduction of junctional permeability in cells infected with a temperature-sensitive mutant of avian sarcoma virus. *Journal of Cell Biology* **91**, 573–578.

Baker K, Chernin M, Wixcon S and Aceto J (1990) Renin angiotensin system involvement in pressure-overload cardiac hypetrophy in rats. *American Journal of Physiology* **259**, H324–H332.

Baker KM, Campanile MP, Trachte GJ and Peach MJ (1984) Identification and characterization of the rabbit angiotensin II myocardial receptor. *Circulation Research* **54**, 286–293.

Bonvalet JP, Alfaidy N, Farman N and Lombes M (1995) Aldosterone intracellular receptors in human heart. *European Heart Journal* **16** (Suppl N), 92–97.

Campbell DJ and Valentin AJ (1994) Identification of vascular renin-binding proteins by chemical cross-linking: inhibition of renin by renin inhibitors. *Journal of Hypertension* **12**, 879–890.

Clausmeyer S, Reinecke A, Farrenkopf R, et al. (2000) Tissue-specific expression of a rat renin transcript lacking the coding sequence for the prefragment and its stimulation by myocardial infarction. *Endocrinology* **141**, 2963–2970.

Cook JL, Zhung Z and Re RN (2001) *In vitro* evidence for an intracellular site of angiotensin action. *Circulation Research* **89**, 1138–1146.

Danser AHJ, van Katz JP, Admiraal PJJ, et al. (1994) Cardiac renin and angiotensins: uptake from plasma versus in situ synthesis. *Hypertension* **24**, 37–48.

Danser AHJ, van Kesteren CAM, Bax WA, et al. (1997) Prorenin, renin, angiotensin and ACE in normal and failing human heart: evidence for renin binding. *Circulation* **96**, 220–222.

De Mello WC (1994) Is an intracellular renin angiotensin system involved in the control of cell communication in heart? *Journal of Cardiovascular Pharmacology* **23**, 640–646.

De Mello WC (1995) Influence of intracellular renin on heart cell communication. *Hypertension* **25**, 1172–1177.

De Mello WC (1996) Renin angiotensin system and cell communication in the failing heart. *Hypertension* **27**, 1267–1272.

De Mello WC (1998) Intracellular angiotensin II regulates the inward calcium current in cardiac myocytes. *Hypertension* **32**, 976–982.

De Mello WC (1999) Cell coupling and impulse propagation in the failing heart. *Journal of Cardiovascular Electrophysiology* **10**, 1409–1430.

De Mello WC (2001) Cardiac arrhythmias; the possible role of the renin angiotensin system. *Journal of Molecular Medicine* **79**, 103–108.

De Mello WC (2002a) Aldosterone modulates the effect of angiotensin II on the electrical properties of adult rat heart. *Journal of Cardiovascular Pharmacology* **40**, 90–95.

De Mello WC (2002b) Cell coupling and impulse propagation in the failing heart. In *Heart Cell Coupling and Impulse Propagation in Health and Disease*, De Mello WC and Janse M (eds), Kluwer Academic Publishers, Boston, pp. 283–320.

De Mello WC (2002c) Electrical activity of the heart and angiotensin converting inhibitors; on the hyperpolarizing action of enalapril. *Journal of Human Hypertension* **16**(Suppl 1), S89–S92.

De Mello WC (2003) Further studies on the effect of intracellular angiotensins on heart cell communication: on the role of endogenous angiotensin II. *Regulatory Peptides* **115**, 31–36.

De Mello WC and Altieri P (1992) The role of the renin angiotensin system in the control of cell communication in the heart; effects of angiotensin II and enalapril. *Journal of Cardiovascular Pharmacology* **20**, 643–651.

REFERENCES

De Mello WC and Crespo MJ (1999) Correlation between changes in morphology, electrical properties and angiotensin converting enzyme activity in the failing heart. *European Journal of Pharmacology* **378**, 187–194.

De Mello WC and Danser AHJ (2000) Angiotensin II and the heart. On the intracrine renin angiotensin system. *Hypertension* **35**, 1183–1188.

De Mello WC and Re RN (2003) Is an intracrine renin angiotensin system involved in the control of cardiovascular function? In *Cardiac Remodeling and Failure*, Pawan K, Sigal I, Dixon MC, *et al.* (eds), Kluwer Academic Publishers, Boston, pp. 365–375.

De Mello WC, Crespo MJ and Altieri PI (1993) Effect of enalapril on intracellular resistance and conduction velocity in rat ventricular muscle. *Journal of Cardiovascular Pharmacology* **22**, 259–263.

De Mello WC, Cherry R and Mannivanan S (1997) Electrophysiologic and morphologic abnormalities in the failing heart; effect of enalapril on the electrical properties. *Cardiac Failure* **3**, 53–62.

Dzau VJ (1987) Implications of local angiotensin production in cardiovascular physiology and pharmacology. *American Journal of Cardiology* **59** (Suppl A), 59A–65A.

Dostal DE (2000) The cardiac renin–angiotensin system: novel signaling mechanisms related to cardiac growth and function. *Regulatory Peptides* **91**, 1–11.

Eto K, Ohya Y, Nakamura Y, *et al.* (2002) Intracellular angiotensin II stimulates voltage-operated Ca^{2+} channels in arterial myocytes. *Hypertension* **39**, 474–478.

Ferrari R (1998) Effect of ACE inhibition on myocardial ischemia. *European Heart Journal* **19** (Suppl J), J30–J35.

Filipenu CM, Henning RH, de Zeeuw D and Nelemans A (2001) Intracellular angiotensin II and cell growth of vascular smooth muscle cells. *British Journal of Pharmacology* **132**, 1590–1596.

Fu ML, Schulze W, Wallukat G, *et al.* (1998) Immunochemical localization of angiotensin II receptor (AT_1) in the heart with anti-peptide antibody showing a positive chronotropic effect. *Receptor Channels* **6**, 99–111.

Haendeler J and Berk B (2000) Tyrosine phosphorylation is involved in Ang II-mediated signal transduction. *Regulatory Peptides* **95**, 1–7.

Harada K, Sugaya T, Murakami K, *et al.* (1999) Angiotensin II type 1A receptor knockout mice display less left ventricular remodeling and improved survival after myocardial infarction. *Circulation* **100**, 2093–2999.

Horiuchi M, Ashita M and Dzau VJ (1999) Recent progress in angiotensin II type 2 receptor research in the cardiovascular system. *Hypertension* **33**, 613–621.

Hunter T (1996) Tyrosine phosphorylation: past, present and future. *Biochemical Society Transactions Hopkins Medal Lecture* **24**, 307–327.

Imanaga I, Hirosawa N, Lin H, *et al.* (2002) Phosphorylation of connexin 43 and regulation of cardiac gap junctions. In *Heart Cell Coupling and Impulse Propagation in Health and Disease*, De Mello WC and Janse M (eds), Kluwer Academic Publishers, Boston, pp. 185–205.

Jin M, Wilhelm MJ, Lang RE, *et al.* (1988) Endogenous tissue renin angiotensin systems. From molecular biology to therapeutics. *American Journal of Medicine* **84** (Suppl 3A), 28–36.

Kang PM, Nakousi A, Simpson T, *et al.* (1996) Role of endogenous renin angiotensin system in c-fos activation and PKC-epsilon translocation in adult rat hearts. *American Journal of Physiology* **270**, H2177–H2183.

Kato A, Sugiura N, Hagiwara H and Hirose S (1994) Cloning, amino acid sequence and tissue distribution of porcine thimet oligopeptidase. A comparison with soluble angiotensin-binding protein. *European Journal of Biochemistry* **221**, 159–165.

Katz SA, Opsahl JA, Lunser MM, et al. (1997) Effect of bilateral nephrectomy on active renin, angiotensinogen and renin glycoforms in plasma and myocardium. *Hypertension* **30**, 259–266.

van Katz JP, Danser AHJ, van Maegen J, et al. (1998) Angiotensin production in the heart: a quantitative study in pigs with the use of radio labeled angiotensin infusions. *Circulation* **98**, 73–81.

van Kesteren CAM, Danser AHJ, Derbx FHM, et al. (1997) Mannose-6 phosphate receptor-mediated internalization and activation of prorenin in cardiac cells. *Hypertension* **30**, 389–396.

van Kesteren CAM, Saris H, Dekkers DHW, et al. (1999) Cultured neonatal rat cardiac myocytes and fibroblasts do not synthesize renin or angiotensinogen: evidence for stretch-induced cardiomyocyte hypertrophy independent of angiotensin II. *Cardiovascular Research* **43**, 148–156.

Koch Weser J (1995) Nature of inotropic action of angiotensin on ventricular myocardium. *Circulation Research* **16**, 230–237.

de Lannoy LM, Danser AHJ, van Katz JP, et al. (1997) Renin angiotensin system components in the interstitial fluid of the isolated perfused rat heart: local production of angiotensin I. *Hypertension* **29**, 1240–1251.

Lee YA, Liang CS, Lee HA and Lindpaintner K (1996) Local stress, not systemic factors regulate gene expression of cardiac renin angiotensin system *in vivo*: a comprehensive study of all its components in the dog. *Proceedings of the National Academy of Sciences of the United States of America* **93**, 11035–11040.

Lee-Kirsch M, Gaudet F, Cardoso M and Lindpaintner K (1999) Distinct renin isoforms generated by tissue specific transcription initiation and alternative splicing. *Circulation Research* **84**, 240–246.

Lindpaintner K, Jin MW, Niedrmaier N, et al. (1990) Cardiac angiotensinogen and its local activation in the isolated perfused beating heart. *Circulation Research* **67**, 564–573.

Malhotra R, Sadoshima J, Broscius FC and Izumo S (1999) Mechanical stretch and angiotensin II differentially upregulated the renin angiotensin system in cardiac myocytes *in vitro*. *Circulation Research* **85**, 137–146.

Mazzolai L, Nussberger J, Aubert JF, et al. (1998) Blood pressure-independent cardiac hypertrophy induced by locally activated renin–angiotensin system. *Hypertension* **31**, 1324–1330.

Mazzolai L, Pedrazzini T, Nicoud F, et al. (2000) Increased cardiac angiotensin II levels induce right and left ventricular hypertrophy in normotensive mice. *Hypertension* **35**, 985–991.

Nicholls MG, Richards AM and Agarwal M (1998) The importance of the renin angiotensin system in cardiovascular disease. *Journal of Human Hypertension* **12**, 295–299.

Passier RCJJ, Smits JFM, Verluyten MJA and Daemen MJAP (1996) Expression and localization of renin and angiotensinogen in rat heart after myocardial infarction. *American Journal of Physiology* **271**, H1040–H1048.

Prescott G, Siversides DW, Chiu SML and Reudelhuber TL (2000) Contribution of circulating renin to local synthesis of angiotensin peptides in the heart. *Physiological Genomics* **4**, 67–73.

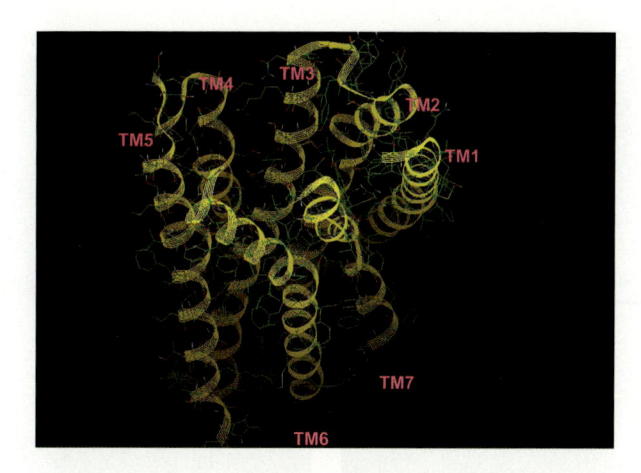

Figure 7.1a

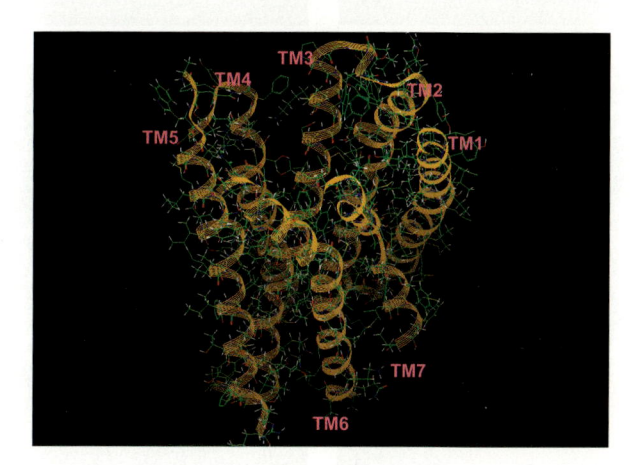

Figure 7.1b

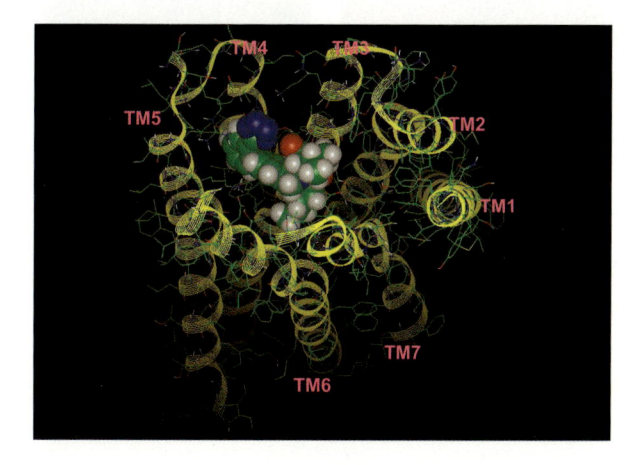

Figure 7.1c

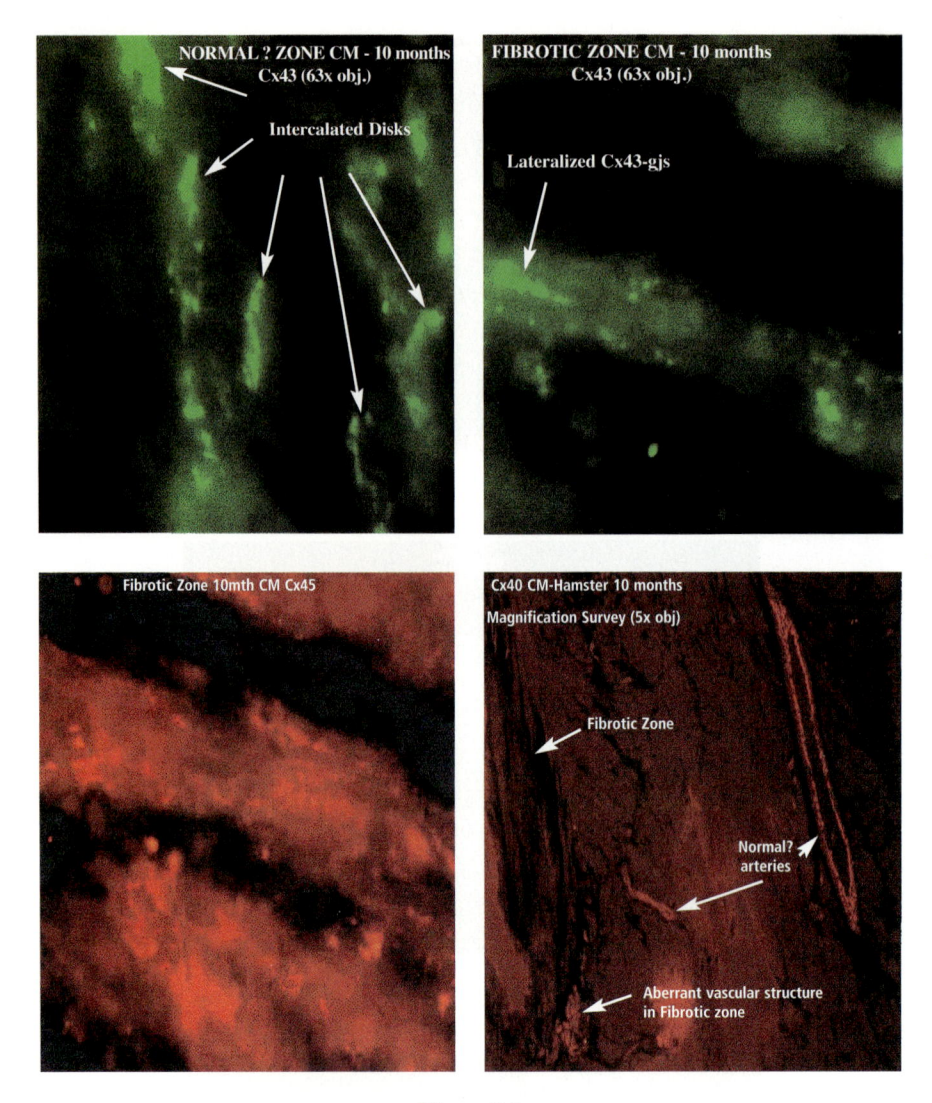

Figure 8.2

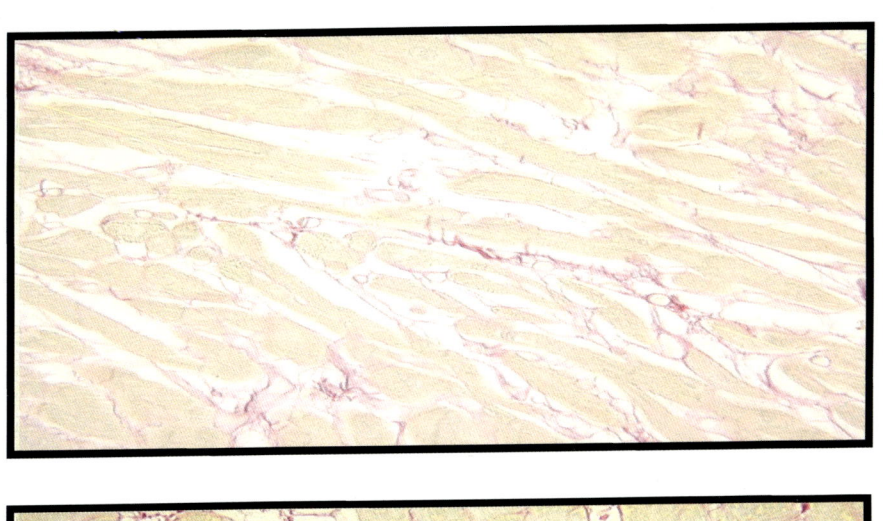

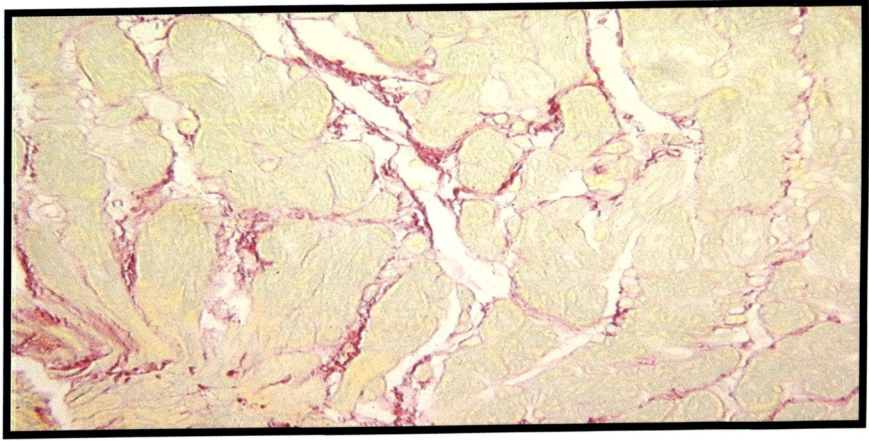

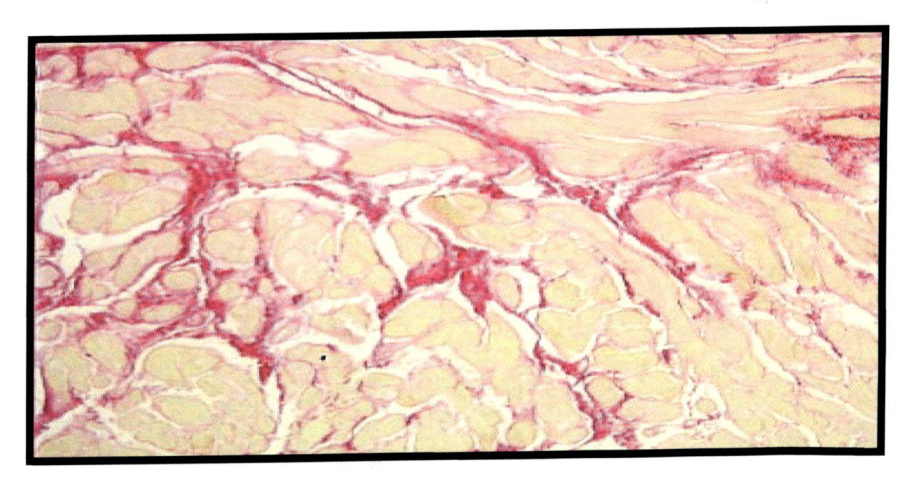

Figure 13.1

Re RN, LaBiche RA and Bryan SE (1983) Nuclear-hormone mediated changes in chromatin solubility. *Biochemical and Biophysical Research Communications* **110**, 61–68.

Ruch RJ (1994) The role of gap junction intercellular communication in neoplasia. *Annals of Clinical Laboratory Science* **24**, 216–231.

Sen I and Rajasekaran AK (1991) Angiotensin II-binding protein in adult and neonatal rat heart. *Journal of Molecular and Cellular Cardiology* **23**, 563–572.

Silvestre JS, Heymans C, Oubenaissa A, *et al.* (1999) Activation of cardiac aldosterone production in rat myocardial infarction. *Circulation* **99**, 2694–2701.

Sosinsky G (2000) Gap junction structure: new structures and new insights. In *Gap Junctions*, Peracchia C (ed), Academic Press, San Diego, pp. 1–22.

Soubrier F, Alhenc-Gelas F, Hubert C, *et al.* (1988) Two putative active centers in human angiotensin I-converting enzyme revealed by molecular cloning. *Proceedings of the National Academy of Science of the United States of America* **85**, 9386–9390.

Takeda Y, Takashi Y, Masashi D, *et al.* (2000) Cardiac aldosterone production in genetic hypertensive rats. *Hypertension* **36**, 495–500.

Tamura K, Umemura S, Nyui N, *et al.* (1998) Activation of angiotensinogen gene in cardiac myocytes by angiotensin II and mechanical stretch. *American Journal of Physiology* **44**, R1–R9.

Toyofuku T, Yabuki M, Otsu K, *et al.* (1999) Functional role of c-src in gap junctions of the cardiomyopathic hamster heart. *Circulation Research* **85**, 672–681.

Trosko JE, Chia-Chang CC, Madhukaar BV and Oh SY (1990) Chemical, oncogene and growth. Regulator modulation of extracellular, intracellular and intercellular communication. In *Intercellular Communication*, De Mello WC (ed), CRC Press, Boca Raton FL, pp. 111–126.

Warn-Cramer BJ, Cotrell GT, Burt JM and Lau AF (1998) Regulation of connexin 43 gap junctional communication by mitogen-activated protein kinase. *Journal of Biological Chemistry* **273**, 9188–9196.

Wilgenbus KK, Kirkpatrik CJ, Kmechem R, *et al.* (1992) Expression of Cx26, Cx32 and Cx43 gap junction proteins in normal and neoplastic human tissues. *International Journal of Cancer* **51**, 522–529.

Yamada H, Fabris B, Allen AM, *et al.* (1991) Localization of angiotensin converting enzyme in rat heart. *Circulation Research* **68**, 141–149.

Zhou L, Kasperek EM and Nicholson BJ (1999) Dissection of the molecular basis of Pp60-src induced gating of connexin 43 gap junctions. *Journal of Cell Biology* **144**, 1033–1045.

9

ACE2: Its Role in the Counter-regulatory Response to Heart Failure

Lawrence S. Zisman

Introduction

Angiotensin II (Ang II), plays a critical role in the pathophysiology of heart failure and inhibition of angiotensin-converting enzyme (ACE) and is a mainstay of therapeutics for heart failure. Great attention has been given to elucidating pathways for both Ang II generation and degradation over the past 30 years. While many enzymes have been described which are capable of hydrolyzing Ang II to smaller peptides, very little is known regarding the relative importance of these enzymes in the intact nonfailing and failing human heart. A newly described enzyme with high homology to ACE, termed ACE2 or ACEH, has been shown to hydrolyze Ang II to the bioactive peptide Ang-(1-7). Because Ang-(1-7) opposes many of the signal transduction events mediated by Ang II, this pathway for Ang II degradation and Ang-(1-7) generation is of great potential importance. This chapter will review what is currently known about ACE2 and its potential role as a counter-regulatory, cardioprotective enzyme in the failing human heart.

Renin Angiotensin System and the Heart Edited by Walmor De Mello
© 2004 by John Wiley & Sons Ltd. ISBN 0 470 86292 0

A paradigm of human heart failure: secondary activation of neurohormonal systems and a counterbalancing response

The neurohormonal model has guided the development of pharmacologic treatment for heart failure over the past two decades. In this model, secondary activation of the renin angiotensin, endothelin, and adrenergic systems after an initial insult to the myocardium plays a major role in the progression of ventricular dysfunction. This model, depicted schematically in Figure 9.1, proposes that activation of a local cardiac renin angiotensin system (RAS) modulates the chronic trophic response of the cardiac myocyte to increased stress. The RAS is an endocrine cascade that results in the conversion of the inactive prohormone angiotensin I (Ang I) to the active peptide hormone Ang II, and may also function as an autocrine/paracrine system to modulate cardiac function and growth. Renin, the initial enzyme of this cascade, cleaves the amino terminus of the preprohormone angiotensinogen (338 amino acids), releasing the decapeptide prohormone Ang I. ACE removes two additional amino acids to yield the active octapeptide

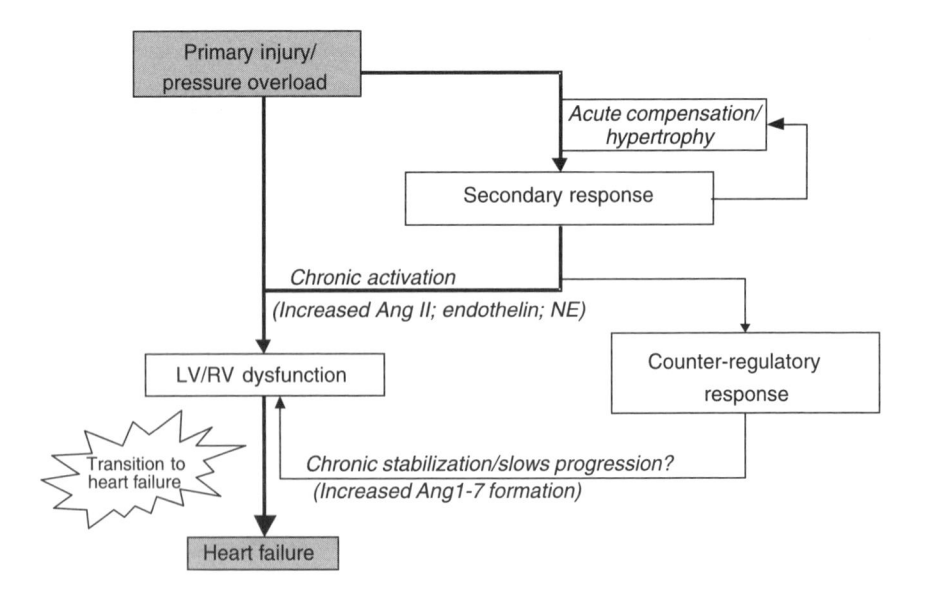

Figure 9.1 A general model of human heart failure: importance of secondary RAS activation and a proposed tertiary (counter-regulatory) response. It is proposed that a counter-regulatory response slows the progression of ventricular dysfunction but, as represented by the weight of the arrows, is insufficient to prevent the transition to heart failure. LV, left ventricle; Ang1-7, Angiotensin-(1-7); NE, norepinephrine

hormone Ang II. Ang II, acting through the Ang II type 1 plasma membrane receptor (AT$_1$) is a potent vasoconstrictor and stimulates cardiac growth. This cardiac growth may be related to myocyte hypertrophy and/or fibroblast proliferation with a concomitant alteration in the extracellular matrix (ECM) (Sadoshima *et al.*, 1993; Sabbah *et al.*, 1995). In addition, Ang II, by interaction with the neuroadrenergic and endothelin systems may cause an increase in local norepinephrine and endothelin levels which in turn may have direct trophic and toxic effects on the cardiac myocyte. The cellular events triggered by increased Ang II formation, while initially compensatory, may lead to eventual loss of cellular function (contractility) and/or viability. ACE inhibitor therapy has been shown to improve survival and cardiac function in patients with left heart failure (SOLVD Investigators, 1991; Konstam *et al.*, 1992). Presumably, a significant benefit of this therapy results from a reduction of Ang II concentration in the heart.

The neurohormonal model also proposes that there is a tertiary, counter-regulatory response to RAS activation. It is proposed that, in response to RAS activation, there is an increase both at the level of gene and protein expression of components that decrease the local concentration of Ang II, and which generate bioactive compounds that counteract Ang II mediated effects. Potentially novel counter-regulatory responses to cardiac RAS activation, have recently received increased attention. One such response is the increased metabolism of Ang II to the smaller bioactive peptide Ang-(1-7).

Angiotensin metabolites

Both Ang I and Ang II may be hydrolyzed to form other angiotensin peptides (Figure 9.2). Other angiotensin metabolites with known biological activity include Ang III, Ang IV, and Ang-(1-7). Ang III is formed by

	1	2	3	4	5	6	7	8	9	10
Ang I	Asp	Arg	Val	Tyr	Ile	His	Pro	Phe	His	Leu
Ang1-9	Asp	Arg	Val	Tyr	Ile	His	Pro	Phe	His	
Ang II	Asp	Arg	Val	Tyr	Ile	His	Pro	Phe		
Ang1-7	Asp	Arg	Val	Tyr	Ile	His	Pro			
Ang III		Arg	Val	Tyr	Ile	His	Pro	Phe		
Ang IV			Val	Tyr	Ile	His	Pro	Phe		
Ang1-5	Asp	Arg	Val	Tyr	Ile					

Figure 9.2 Angiotensin metabolites and their nomenclature

hydrolysis of the Asp–Arg bond, a reaction catalyzed by aminopeptidase A (Reaux et al., 2000). Ang III in turn may be hydrolyzed by aminopeptidase N to form Ang IV (Reaux et al., 2000). Ang III has been shown to bind the AT_1 receptor as an agonist, and Ang IV may bind its own unique AT_4 receptor (Hall et al., 1995; Bernier et al., 1998; Briand et al., 1998; Coleman et al., 1998; Fitzgerald et al., 1999).

In contrast to Ang III which appears to be an agonist for the AT_1 receptor, it has been proposed that Ang-(1-7) counteracts the effects of Ang II (Ferrario et al., 1997). During combined therapy with an ACE inhibitor and an AT_1 receptor antagonist, administration of a specific antibody to Ang-(1-7) increased blood pressure in SHR rats (Iyer et al., 1998). It has also been shown in the rat that Ang-(1-7) lowered blood pressure by a mechanism that may involve cross-talk with the bradykinin type 2 receptor (Abbas et al., 1997). It has been demonstrated that Ang-(1-7) stimulates the release of nitric oxide from porcine coronary endothelium (Porsti et al., 1994). Ang-(1-7) inhibited vascular smooth muscle cell growth; this effect was not blocked by selective AT_1 or AT_2 receptor antagonists (Freeman et al., 1996). These data provide indirect evidence for a novel Ang-(1-7) receptor. The finding of specific and saturable binding of ^{125}I-Ang-(1-7) to bovine endothelial cells provided the first direct evidence for a unique Ang-(1-7) receptor. The Ang-(1-7) antagonist D-alanine-7-Ang-(1-7) completely blocked ^{125}I-Ang-(1-7) binding with an IC_{50} of 19.8 nmol/l. Neither the AT_1 selective antagonist losartan, nor the AT_2 receptor antagonist PD 123319 competed with ^{125}I-Ang-(1-7) binding to these cells (Tallant et al., 1997).

Overview of peptidases

Enzymes which hydrolyze peptides may be classified according to characteristics of the active site and peptide hydrolysis site preference. Five major groups of peptidases based on active site characteristics have been described: (1) metalloproteases; (2) serine proteases; (3) cysteine proteases; (4) aspartyl proteases; and (5) furin convertases. Metalloproteases are characterized by the presence of one or more metal ion binding motifs; for example, neutral endopeptidase, ACE, and endothelin-converting enzyme (ECE) are all zinc-binding metalloproteases. Alternatively, peptidases have been classified based on the region of the peptide subject to hydrolysis, and/or whether the enzyme has specificity for a particular amino acid. Thus peptidases may be classified in three broad categories based on the region of the peptide hydrolyzed: (1) aminopeptidases; (2) carboxypeptidases; and (3) endopeptidases.

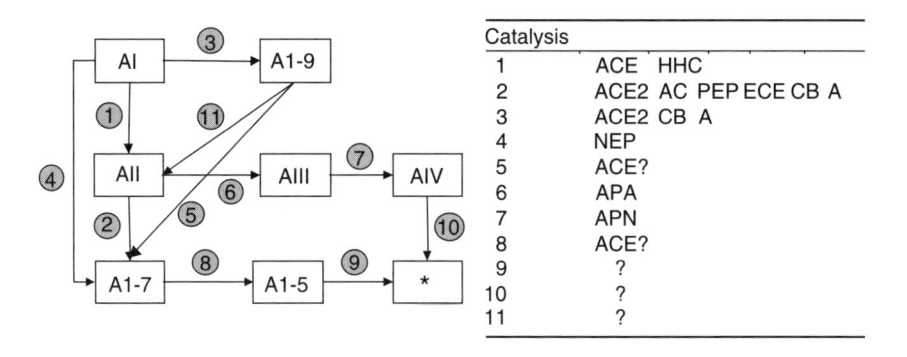

Catalysis	
1	ACE HHC
2	ACE2 AC PEP ECE CB A
3	ACE2 CB A
4	NEP
5	ACE?
6	APA
7	APN
8	ACE?
9	?
10	?
11	?

Figure 9.3 Pathways for angiotensin metabolism. Enzymes which may catalyze the hydrolysis of angiotensin peptides are shown in the right panel. AI, angiotensin I; AII, angiotensin II; AIII, angiotensin III; AIV, angiotensin IV; A1-7, angiotensin 1-7; A1-9, angiotensin 1-9; A1-5, angiotensin 1-5. Enzymes which may catalyze the hydrolysis of angiotensin peptides are shown in the accompanying figure. ACE, angiotensin-converting enzyme; ACE2, angiotensin-converting enzyme homolog; HHC, human heart chymase; NEP, neutral endopeptidase; PEP, prolylendopeptidase; AC, angiotensinase C; ECE, endothelin-converting enzyme; AP A, aminopeptidase A; APN, aminopeptidase N; CB A, carboxypeptidase A

The enzymes that catalyze the formation of nonAng I/nonAng II fragments have been studied in the human kidney, endothelial cells, and in various tissues of the rat (Santos et al., 1992; Campbell et al., 1994). The specific angiotensin fragments that have been described are angiotensin 3-8 (Ang III), angiotensin 3-7 (Ang IV), and angiotensin II fragment 1-7 (Ang-(1-7)). Enzymes that hydrolyze Ang I and II to smaller fragments are called angiotensinases (Figure 9.3). A prolylcarboxypeptidase called angiotensinase C (Angase C) that hydrolyzes the Pro–Phe bond in Ang II to form Ang-(1-7) was first described over 30 years ago (Yang et al., 1968; Odya et al., 1978), although the cDNA sequence was only reported in 1993 (Tan et al., 1993). Another class of enzymes, the prolylendopeptidases (PEPs), also hydrolyze the Pro–Phe bond, and may contribute to Ang-(1-7) formation. A PEP has been purified from porcine skeletal muscle and has high substrate specificity for both Ang I and Ang II (Moriyama et al., 1988). Shirasawa et al. (1994) cloned a PEP from human T cells and demonstrated PEP mRNA in human brain, heart, skeletal muscle, and kidney. The human T cell PEP nucleotide sequence showed 91 percent homology to the porcine PEP. Western blot analysis demonstrated a molecular size of approximately 80 kDa for the human T cell PEP, compared to 74 kDa for the porcine PEP. In contrast, Angase C had a molecular weight of 58 kDa on sodium dodecyl sulfate–polyacrylamide gel electrophoresis, and only 29 percent amino acid sequence homology to human PEP. Both enzymes were inhibited by Z-Pro-Prolinal. However, porcine and, presumably, human PEP were inhibited by *p*-chloromercuriphenylsulfonate (*p*-CMPS) with an IC$_{50}$ of 2.6×10^{-7} M whereas Angase C was not inhibited by this compound (Shirasawa *et al.*, 1994). These data indicate significant differences between the Angase C first cloned and purified from human kidney and the PEP cloned from human T cells.

Neutral endopeptidase (NEP) has also been shown to break down Ang I to Ang-(1-7), and has been described in heart and endothelial cells (Llorens-Cortes *et al.*, 1992; Piedimonte *et al.*, 1994). ECE-1 was first described as a metalloprotease which hydrolyzes the 38 amino acid endothelin-1 (ET1) precursor, big ET1, at Trp21–Val22 to form the active peptide ET1. The importance of ECE-1 is highlighted by the observation that ET1 is the most potent vasoconstrictive peptide known. Interestingly, ECE-1 has 37 percent homology to neutral endopeptidase 24.11, and may hydrolyze Ang I as efficiently as big ET-1 (Johnson *et al.*, 1999). Thus, its name notwithstanding, ECE-1 may function as an angiotensinase. It has been reported that Ang II increased functional ECE activity in WYK rats *in vivo* and that ACE inhibition prevented upregulation of ECE-1 in failing human atrial tissue (Barton *et al.*, 1997; Morawietz *et al.*, 2002). These reports provide evidence for cross-regulation between the renin angiotensin and endothelin systems.

Carboxypeptidases

Several carboxypeptidases have been described, and their nomenclature makes liberal use of the alphabet. Thus, carboxypeptidase A, B, C, D, E, H, N, M, R, X, Y, and Z have been reported. For the most part these carboxypeptidases are metallopeptidases which co-ordinate Zn^{2+} at their active sites. The initial nomenclature for metallocarboxypeptidases was derived from the characteristics of the C-terminal amino acid cleaved. Thus, carboxypeptidase A cleaves C-terminal *acidic* amino acids, whereas carboxypeptidase B cleaves C-terminal *basic* amino acids (i.e., Arg or Lys) (Skidgel *et al.*, 1998). Originally, carboxypeptidase A and B were purified from pancreatic tissue, and generally considered to play a role in digestion. A lysosomal carboxypeptidase A, also known as lysosomal protective protein, or cathepsin A has been shown to hydrolyze Ang I to Ang-(1-9) at acidic pH, and to be present in human heart atrial and ventricular tissue (Jackman *et al.*, 2002). Because of its location in the lysosome, and its optimal activity at acidic pH, the importance of cathepsin A in the intact human heart remains unclear.

ACE2, a novel homologue of ACE, functions as a carboxypeptidase and angiotensinase

Two groups simultaneously described a novel carboxypeptidase with 40 percent identity to ACE but which was not inhibited by captopril or other 'classical' ACE inhibitors, including enalaprilat and lisinopril. This enzyme, called ACE2 (Donoghue et al., 2000) or ACEH (Tipnis et al., 2000), was first reported to hydrolyze the His–Leu bond in Ang I to release Ang-(1-9). It was reported that Ang-(1-9) was a substrate for ACE which hydrolyzed it to Ang-(1-7). ACE2 did not hydrolyze Ang-(1-9) to form Ang II (Donoghue et al., 2000). However, ACEH was found to hydrolyze Ang II to produce Ang-(1-7) (Tipnis et al., 2000). Thus, ACEH/ACE2 should, theoretically, function to decrease Ang II concentration where it is present and active. ACE2 contains a single HEXXH zinc-binding domain which is essentially homologous to the active site of ACE (although ACE is known to have two active sites; Figure 9.4). A conserved glutamic acid residue, 24 amino acids downstream of the HEXXH motif corresponds to the glutamate in ACE which is required for catalytic activity. ACE2 contains eight cysteine residues of which six are conserved in the N and C terminal domains of ACE (Tipnis et al., 2000). The cDNA for ACE2 consists of 3405 nucleotides (2418 bp open reading frame resulting in a protein of 805 amino acids.) Based on this it is predicted to have a molecular weight of 92.4 kDa. When expressed in Chinese hamster ovary cells as a recombinant protein without the transmembrane and cytosolic domains its apparent molecular weight was 120 kDa. However, when deglycosylated its molecular weight was more consistent with that predicted from its sequence. A hydrophobic region at the C-terminus suggests that ACE2 is membrane bound. Northern blot analysis demonstrated ACE2 gene expression in the heart, kidney, and testes. By quantitative RT–PCR ACE2 gene expression was also detected in the duodenum and ileum (Harmer et al., 2002). Immunohistochemistry demonstrated that ACE2 protein was present predominantly in endothelium of the microvasculature in human heart ventricle. The predominant expression of ACE2 to heart, kidney, and testes contrasts to the near ubiquitous expression of ACE in endothelial cells of multiple organs including skeletal muscle, heart, kidney, testes and lung (Donoghue et al., 2000). The activity of ACE2 was quenched by EDTA, consistent with its predicted function as a metallopeptidase. More recently, recombinant soluble ACE2 expressed in Sf9 cells was shown to have substrate preference for Ang II ($K_m = 2\,\mu M$, $k_{cat} = 3.5\,s^{-1}$) compared to Ang I ($K_m = 7\,\mu M$, $k_{cat} = 0.034\,s^{-1}$).

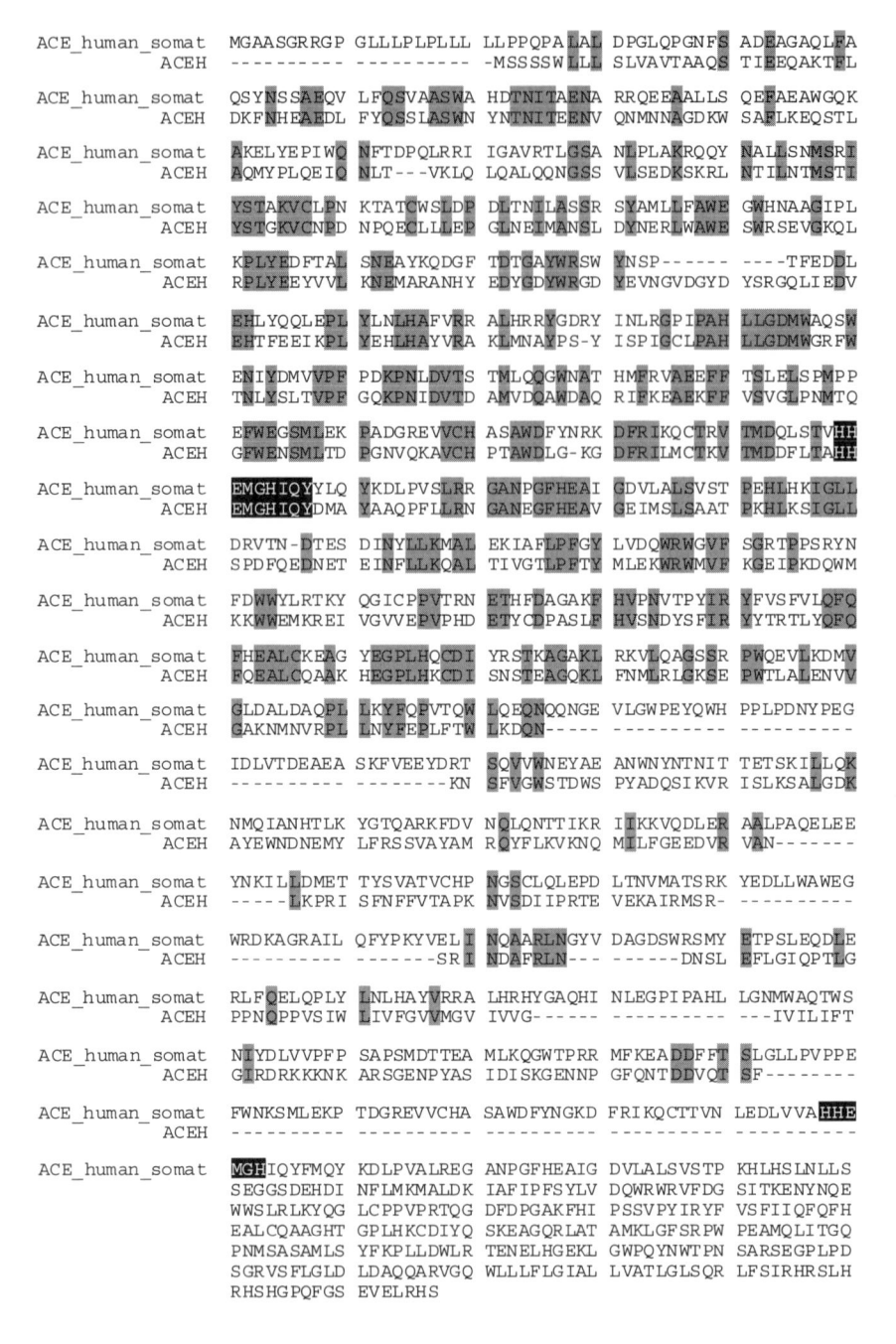

```
ACE_human_somat  MGAASGRRGP GLLLPLPLLL LLPPQPALAL DPGLQPGNFS ADEAGAQLFA
          ACEH  ---------- ---------- -MSSSSWLLL SLVAVTAAQS TIEEQAKTFL

ACE_human_somat  QSYNSSAEQV LFQSVAASWA HDTNITAENA RRQEEAALLS QEFAEAWGQK
          ACEH  DKFNHEAEDL FYQSSLASWN YNTNITEENV QNMNNAGDKW SAFLKEQSTL

ACE_human_somat  AKELYEPIWQ NFTDPQLRRI IGAVRTLGSA NLPLAKRQQY NALLSNMSRI
          ACEH  AQMYPLQEIQ NLT---VKLQ LQALQQNGSS VLSEDKSKRL NTILNTMSTI

ACE_human_somat  YSTAKVCLPN KTATCWSLDP DLTNILASSR SYAMLLFAWE GWHNAAGIPL
          ACEH  YSTGKVCNPD NPQECLLLEP GLNEIMANSL DYNERLWAWE SWRSEVGKQL

ACE_human_somat  KPLYEDFTAL SNEAYKQDGF TDTGAYWRSW YNSP------ ----TFEDDL
          ACEH  RPLYEEYVVL KNEMARANHY EDYGDYWRGD YEVNGVDGYD YSRGQLIEDV

ACE_human_somat  EHLYQQLEPL YLNLHAFVRR ALHRRYGDRY INLRGPIPAH LLGDMWAQSW
          ACEH  EHTFEEIKPL YEHLHAYVRA KLMNAYPS-Y ISPIGCLPAH LLGDMWGRFW

ACE_human_somat  ENIYDMVVPF PDKPNLDVTS TMLQQGWNAT HMFRVAEEFP TSLELSPMPP
          ACEH  TNLYSLTVPF GQKPNIDVTD AMVDQAWDAQ RIFKEAEKFF VSVGLPNMTQ

ACE_human_somat  EFWEGSMLEK PADGREVVCH ASAWDFYNRK DFRIKQCTRV TMDQLSTVHH
          ACEH  GFWENSMLTD PGNVQKAVCH PTAWDLG-KG DFRILMCTKV TMDDFLIAHH

ACE_human_somat  EMGHIQYYLQ YKDLPVSLRR GANPGFHEAI GDVLALSVST PEHLHKIGLL
          ACEH  EMGHIQYDMA YAAQPFLLRN GANEGFHEAV GEIMSLSAAT PKHLKSIGLL

ACE_human_somat  DRVTN-DTES DINYLLKMAL EKIAFLPFGY LVDQWRWGVF SGRTPPSRYN
          ACEH  SPDFQEDNET EINFLLKQAL TIVGTLPFTY MLEKWRWMVF KGEIPKDQWM

ACE_human_somat  FDWWYLRTKY QGICPPVTRN ETHFDAGAKF HVPNVTPYIR YFVSFVLQFQ
          ACEH  KKWWEMKREI VGVVEPVPHD ETYCDPASLF HVSNDYSFIR YYTRTLYQFQ

ACE_human_somat  FHEALCKEAG YEGPLHQCDI YRSTKAGAKL RKVLQAGSSR PWQEVLKDMV
          ACEH  FQEALCQAAK HEGPLHKCDI SNSTEAGQKL FNMLRLGKSE PWTLALENVV

ACE_human_somat  GLDALDAQPL LKYFQPVTQW LQEQNQQNGE VLGWPEYQWH PPLPDNYPEG
          ACEH  GAKNMNVRPL LNYFEPLFTW LKDQN----- ---------- ----------

ACE_human_somat  IDLVTDEAEA SKFVEEYDRT SQVVWNEYAE ANWNYNTNIT TETSKILLQK
          ACEH  ---------- --------KN SFVGWSTDWS PYADQSIKVR ISLKSALGDK

ACE_human_somat  NMQIANHTLK YGTQARKFDV NQLQNTTIKR IIKKVQDLER AALPAQELEE
          ACEH  AYEWNDNEMY LFRSSVAYAM RQYFLKVKNQ MILFGEEDVR VAN-------

ACE_human_somat  YNKILLDMET TYSVATVCHP NGSCLQLEPD LTNVMATSRK YEDLLWAWEG
          ACEH  -----LKPRI SFNFFVTAPK NVSDIIPRTE VEKAIRMSR- ----------

ACE_human_somat  WRDKAGRAIL QFYPKYVELI NQAARLNGYV DAGDSWRSMY ETPSLEQDLE
          ACEH  ---------- -------SRI NDAFRLN--- ------DNSL EFLGIQPTLG

ACE_human_somat  RLFQELQPLY LNLHAYVRRA LHRHYGAQHI NLEGPIPAHL LGNMWAQTWS
          ACEH  PPNQPPVSIW LIVFGVVMGV IVVG------ ---------- ---IVILIFT

ACE_human_somat  NIYDLVVPFP SAPSMDTTEA MLKQGWTPRR MFKEADDFFT SLGLLPVPPE
          ACEH  GIRDKKKNK ARSGENPYAS IDISKGENNP GFQNTDDVQT SF--------

ACE_human_somat  FWNKSMLEKP TDGREVVCHA SAWDFYNGKD FRIKQCTTVN LEDLVVAHHE
          ACEH  ---------- ---------- ---------- ---------- ----------

ACE_human_somat  MGHIQYFMQY KDLPVALREG ANPGFHEAIG DVLALSVSTP KHLHSLNLLS
                 SEGGSDEHDI NFLMKMALDK IAFIPFSYLV DQWRWRVFDG SITKENYNQE
                 WWSLRLKYQG LCPPVPRTQG DFDPGAKFHI PSSVPYIRYF VSFIIQFQFH
                 EALCQAAGHT GPLHKCDIYQ SKEAGQRLAT AMKLGFSRPW PEAMQLITGQ
                 PNMSASAMLS YFKPLLDWLR TENELHGEKL GWPQYNWTPN SARSEGPLPD
                 SGRVSFLGLD LDAQQARVGQ WLLLFLGIAL LVATLGLSQR LFSIRHRSLH
                 RHSHGPQFGS EVELRHS
```

Figure 9.4 Homology of ACE2 protein to ACE protein. The active site HHEMGH which is identical in ACE2 and ACE is highlighted in black. The second active site of ACE, which has no counterpart in ACE2 is also shown. Gray highlighted areas indicate identical amino acids between ACE and ACE2

The recombinant ACE2 had an apparent molecular weight of 89 kDa and pH optimum of 6.5 (Vickers et al., 2002).

ACE2-mediated hydrolysis of biological peptides

Michaelis–Menten kinetics performed with recombinantly expressed ACE2 and Ang II as substrate demonstrated a $K_m = 2\,\mu M$ and $k_{cat}/K_m = 1.9 \times 10^6\,M^{-1}\,s^{-1}$ for the formation of Ang-(1-7). In contrast, with Ang I as substrate the K_m was higher (6.9 μM) indicating lower affinity of ACE2 for Ang I, and the k_{cat}/K_m was substantially lower ($k_{cat}/K_m = 4.9 \times 10^3\,M^{-1}\,s^{-1}$) for the formation of Ang-(1-9). ACE2 has been shown to hydrolyze two other peptides with high efficiency: apelin-13 ($k_{cat}/K_m = 2.1 \times 10^6\,M^{-1}\,s^{-1}$), and dynorphin A 1-13 ($k_{cat}/K_m = 3.1 \times 10^6\,M^{-1}\,s^{-1}$). In addition, ACE2 shows catalytic activity with des-Arg9-bradykinin, but does not hydrolyze bradykinin (Vickers et al., 2002). Other substrates for which ACE2 shows intermediate catalytic activity include, β-casmophorin ($k_{cat}/K_m = 2.2 \times 10^5\,M^{-1}\,s^{-1}$) and neurotensin 1-8 ($k_{cat}/K_m = 1.9 \times 10^5\,M^{-1}\,s^{-1}$). The consensus sequence for ACE2-mediated hydrolysis consists of a proline followed by a hydrophobic amino acid (Vickers et al., 2002).

Genetics and cross-species homology

Two forms of ACE (AnCE and ACEr) have been described in Drosophila, and two forms of ACE have been described in mammals. The mammalian forms of ACE consist of a somatic form with two active sites, and a testicular form (tACE) with one active site. tACE is derived from alternative splicing of the somatic ACE gene. The ACE gene maps to chromosome 17q23 (NM 000789). The ACEH gene consists of 18 exons within 41572 bp located on the X chromosome (Xp22, Accession AY217547). Phylogenetic analysis of ACEH by the Clustal V method showed early divergence of the ACE drosophila homolog from mammalian forms of ACE. Relative conservation of the exon/intron organization between ACE2 and mammalian ACE suggests that these genes arose by duplication of a common ancestor (Donoghue et al., 2000). In three models of hypertensive rats ACE2 mapped to a quantitative trait locus for hypertension on the X chromosome (Crackower et al., 2002), and has, therefore, been proposed as a candidate gene for hypertension.

Recently, a protein, collectrin, with 47.8 percent identity to ACE2 was found. Collectrin, although homologous to ACE2, contained no catalytic domain. It consists of 222 amino acids and has a predicted molecular weight of approximately 32 kDa. The gene expression of Collectrin was restricted to the kidney, and immunohistochemistry demonstrated presence of protein in the ureteric bud of the embryonic mouse kidney. Based on these findings it has been proposed that collectrin may play a role in renal organogenesis independent of peptidase activity (Zhang et al., 2001).

The ACE2 knockout mouse

The ACE2 gene was disrupted by homologous recombination in a mouse model and absence of ACE2 mRNA and protein verified. In contrast to a previously developed ACE knockout mouse, the ACE2 knockout did not demonstrate altered systemic blood pressure regulation to the age of 3 months. Significant effects on cardiac morphology and function not observed in the ACE knockout mouse occurred in the ACE2 knockout model. These changes consisted of mild left ventricular wall thinning, dilation, and significantly decreased contractility as demonstrated by echocardiography and invasive hemodynamics (Crackower et al., 2002). Both fractional shortening and dP/dt were significantly decreased in ACE2 knockout mice. Other characteristics of dilated cardiomyopathy were not observed: there was no evidence for interstitial fibrosis, no upregulation of atrial natriuretic factor, and no myosin heavy chain isoform switch. There was no significant effect on left ventricular mass and no evidence for hypertrophy of individual cardiac myocytes. The decrease in contractility was more pronounced in 6 month-old male mice compared to age-matched female mice, and less severe in 3 month-old males. The systemic blood pressure in the 6 month-old ACE2 knockout mice was significantly lower than in the age-matched female mice or the 3 month-old males. Gene expression of the hypoxia-inducible genes *BNIP3* and *PAI-1* were upregulated in ACE2 null mice compared to wild-type littermates. This finding suggests that a loss of ACE2 resulted in impaired oxygen delivery to the myocardium (Crackower et al., 2002).

Design and characteristics of ACE2-specific inhibitors

ACE2 peptide inhibitors with K_i values in the nanomolar range have been identified from screening constrained phage libraries (Huang et al.,

2003). Peptides with the motif CXPXRXXPWXXC showed the greatest inhibition with K_i values ranging from 2.8 to 139 nM. Rational drug design has also been used to synthesize a highly potent and selective inhibitor of ACE2 ($IC_{50} = 0.44$ nM, IC_{50} for ACE, $>100 \mu M$, and for carboxypeptidase A, 27 μM; Dales et al., 2002).

Regulation of Ang-(1-7) formation in human heart failure

It has recently been demonstrated that ACE2 is a major pathway for Ang-(1-7) formation in the failing human heart (Figure 9.5). In failing human heart ventricles from subjects with idiopathic dilated cardiomyopathy, ACE2 activity with Ang II substrate, was significantly increased compared to nonfailing hearts. ACE2-mediated Ang-(1-7) formation has been shown to be significantly increased in both the left and right ventricles of hearts from subjects with idiopathic dilated cardiomyopathy, and to be selectively increased in the failing right ventricles from

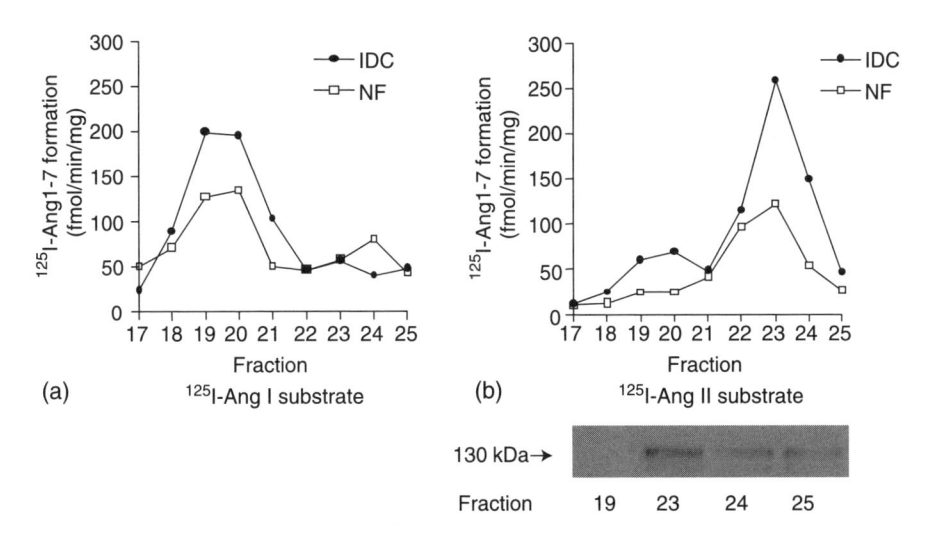

Figure 9.5 Separation of NEP from ACE2 by column chromatography demonstrated that the Ang-(1-7) forming activity of NEP (fraction 19) had substrate preference for Ang I, whereas ACE2 (fraction 23) had substrate preference for Ang II. Peak angiotensinase activity in fraction 19 with Ang I substrate was higher in the IDC preparation, whereas peak angiotensinase activity with Ang II was higher in fraction 23 of the IDC compared to the NF preparation. Immunoblotting with an anti-ACE2 antibody demonstrated presence of ACE2 in the fractions with peak angiotensinase activity (Ang II substrate). Reproduced with permission by Lippincott, Williams and Wilkins

subjects with primary pulmonary hypertension. In addition, ACE2 activity in the right ventricles from subjects with idiopathic dilated cardiomyopathy was higher than in the left ventricles (Zisman et al., 2003) (Figure 9.6). Therefore, it is likely that right ventricular pressure overload results in increased expression of ACE2 protein and/or post-translational modifications which lead to increased ACE2 activity. With Ang I as substrate, the major pathway for direct hydrolysis of

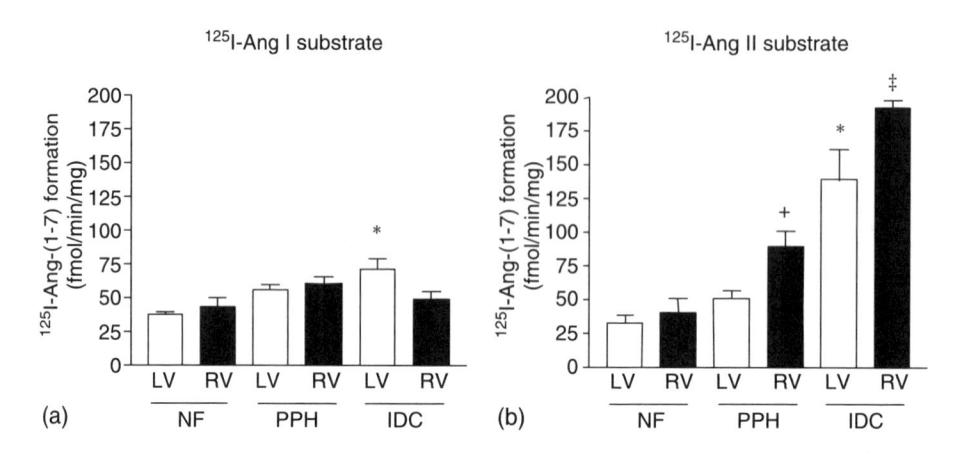

Figure 9.6 (a) ^{125}I-Ang-(1-7) forming activity with ^{125}I-Ang I as substrate was increased in the failing IDC LVs compared to the NF LVs. (b) ^{125}I-Ang-(1-7) forming activity with ^{125}I-Ang II substrate was increased in the IDC LVs compared to NF LVs, the IDC RVs compared to the NF RVs, the PPH RV compared to the NF RV, and the PPH RV compared to the PPH LV. In addition, angiotensinase activity with ^{125}I-Ang II substrate was higher in the IDC RVs compared to the IDC LVs ($P < 0.05$). *$P < 0.001$ vs. NF LV; +$P < 0.05$ vs. NF RV and PPH LV; ‡$P < 0.001$ vs. NF RV (Reproduced from Zisman et al., 2003)

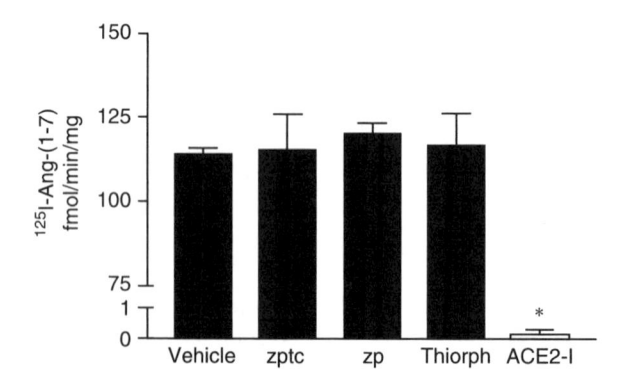

Figure 9.7 An ACE2 specific inhibitor virtually prevented ^{125}I-Ang-(1-7) formation from ^{125}I-Ang II in failing IDC LVs. (Angiotensinase inhibitor abbreviations: ZP: Z-pro-prolinal; C: pCMPS and carboxypeptidase A inhibitor; T, thiorphan; ACE2-I: ACE2 specific inhibitor. *$P < 0.001$) (Reproduced from Zisman et al., 2003)

Ang I to Ang-(1-7) was found to be neutral endopeptidase. Ang-(1-7) formation with Ang I as substrate was increased in left ventricular membranes from idiopathic dilated cardiomyopathy hearts, but not in right ventricles of these hearts. Neither was neutral endopeptidase activity increased in the failing right ventricles from primary pulmonary hypertension hearts. Total Ang-(1-7) formation in failing human heart membrane preparations correlated with Ang II formation, indicating greater efficiency of ACE2-mediated activity with Ang II substrate, compared to neutral endopeptidase activity for the generation of Ang-(1-7) (Zisman *et al.*, 2003). Based on inhibition studies, there did not appear to be a significant contribution of Angase C or PEP to Ang-(1-7) formation from Ang II in failing human heart (Figure 9.7).

Ang II-mediated signal transduction

The AT_1 receptor has been shown to be down-regulated at both the level of protein and gene expression in the failing human heart (Asano *et al.*, 1997; Haywood *et al.*, 1997). It is reasonable to argue that down-regulation of the AT_1 receptor is the result of chronic stimulation by its agonist, Ang II, and that Ang II formation is increased because cardiac tissue ACE is up-regulated in human heart failure. Previous studies have shown that ACE mRNA abundance is increased in failing compared to nonfailing human heart (Studer *et al.*, 1994). Although alternative pathways for Ang II formation have been described (i.e., human heart chymase), it appears that ACE is the major pathway for Ang II formation in the intact human heart (Zisman *et al.*, 1995). Furthermore, ACE protein density is increased in both the left and right ventricles of myocardium from failing IDC hearts (Zisman *et al.*, 1998).

ACE protein levels and activity have also been reported in hearts from patients with primary pulmonary hypertension (PPH). In these hearts the phenotype is that of selective failure of the right ventricle with preservation of left ventricular systolic function. It was found that ACE protein was up-regulated in both the failing right ventricle and the nonfailing left ventricle of the PPH hearts. These data suggested that, in PPH, systemic factors influenced ACE regulation. In contrast ACE2 activity was selectively increased only in the failing right ventricle of the PPH hearts. This finding suggests that the regulation of ACE2 activity is under local control and its expression at the protein level is influenced by pressure overload. It also suggests that, although there is high homology between ACE and ACE2, the two proteins are regulated differently (Zisman *et al.*, 1998, 2003).

A direct correlation between Ang-(1-7) formation and total angiotensin receptor membrane concentration in the PPH right ventricles was found; furthermore, this correlation was the result of a direct relationship between Ang-(1-7) forming activity and AT_2 receptor density. However, Ang-(1-7) is not a ligand for this receptor. A growing body of evidence suggests that there is a distinct Ang-(1-7) receptor (Tallant *et al.*, 1997). The correlation between Ang-(1-7) formation and AT_2 receptor density in PPH right ventricles suggests cross-regulation between the AT_2 receptor and the Ang-(1-7) receptor (Zisman *et al.*, 2003).

Summary

ACE2 is a recently discovered homolog of ACE which has high catalytic activity for the hydrolysis of Ang II to Ang-(1-7). The predominant gene expression of ACE2 is in the heart and kidneys. Ablation of ACE2 gene expression resulted in a heart failure phenotype with decreased contractility and up-regulation of hypoxia induced genes. In human heart failure, ACE2 activity was selectively increased in the failing right ventricles from patients with primary pulmonary hypertension, and in failing right and left ventricles from patients with idiopathic dilated cardiomyopathy. Ang-(1-7) has been shown to be a ligand for a unique Ang-(1-7) receptor. Ang-(1-7) causes vasodilation and counteracts Ang II mediated effects. Accordingly, an increase in ACE2 activity may represent a counter-regulatory response to heart failure. Further investigations will be required to determine if augmentation of ACE2 activity by pharmogologic means or through genetic manipulation will be a therapeutic modality for this disease.

References

Abbas AG, Gorelik L and Carbini SA (1997) Angiotensin-(1-7) induces bradykinin-mediated hypotensive responses in anesthetized rats. *Hypertension* **30**, 217–221.

Asano K, Dutcher D, Port J, *et al.* (1997) Selective downregulation of the angiotensin II AT_1-receptor subtype in failing human ventricular myocardium. *Circulation* **95**, 1193–1200.

Barton M, Shaw S, d'Uscio L, *et al.* (1997) Angiotensin II increases vascular and renal endothelin-1 and functional endothelin converting enzyme activity *in vivo*: role of ETA receptors for endothelin regulation. *Biochemical and Biophysical Research Communications* **238**, 861–865.

REFERENCES

Bernier SG, Bellemare JM, Escher E and Guillemette G (1998) Characterization of AT$_4$ receptor from bovine aortic endothelium with photosensitive analogues of angiotensin IV. *Biochemistry* **37**, 4280–4287.

Briand SI, Bellemare JM, Bernier SG and Guillemette G (1998) Study on the functionality and molecular properties of the AT$_4$ receptor. *Endocrinology Research* **24**, 315–323.

Campbell DJ, Kladis A and Duncan AM (1994) Effects of converting enzyme inhibitors on angiotensin and bradykinin peptides. *Hypertension* **23**, 439–449.

Coleman JK, Krebs LT, Hamilton TA, et al. (1998) Autoradiographic identification of kidney angiotensin IV binding sites and angiotensin IV-induced renal cortical blood flow changes in rats. *Peptides* **19**, 269–277.

Crackower MA, Sarao R, Oudit GY, et al. (2002) Angiotensin-converting enzyme 2 is an essential regulator of heart function. *Nature* **417**, 799–802.

Dales NA, Gould AE, Brown JA, et al. (2002) Substrate-based design of the first class of angiotensin-converting enzyme-related carboxypeptidase (ACE2) inhibitors. *Journal of the American Chemical Society* **124**, 11852–11853.

Donoghue M, Hsieh F, Baronas E, et al. (2000) A novel angiotensin-converting enzyme-related carboxypeptidase (ACE2) converts angiotensin I to angiotensin 1-9. *Circulation Research* **87**, E1–E9.

Ferrario C, Chappell M, Tallant EK, et al. (1997) Counterregulatory actions of angiotensin-(1-7). *Hypertension* **30**, 535–541.

Fitzgerald SM, Evans RG, Bergstrom G and Anderson WP (1999) Renal hemodynamic responses to intrarenal infusion of ligands for the putative angiotensin IV receptor in anesthetized rats. *Journal of Cardiovascular Pharmacology* **34**, 206–211.

Freeman E, Chisolm G, Ferrario C and Tallant E (1996) Angiotensin-(1-7) inhibits vascular smooth muscle cell growth. *Hypertension* **28**, 104–108.

Hall KL, Venkateswaran S, Hanesworth JM, et al. (1995) Characterization of a functional angiotensin IV receptor on coronary microvascular endothelial cells. *Regulatory Peptides* **58**, 107–115.

Harmer D, Gilbert M, Borman R and Clark KL (2002) Quantitative mRNA expression profiling of ACE2, a novel homologue of angiotensin converting enzyme. *FEBS Letters* **532**(1–2), 107–110.

Haywood GA, Gullestad L, Katsuya T, et al. (1997) AT$_1$ and AT$_2$ angiotensin receptor gene expression in human heart failure. *Circulation* **95**, 1201–1206.

Huang L, Sexton DJ, Skogerson K, et al. (2003) Novel peptide inhibitors of angiotensin-converting enzyme 2. *Journal of Biological Chemistry* **278**, 15532–15540.

Iyer S, Chappell M, Averill D, et al. (1998) Vasodepressor actions of angiotensin-(1-7) unmasked during combined treatment with lisinopril and losartan. *Hypertension* **31**, 699–705.

Jackman HL, Massad MG, Sekosan M, et al. (2002) Angiotensins 1-9 and 1-7 release in human heart: role of cathepsin A. *Hypertension* **39**, 976–981.

Johnson G, Stevenson T and Ahn K (1999) Hydrolysis of peptide hormones by endothelin-converting enzyme-1. A comparison with neprilysin. *Journal of Biological Chemistry* **274**, 4053–4058.

Konstam MA, Rousseau MF, Kronenberg MW, et al. (1992) Effects of the angiotensin converting enzyme inhibitor enalapril on the long-term progression of left ventricular dysfunction in patients with heart failure. *Circulation* **86**, 431–438.

Llorens-Cortes C, Huang H, Vicart P, et al. (1992) Identification and characterization of neutral endopeptidase in endothelial cells from venous or arterial origins. *Journal of Biological Chemistry* **267**, 14012–14018.

Morawietz H, Goettsch W, Szibor M, et al. (2002) Angiotensin-converting enzyme inhibitor therapy prevents upregulation of endothelin-converting enzyme-1 in failing human myocardium. *Biochemical and Biophysical Research Communications* **295**, 1057–1061.

Moriyama A, Nakanishi M and Sasaki M (1988) Porcine muscle prolyl endopeptidase and its endogenous substrates. *Journal of Biochemistry* **104**, 112–117.

Odya C, Marinkovic D, Hammon K, et al. (1978) Purification and properties of prolylcarboxypeptidase (angiotensinase C) from human kidney. *Journal of Biological Chemistry* **253**, 5927–5931.

Piedimonte G, Nadel J, Long C and Hoffman J (1994) Neutral endopeptidase in the heart: neutral endopeptidase inhibition prevents isoproterenol-induced myocardial hypoperfusion in rats by reducing bradykinin degradation. *Circulation Research* **75**, 770–779.

Porsti I, Bara AT, Busse R and Hecker M (1994) Release of nitric oxide by angiotensin-(1-7) from porcine coronary endothelium: implications for a novel angiotensin receptor. *British Journal of Pharmacology* **111**, 652–654.

Reaux A, Iturrioz X, Vazeux G, et al. (2000) Aminopeptidase A, which generates one of the main effector peptides of the brain renin–angiotensin system, angiotensin III, has a key role in central control of arterial blood pressure. *Biochemical Society Transactions* **28**, 435–440.

Sabbah HN, Sharov VG, Lesch M and Goldstein S (1995) Progression of heart failure: a role for interstitial fibrosis. *Molecular and Cellular Biochemistry* **147**, 29–34.

Sadoshima J-I, Xu Y, Slayter H and Izumo S (1993) Autocrine release of angiotensin II mediates stretch-induced hypertrophy of cardiac myocytes *in vitro*. *Cell* **75**, 977–984.

Santos RAS, Brosnihan KB, Jacobsen DW, et al. (1992) Production of angiotensin-(1-7) by human vascular endothelium. *Hypertension* **19**, II56–II61.

Shirasawa Y, Osawa T and Hirashima A (1994) Molecular cloning and characterization of prolyl endopeptidase from human T cells. *Journal of Biochemistry* **115**, 724–729.

Skidgel RA and Erdos EG (1998) Cellular carboxypeptidases. *Immunological Reviews* **161**, 129–141.

SOLVD Investigators (1991) Effect of enalapril on survival in patients with reduced left ventricular ejection fractions and congestive heart failure. *New England Journal of Medicine* **325**, 293–302.

Studer R, Reinecke H, Muller B, et al. (1994) Increased angiotensin-I converting enzyme gene expression in the failing human heart. *Journal of Clinical Investigation* **94**, 301–310.

Tallant E, Lu X, Weiss R, et al. (1997) Bovine aortic endothelial cells contain an angiotensin-(1-7) receptor. *Hypertension* **29**, 388–393.

Tan F, Morris P, Skidgel RA and Erdos EG (1993) Sequencing and cloning of human prolylcarboxypeptidase (angiotensinase C). Similarity to both serine carboxypeptidase and prolylendopeptidase families. *Journal of Biological Chemistry* **268**, 16631–16638.

Tipnis SR, Hooper NM, Hyde R, et al. (2000) A human homolog of angiotensin-converting enzyme. Cloning and functional expression as a captopril-insensitive carboxypeptidase. *Journal of Biological Chemistry* **275**, 33238–33243.

Vickers C, Hales P, Kaushik V, et al. (2002) Hydrolysis of biological peptides by human angiotensin-converting enzyme-related carboxypeptidase. *Journal of Biological Chemistry* **277**, 14838–14843.

Yang H, Erdos E and Chiang T (1968) New enzymatic route for the inactivation of angiotensin. *Nature* **218**, 1224–1226.

Zhang H, Wada J, Hida K, et al. (2001) Collectrin, a collecting duct-specific transmembrane glycoprotein is a novel homolog of ACE2 and is developmentally regulated in embryonic kidneys. *Journal of Biological Chemistry* **276**, 17132–17139.

Zisman LS, Abraham WT, Meixell GE, et al. (1995) Angiotensin II formation in the intact human heart: predominance of the angiotensin converting enzyme pathway. *Journal of Clinical Investigation* **95**, 1490–1498.

Zisman LS, Asano K, Dutcher DL, et al. (1998) Differential regulation of cardiac angiotensin converting enzyme (ACE) binding sites and AT_1 receptor density in primary pulmonary hypertension (PPH). *Circulation* **98**, 1735–1741.

Zisman LS, Keller RS, Weaver B, et al. (2003) Increased angiotensin-(1-7) forming activity in failing human heart ventricles: evidence for upregulation of the angiotensin converting enzyme homolog, ACE2. *Circulation* **108**, 1707–1712.

10

Wound Healing and the Tissue Renin Angiotensin Aldosterone System

Yao Sun and Karl T. Weber

Introduction

The circulating renin angiotensin aldosterone system (cRAAS) is integral to maintaining cardiovascular homeostasis, including vascular tonicity and salt and water balance (Chappell et al., 2000; Erdös, 2001). Pharmacologic inhibition of angiotensin-converting enzyme (ACE) and antagonism of angiotensin (Ang) II and aldosterone receptors have proven effective strategies for the management of hypertension and heart failure. These agents have provided important insights into the pivotal contribution of cRAAS activation to the pathophysiologic expression of these cardiovascular disorders (Francis et al., 1990; Swedberg et al., 1990; Anon, 1991; Rouleau et al., 1993; Pitt et al., 1999, 2003; Weber, 2001). In patients without cRAAS activation, ACE inhibition is also accompanied by risk reduction for morbid and mortal events, including the progressive nature of heart failure (Anon, 1992). These results call into question the presence and function of a tissue renin angiotensin aldosterone system (tRAAS). In recent years, the generation of RAAS components within the cardiovasculature has been documented (*vide infra*). The identification of auto-paracrine properties of *de novo* Ang II and aldosterone production represents an area of considerable research interest. This is nowhere more evident than the role of tRAAS in regulating tissue repair, such as collagen turnover in

Renin Angiotensin System and the Heart Edited by Walmor De Mello
© 2004 by John Wiley & Sons Ltd. ISBN 0 470 86292 0

heart valve leaflets and fibrous tissue formation that appears at and remote to myocardial infarction. This review focuses on the tRAAS and repair of extracellular matrix in the normal and diseased cardiovasculature. The fibrillar collagen scaffolding found in the extracellular matrix of the heart and vasculature is integral to preserving the structural integrity and functional behavior of these tissues (Weber, 1989; Weber et al., 1993; Baicu et al., 2003).

Expression of tRAAS

Normal heart

Valve leaflets, an exteriorized portion of the heart's extracellular matrix, are composed of valvular interstitial cells residing in a fibrillar collagen scaffolding and whose phenotype resembles contractile myofibroblasts (myoFb) (Filip et al., 1986; Messier et al., 1994; Chester et al., 2000; Taylor et al., 2000). Leaflet myoFb express (mRNA and protein) type I and III fibrillar collagens (Katwa et al., 1995, 1996). As seen in Figure 10.1, they also express renin and are a site of high-density autoradiographic binding for ACE and Ang II receptors (Pinto et al., 1991; Yamada et al., 1991; Sun et al., 1994a). High-density binding is also found within the endothelium and adventitia of aorta, pulmonary artery and intramural coronary arteries (Pinto et al., 1991; Yamada et al., 1991; Sun et al., 1994a). Throughout the myocardium of the right and left ventricles and right and left atria of the adult rat heart binding densities for ACE and Ang II receptors are low. Autoradiography further identifies leaflets as sites of high-density receptor binding for the fibrogenic cytokine transforming growth factor-β1 (TGF-β1; Sun et al., 1994a, 1998). Such anatomic concordance between ACE, receptors for Ang II and TGF-β, and type I collagen expression in valve leaflets, composed predominantly of fibroblast-like cells, implicates de novo generation of Ang II in governing myoFb connective tissue turnover via auto-/paracrine-based expression of the fibrogenic cytokine TGF-β. Indeed, cultured leaflet myoFb express (mRNA and protein) requisites to angiotensin peptide formation, including angiotensinogen, an aspartyl protease (cathepsin D), and ACE (Katwa et al., 1995, 1996). Their ACE and kininase activities include conversion of such substrates as Ang I, bradykinin and substance P, respectively. Ang II generated by these cells is involved in the autocrine induction of type I collagen expression via upregulation of TGF-β1 expression (Campbell and Katwa, 1997; Katwa et al., 1997). This is an AT_1 receptor-mediated event. Contraction of

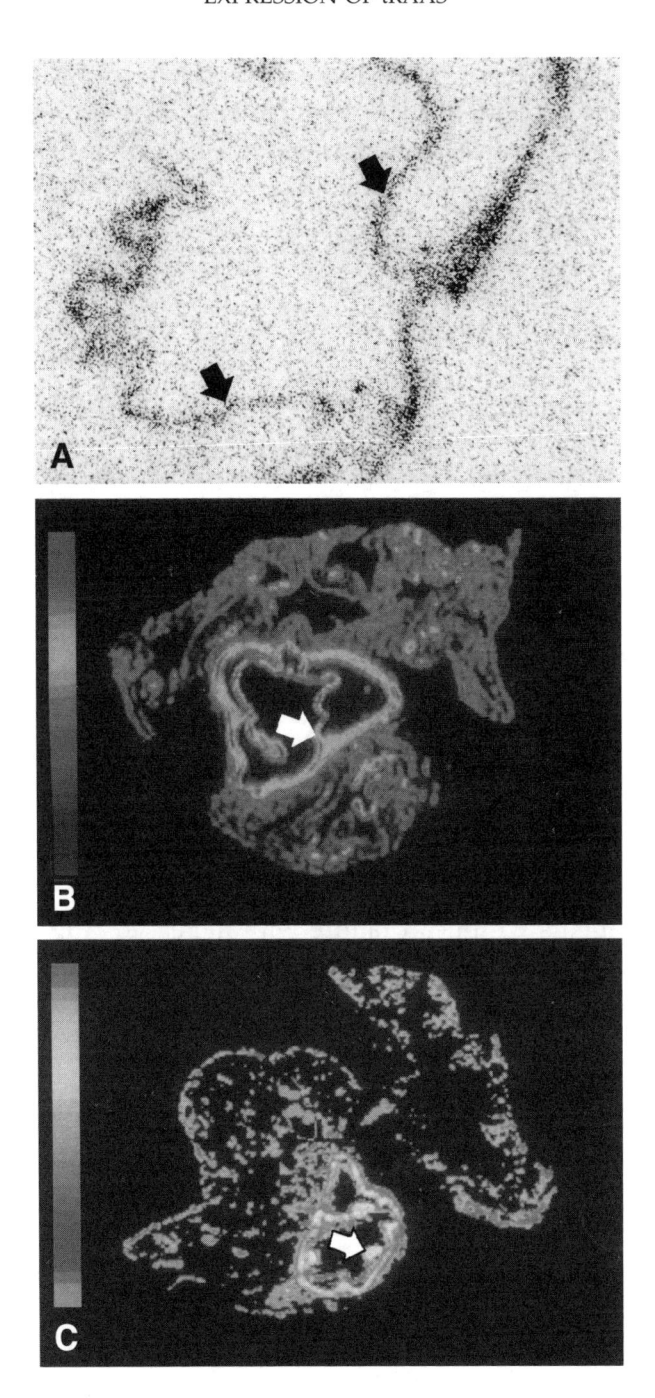

Figure 10.1 tRAAS and heart valve leaflets (arrows). As shown by *in situ* hybridization, renin mRNA (A) expression is markedly increased in leaflets as contrasted to surrounding tissue. The tricuspid valve of the rat heart is shown. Using *in vitro* autoradiography, high-density binding for ACE (B) and Ang II receptors (C) are found in valve leaflets. The aortic valve of the normal rat heart is shown. Reproduced from Sun Y and Weber KT (2003) *International Journal of Biochemistry and Cell Biology* **35**, 919–931, with permission from Elsevier

leaflet myoFb grown on a flexible substratum and mediated by α-smooth muscle actin (α-SMA) microfilaments in these myoFb can be induced by Ang II, catecholamines, endothelin-1 or serotonin through their respective receptor–ligand binding; papaverine induces relaxation (Chester et al., 2000).

Diseased hearts

Compared to nonfailing donor heart tissue, the number of ACE transcripts is increased in tissue homogenates prepared from explanted failing human hearts (Studer et al., 1994). ACE and TGF-β1 expression is likewise increased in myocardium obtained from patients undergoing aortic valve replacement for aortic stenosis and correlate with the extent of fibrosis found in these tissue samples (Hein et al., 2003). ACE and Ang II are present in the fibrous tissue that contributes to the sclerosis and the stenosis of diseased human aortic valves (O'Brien et al., 2002). In keeping with the expression of ACE in heart valve leaflets and Ang II in regulating leaflet collagen turnover, Atalar et al. (2003) have recently suggested the ACE-DD genotype is associated with a greater risk of valve deformity following a bout of acute rheumatic fever.

The aorta–coronary sinus concentration gradient for Ang II is decreased in patients with heart failure with increased Ang II appearing in this venous effluent and accompanied by increased mRNA expression of angiotensinogen and ACE in noncardiomyocyte cells of explanted failing hearts (Serneri et al., 2001). ACE-dependent Ang II formation is increased in the infarcted segment of scarred myocardium in autopsied hearts (Ihara et al., 2000), while it has also been reported that expression of angiotensinogen, renin, ACE and Ang II receptor genes is present in adult cardiomyocytes and upregulated in response to myocardial ischemia (Anversa et al., 2000).

Temporal and spatial responses in autoradiographic ACE binding have been assessed in a rat heart model of myocardial infarction. Other forms of injury involving various tissues are also present in this model. They include the heart, visceral pericardium, kidneys and skin. Each serve as positive controls in the analysis of ACE and tissue repair. Low-density ACE binding is present in normal rat myocardium, where renin mRNA expression is not found (Sun et al., 2001). High-density ACE binding and renin mRNA expression appear at the site of transmural anterior myocardial infarction on day 7 following left coronary artery ligation and are coincident with the appearance of fibrillar collagen. As a fibrillar collagen network forms scar tissue over 8 weeks, the density of ACE binding and renin expression (see Figures 10.2A and B) at this site increase progressively. A large transmural myocardial infarction in the rat heart is associated with high-density ACE binding and the appearance of fibrosis at sites remote to the infarct, including the noninfarcted left ventricle, interventricular septum and right ventricle (see Figure 10.2B). The appearance of fibrosis at these remote sites is directly related to the extent of infarct injury (van Krimpen et al., 1991a; Smits et al., 1992; Volders et al., 1993). When infarct injury is extensive, the entire myocardium, including infarcted and noninfarcted ventricular tissue, is involved with tissue repair and subsequent structural remodeling by fibrosis tissue.

Noninfarct-related sites of injury serve to further address the relationship between the appearance of ACE and repair. Sham operation includes: manual handling of the heart, and this leads to inflammation and subsequent fibrosis of visceral pericardium; and a silk ligature placement around the left coronary artery or within skin to close the surgical incision, with each site associated with a foreign body fibrosis. The appearance of a mural thrombus in the infarcted left ventricle is associated with subsequent endocardial fibrosis and on occasion leads to thromboembolic renal infarction. At each of these sites of injury and repair, high-density autoradiographic ACE binding is temporally and spatially concordant with fibrous tissue formation. Angiotensinogen, renin, ACE and TGF-β1 mRNA levels are increased in the rat right ventricle at 3 and 6 weeks after monocrotaline-induced pulmonary injury (Park et al., 2001). In mice with desmin-deficient cardiomyopathy, areas of cardiac fibrosis are co-localized with upregulated expression of ACE and TGF-β1 (Mavroidis and Capetanaki, 2002).

Potential differences in healing and thereby ACE expression could occur as a result of ischemic vs. nonischemic injury. Permanent coronary artery ligation, for example, can impede the delivery of circulating cells and signals to the site of injury and limit same to that provided by collateral vessels. Nonischemic models of cardiac myocyte necrosis have been examined. They include: endogenous release of catecholamines that accompanies Ang II infusion from implanted mini-pump (Ratajska et al., 1994) or exogenous administration of isoproterenol (Benjamin et al., 1989); chronic (>3 weeks) administration of aldosterone by mini-pump in uninephrectomized rats on a high salt diet and which is accompanied by enhanced urinary potassium excretion and subsequent cardiac myocyte potassium depletion with cell necrosis (Darrow and Miller, 1942; Campbell et al., 1993); and subcutaneous pouch tissue formation in response to croton oil instillation (Sun et al.,

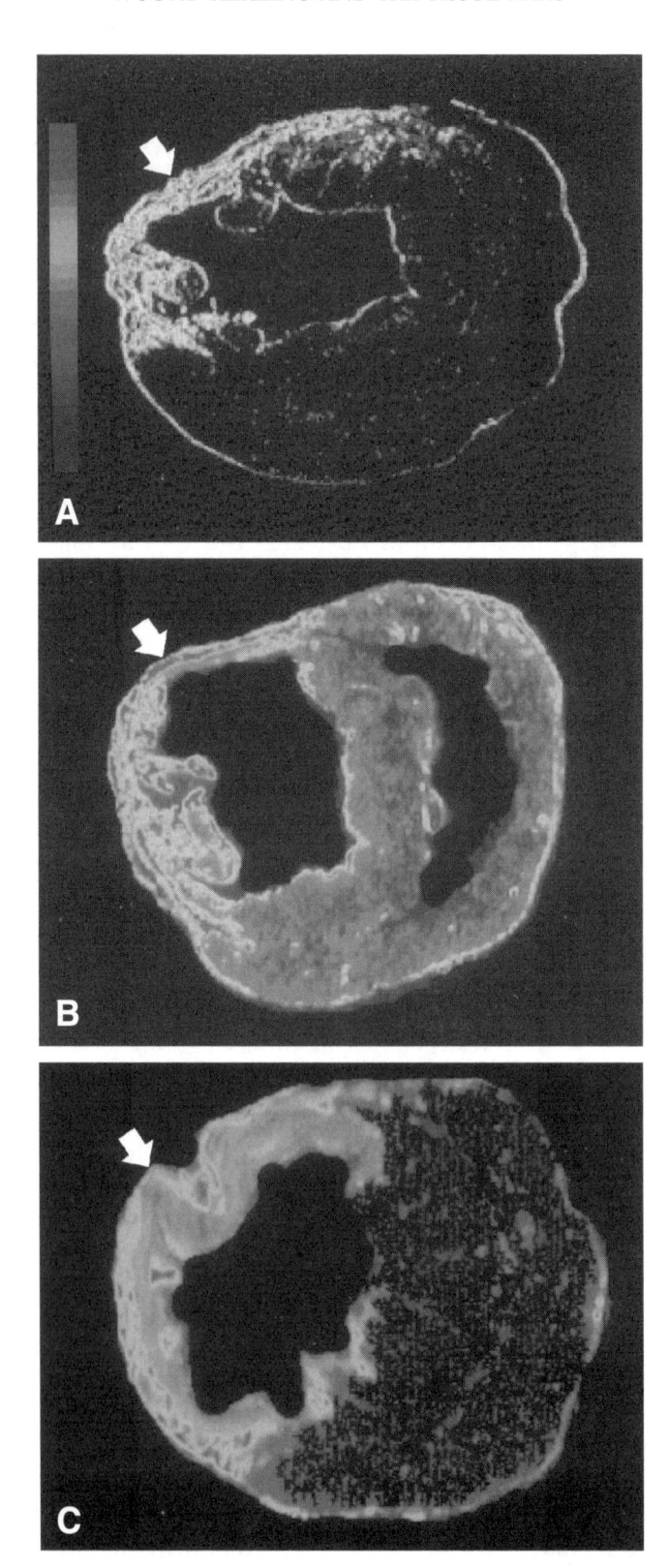

142 WOUND HEALING AND THE TISSUE RAAS

1997b). At each site involving nonischemic myocyte loss or simply fibrous tissue formation independent of myocyte loss, and irrespective of its etiologic basis, the temporal and spatial appearance of high-density ACE binding is coincident with the deposition of fibrous tissue (Sun et al., 1993; Sun and Weber, 1996b) and resembles the aforementioned responses observed in the infarcted heart following permanent coronary artery ligation. Marked autoradiographic ACE binding is coincident with fibrous tissue formation irrespective of the etiologic basis of injury, the tissue involved in repair, the presence of ischemic vs. nonischemic repair, or the presence or absence of cardiomyocyte death. Furthermore, examination of serial heart sections of the infarcted rat heart demonstrates high-density ACE binding to be spatially concordant with marked autoradiographic Ang II (see Figure 10.2c) and TGF-β receptor binding densities and mRNA expression of renin, TGF-β1 and type I collagen by *in situ* hybridization at these sites of fibrosis (Sun et al., 2001). Collectively, these findings in various injured tissues implicate both Ang II and TGF-β1 as a common signaling pathway involved in promoting repair (Weber, 1997a).

The mRNA expression of aldosterone synthase (CYP11B2), integral to the biosynthesis of aldosterone (Hatakeyama et al., 1994; Takeda et al., 1995, 1996; Silvestre et al., 1998), and aldosterone production have each been demonstrated in rodent heart and vascular tissue. Extra-adrenal aldosterone generation is regulated by Ang II (via AT_1 receptor ligand binding), a low Na^+ or high K^+ diet, or adrenocorticotropin (Silvestre et al., 1998; Delcayre and Swynghedauw, 2002). Aldosterone is extracted by the heart following myocardial infarction and the transcardiac aldosterone gradient (between aorta and coronary sinus) correlates with a serologic marker of collagen turnover (i.e., procollagen type III aminoterminal peptide) found in coronary venous effluent and which is associated with LV dilatation and impaired function (Hayashi et al., 2001). Aldosterone is extracted by the chronically failing human heart of diverse etiologic origins, a response blocked by spironolactone (Tsutamoto et al., 2000). Others have reported (Mizuno et al., 2001) that

---

Figure 10.2 Renin, ACE and Ang II receptor expression in the infarcted rat heart (arrows). Following myocardial infarction, high-density renin mRNA expression is observed at the site of myocardial infarction, as well as inflamed pericardium and endocardium at week 1 (A) and which remains elevated over the course of 4 weeks (not shown). ACE and Ang II receptor binding density was also markedly increased at the same sites. ACE (B) and Ang II (C) receptor binding densities in the infarcted heart at week 4 post myocardial infarction. Reproduced from Sun Y and Weber KT (2003) *International Journal of Biochemistry and Cell Biology* **35**, 919–931, with permission from Elsevier

aldosterone production is increased in the failing human left ventricle based on coronary sinus levels of aldosterone that exceed those found in the aorta. There exists an upregulated expression of CYP11B2 in the left ventricle of the failing human heart of diverse etiologic origins (Yoshimura et al., 2002). Additionally, 11β-hydroxysteroid dehydrogenase, an enzyme critical to maintaining the specificity of the mineralocorticoid receptor, given its equal affinity for mineralo- and glucocorticoids, has been found in human cardiac tissue (Slight et al., 1996).

Cells expressing tRAAS

Normal heart

Cells expressing ACE in normal rat heart valve leaflets have been identified by immunolabeling with a monoclonal antibody. They include: endothelial cells lining atrial and ventricular leaflet surfaces; and myoFb residing within leaflet matrix (Filip et al., 1986; Messier et al., 1994; Katwa et al., 1995). TGF-β1 induces ACE synthesis in cultured rat heart interstitial fibroblasts and which is accompanied by their differentiation into myoFb (Petrov et al., 2000).

Diseased hearts

The identity and temporal response in renin expression of ACE-positive cells seen at and remote to the infarct site include macrophages that invade the infarct site and myoFb (Falkenhahn et al., 1995; Sun and Weber, 1996c; Sun et al., 2001). Within 24 h of myocardial infarction, macrophages appear at the interface between viable and necrotic myocardium; by day 3, stromal fibroblasts co-aggregate with macrophage clusters bordering on the infarct site. Thereafter, fibroblast differentiation follows resulting in α-SMA positive myoFb phenotype that then proliferates and migrates into the site of necrosis during the remainder of week 1. A combination of cell growth with spatial control of growth and fibrillar collagen assembly governs rebuilding of infarcted tissue.

Macrophages and myoFb found at the infarct site also express Ang II receptors, TGF-β1 and its receptors (Sun et al., 2001). Beyond day 14, only myoFb and endothelial cells are renin- and ACE-positive coincident with the gradual disappearance of macrophages from the infarct site. Persistent renin expression and high-density ACE and Ang II receptor binding are present at the infarct site in rat hearts for 8 weeks or more postmyocardial infarction (Lefroy et al., 1996; Sun et al., 2001). This is primarily due to α-SMA-positive myoFb, which remain in infarct scar tissue for prolonged periods of time. In the infarcted human heart these myoFb persist at the site of myocardial infarction for years (Willems et al., 1994).

MyoFb have considerable phenotypic and functional diversity (Sappino et al., 1988; Skalli et al., 1989). Immunolabeling with α-SMA, vimentin and desmin defines their phenotype at the infarct site. Fibroblast-like cells express vimentin. ACE-labeled fibroblasts found in the infarct scar and involved in the expression of fibrillar collagen mRNA are positive for cytoskeletal proteins α-SMA and vimentin. These vimentin-positive myoFb, instrumental to tissue repair including wound contraction, are likewise found in the connective tissue that comprises endocardial fibrosis, pericardial fibrosis, renal infarction and sites of foreign-body fibrosis. Unlike incised skin, where myoFb contribute to tissue repair and then progressively disappear through programmed cell death (apoptosis) coincident with wound closure and scar tissue formation at week 4 (Desmouliére et al., 1995), the vimentin phenotype at the infarct site remain for prolonged periods (Sun and Weber, 1996c). Whether pathologic fibrosis at and remote to myocardial infarction found in the infarcted heart is related to its persistent myoFb is presently uncertain.

In vitro emulsion autoradiography identifies vimentin-positive myoFb as expressing Ang II receptors (Sun and Weber, 1996a). Together with displacement studies using either an AT_1 receptor antagonist, losartan, or AT_2 receptor antagonist, PD123177, the great majority of these receptors in the infarcted rat heart are of the AT_1 subtype (Sun and Weber, 1994, 1996a; Sun et al., 1994b; Lefroy et al., 1996; Passier et al., 1996). MyoFb found at sites of microscopic scarring involving both infarcted and noninfarcted tissue also express mRNA for the fibrogenic cytokine TGF-β1 and TGF-β receptors (Sun et al., 1998). This has implicated locally produced Ang II at sites of injury in regulating collagen turnover, which has been further suggested by the cardioprotective actions of losartan, an AT_1 receptor antagonist, in attenuating fibrous tissue formation at and remote to the infarction (Sun et al., 1998). Locally produced Ang II is also involved in regulating *de novo* aldosterone production in the infarcted heart (Silvestre et al., 1999), which likewise may contribute to tissue repair. Increased expression of aldosterone synthase and aldosterone tissue levels, together with increased concentrations of Ang II, have been observed in noninfarcted rat myocardium following coronary artery ligation (Silvestre et al., 1999; Delcayre et al., 2000). Treatment with losartan prevented these responses related to *de novo* aldosterone production.

tRAAS and wound healing

Normal heart

ACE imparts connective tissue with metabolic activity (Weber *et al.*, 1995). Its substrate utilization involves factors participating in a reciprocal regulation of cell behavior – stimulators or inhibitors of cell growth and functions integral to formation and degradation of fibrillar collagen (Weber *et al.*, 1995). Loose and dense connective tissue formation is a dynamic process during early growth and development of newborn rats. The contribution of Ang II to this process has been examined in young rats, where treatment of 4-week-old rats with enalapril attenuated cardiac and vascular accumulation of collagen involving the right and left ventricles, aorta and systemic arteries compared to untreated, age matched control rats (Keeley *et al.*, 1992). No such study has yet been conducted with an Ang II receptor antagonist. In rats with a genetic predisposition to hypertension, treatment with either quinapril or hydralazine during early growth and development each prevented the appearance of hypertension in adulthood. However, only quinapril attenuated the expected development of connective tissue seen in age-matched hypertensive controls (Albaladejo *et al.*, 1994).

Diseased hearts and cardiovasculature

High-density ACE binding in connective tissue that appears in response to tissue repair implies marked ACE activity at such sites. ACE activity has been examined in tissue obtained from the failing, infarcted and noninfarcted human heart tissue (Hokimoto *et al.*, 1995). Homogenates of transmural tissue blocks adjacent to visible scar tissue and obtained at the time of aneurysmectomy were prepared for analysis. Such samples, it was noted, may have contained scar tissue. ACE activity of this homogenate was compared to that prepared from noninfarcted ventricular tissue obtained at necropsy from persons dying of noncardiac causes. Infarct tissue ACE activity exceeded that of such control tissue several-fold and the extent of activity was related to the severity of tissue damage. In rat heart tissue homogenates prepared from sites remote to a large transmural anterior myocardial infarction, ACE activity is increased and the extent to which substrate conversion is increased correlates with infarct size (Hirsch *et al.*, 1991). The importance of fibrous vs. nonfibrous tissue ACE in determining this heightened

ACE activity in infarcted and remote sites could not be addressed from these studies.

A paradigm of tissue repair in which ACE and local Ang II are integral to the orderly and sequential nature of repair that eventuates in fibrosis has been proposed (Weber, 1997b). As shown in Figure 10.3, ACE is involved in a two-part *de novo* generation of Ang II within granulation tissue that forms at sites of injury. The first component to local Ang II generation is provided by macrophages. In an autocrine manner, it regulates expression of the fibrogenic cytokine TGF-β1 that determines phenotype conversion of coaggregating stromal fibroblasts. Vimentin-positive myoFb next generate Ang II whose autocrine induction of TGF-β1 regulates collagen turnover at sites of fibrous tissue formation, including infarcted and noninfarcted myocardium. It is suggested that Ang II generation at the infarct site is related to the extent of the myoFb response, and accordingly the degree of myocyte necrosis and subsequent healing response. An extensive transmural myocardial infarction and accompanying inflammatory cell response generates a

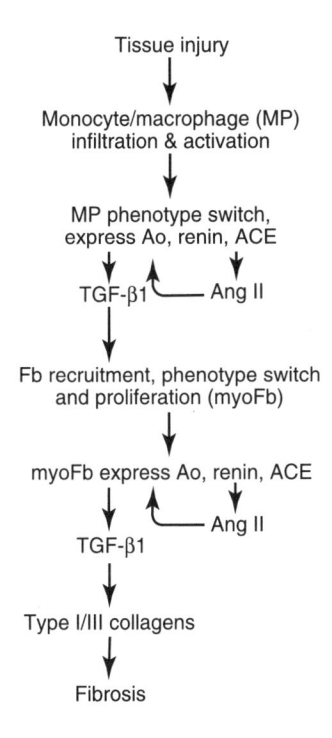

Tissue injury
↓
Monocyte/macrophage (MP) infiltration & activation
↓
MP phenotype switch, express Ao, renin, ACE
↓   ↓
TGF-β1 ⸺ Ang II
↓
Fb recruitment, phenotype switch and proliferation (myoFb)
↓
myoFb express Ao, renin, ACE
↓   ↓
TGF-β1 ⸺ Ang II
↓
Type I/III collagens
↓
Fibrosis

Figure 10.3 A schematic representation of the two-part *de novo* generation of Ang II involved in tissue repair following myocardial infarction. See text for discussion and abbreviations. Adapted from Weber KT (1997) *Circulation* **96**, 4065–4082, with permission

large amount of Ang II, which reaches distant or remote sites via its diffusion through tissue fluid to promote fibrosis. Accordingly, activation of fibrogenesis is greatest at sites closest to the anterior myocardial infarction (e.g., interventricular septum) and less so at more remote sites (e.g., right ventricle). Expression of type I and III collagens is greater and persists longer in the septum compared to right ventricle in rat hearts following left coronary artery ligation (Cleutjens *et al.*, 1995). The autocrine properties of Ang II produced locally at sites of repair may be linked to the Jak-STAT pathway whose blockade has proven efficacious in preventing structural remodeling (El-Adawi *et al.*, 2003).

The generation of fibrogenic signals at a site of myocardial infarction are transferred to remote sites through the heart's common interstitial space. These signals (e.g., Ang II) promote postinfarct remodeling at and remote to the site of infarct. A persistence of vimentin-positive, active myoFb perpetuates such remodeling. Circulating and locally generated Ang II contribute to myocardial remodeling postmyocardial infarction (van Kats *et al.*, 2000). Elevations in circulating Ang II, due to RAAS activation, represent a signal that gains entry to tissue where it further promotes post-infarct fibrosis by AT_1 receptor binding. Diastolic dysfunction is an outcome to such exuberant, unbridled tissue fibrosis. Ang II, whether derived locally or from the circulation, may further contribute to abnormal tissue stiffness through its induction of myoFb and thereby fibrous tissue contraction.

MyoFb persist in the infarct scar. Furthermore, these cells remain active expressing ACE, Ang II and TGF-β receptors, and type I collagen and TGF-β1. Prolonged stimulation of collagen production and adverse myocardial remodeling by fibrosis long after the acute phase of healing post myocardial infarction, is reminiscent of progressive valvular sclerosis that appears years after acute rheumatic valvulitis (Henney *et al.*, 1982) and where valvular deformity (e.g., leaflet and chordal shortening) is related to contractile myoFb (Majno *et al.*, 1971). Persistence of myoFb in injured kidneys is accompanied by progressive interstitial fibrosis, renal dysfunction and poor prognosis (Goumenos *et al.*, 1994; Zhang *et al.*, 1995; Roberts *et al.*, 1997).

Either AT_1 receptor or aldosterone receptor antagonism prevents the accompanying accumulation of collagen at sites remote to the infarct suggesting the involvement of Ang II-driven local aldosterone production in regulating tissue repair (Michel *et al.*, 1988; Sun *et al.*, 1997b; Delyani *et al.*, 2001; Delcayre and Swynghedauw, 2002; Nakamura *et al.*, 2003). Under circumstances where circulating aldosterone may or may not be increased, spironolactone attenuates neointimal thickening following vascular barotrauma (Van Belle *et al.*, 1995) and nephron- and cerebrovascular injury in stroke-prone/SHR rats independent of lowering blood pressure (Rocha et al., 1998, 1999). This pressure-independent effect is also seen for spironolactone in preventing fibrosis of the aorta and conduit vessels in SHR and elderly normotensive rats (Benetos et al., 1997b; Lacolley et al., 2001). In adrenalectomized rats with no circulating aldosterone, spironolactone attenuates fibrous tissue formation in keeping with the *de novo* production of aldosterone and its contribution to repair (Slight et al., 1998). Moreover, these observations further suggest auto-/paracrine-properties of locally produced aldosterone participate in tissue repair.

Salutary clinical responses to ACE inhibition are likely to be multifactoral in origin. One important component relates to a prevention of adverse structural remodeling of infarcted and noninfarcted myocardium by fibrous tissue. Evidence supporting a contribution of locally produced Ang II in regulating myoFb collagen synthesis is obtained using pharmacologic probes that interfere with local Ang II generation (i.e., ACE inhibition) or occupancy of its AT_1 receptor prior to circulating RAAS activation. Captopril or enalapril, begun at or close to the onset of myocardial infarction reduce infarct size, infarct expansion and thinning, and attenuate the rise in hydroxyproline concentration at the infarct site in dogs with permanent coronary artery occlusion (Jugdutt et al., 1992, 1995; Jugdutt, 1995). The potential additional contribution of reduced bradykinin degradation to tissue repair and which would accompany ACE inhibition is under investigation. Bradykinin is released post myocardial infarction (Needleman et al., 1975; Hashimoto et al., 1977; Noda et al., 1993) and a bradykinin-2 receptor antagonist (Hoe140 or icatibant) accentuates collagen accumulation remote to the infarct site (Wollert et al., 1997).

Losartan, begun on day 1 after coronary artery ligation and in a dose that reduced AT_1 receptor binding by 50 percent, reduces infarct scar area (Frimm et al., 1997). Moreover, the expected rise in tissue Ang II concentration found at the infarct site 3 weeks post coronary artery ligation is markedly attenuated by either delapril or TCV-116, an AT_1 receptor antagonist, introduced on postoperative day 1 (Yamagishi et al., 1993). These findings raise the prospect that the number of myoFb or their Ang II-generating activity per cell at sites of repair may be influenced by Ang II. Other studies (Makino et al., 1993; Nio et al., 1995) have not found such antagonists to influence fibrosis post myocardial infarction. An explanation for these divergent findings is presently unclear.

Fibrous tissue formation at sites remote to myocardial infarction is also influenced by these pharmacologic interventions. Perindopril, given 1 week after myocardial infarction, attenuates the endocardial fibrosis that appears in the nonnecrotic segment of the rat left ventricle (Michel et al., 1988). Captopril, commenced at the time of coronary artery ligation, attenuates the expected fibrosis of noninfarcted rat left and right ventricles (van Krimpen et al., 1991b; Bélichard et al., 1994) and proliferation of fibroblasts and endothelial cells that appears at remote sites 1 and 2 weeks following myocardial infarction (van Krimpen et al., 1991b). Under these circumstances, captopril prevents the rise in left ventricle end diastolic pressure that appears in untreated rats and which is not the case in propranolol-treated rats. Captopril also reduces inducibility of ventricular arrhythmias in this model (Bélichard et al., 1994). When initiated 3 weeks post myocardial infarction, well after the tissue repair process has commenced and progressed, captopril does not prevent fibrosis remote to the infarct site or the rise in ventricular stiffness (Litwin et al., 1991). Losartan prevents fibrosis at remote sites (Smits et al., 1992; Schieffer et al., 1994; Frimm et al., 1997), but not the cellular proliferation that appears (Smits et al., 1992). Others did not find an inhibition of types I and III collagen mRNA expression at remote sites (Hanatani et al., 1995; Dixon et al., 1996) and have suggested posttranslational modification in collagen turnover to explain why fibrosis fails to appear at remote sites (Dixon et al., 1996).

These favorable tissue protective effects of ACE inhibition or AT_1 receptor antagonism are not confined to the infarcted heart. These interventions prevent the appearance of fibrosis in diverse organs with experimentally induced or naturally occurring tissue injury and where circulating RAAS is not activated. These include: pericardial fibrosis postpericardiotomy (Sun and Weber, 1994); tubulointerstitial fibrosis associated with unilateral ureteral obstruction (Yanagisawa et al., 1990; Pimentel et al., 1993, 1995; Kaneto et al., 1994; Ishidoya et al., 1995, 1996; Morrissey et al., 1996), toxic nephropathy (Diamond and Anderson, 1990; Lafayette et al., 1993; Cohen et al., 1994), cyclosporine (Burdmann et al., 1995), remnant kidney (Anderson et al., 1986; Ikoma et al., 1991; Tanaka et al., 1995; Shibouta et al., 1996) or renal injury following irradiation (Juncos et al., 1993); cardiovascular and glomerulosclerosis that appear in stroke-prone spontaneously hypertensive rats (Kim et al., 1994, 1995; Nakamura et al., 1994, 1996); interstitial pulmonary fibrosis that follows irradiation (Ward et al., 1989, 1990, 1992) or monocrotaline administration (Molteni et al., 1985); and subcutaneous pouch tissue in response to croton oil (Sun et al., 1997b). Attenuation of fibrous tissue formation by these interventions in diverse organs with various forms of injury supports the importance of local Ang II in promoting fibrosis. A more detailed review of Ang II and tissue repair involving systemic organs can be found elsewhere (Weber, 1997a).

A structural remodeling of the cardiovasculature by fibrous tissue accompanies aldosteronism derived from either endogenous or exogenous sources (Hall and Hall, 1965; Brilla *et al.*, 1990; Sun *et al.*, 1993, 1997a; Robert *et al.*, 1994; Campbell *et al.*, 1995; Nicoletti *et al.*, 1996; Sun *et al.*, 1997a; Rocha *et al.*, 2000; Fiebeler *et al.*, 2001). This fibrogenic phenotype includes intramural arteries of the heart, kidney, pancreas, mesentery and vaso vasorum of aorta and pulmonary artery. Cotreatment with a receptor antagonist (e.g., spironolactone, eplerenone), in either nondepressor or depressor dosage, prevents this remodeling indicating its independence of elevations in blood pressure (Selye, 1960; Robert *et al.*, 1994; Young *et al.*, 1995; Nicoletti *et al.*, 1996; Benetos *et al.*, 1997a; Rocha *et al.*, 2000, 2002; Fiebeler *et al.*, 2001; Lacolley *et al.*, 2002; Martinez *et al.*, 2002). In a substudy to the RALES trial, survival benefit was associated with a reduction in circulating markers of collagen synthesis that presumably reflected an attenuation in ongoing vascular fibrosis (Zannad *et al.*, 2000). In this connection, urinary excretion of hydroxyproline, a marker of collagen turnover, is increased in adrenalectomized rats treated with aldosterone, 1 percent dietary NaCl, and cortisone (Zannad *et al.*, 2000). Glucocorticoids, on the other hand, are known to reduce urinary hydroxyproline excretion and their inhibition of collagen formation in bone is associated with osteoporosis (Thompson *et al.*, 1972).

Summary

The tRAAS serves to regulate local concentrations of various mediators of inflammation and tissue repair in the heart and other organs. MyoFb-bound ACE is integral to *de novo* generation of Ang II that modulates expression of TGF-β1 and whose auto-/paracrine-properties regulate collagen turnover in heart valve leaflets, an exteriorized portion of the normal extracellular matrix, and at sites of fibrous tissue formation that appear in response to various forms of injury involving diverse tissues. Persistent myoFb and their ACE at the infarct site or diseased heart valve leaflets contribute to a sustained metabolic activity that can account for a progressive fibrosis at these sites. It is such adverse structural remodeling by fibrous tissue that eventuates in ischemic cardiomyopathy, a major etiologic factor in the appearance and progressive nature of chronic cardiac failure, or in heart valve deformity, a major cause of chronic circulatory failure.

References

Albaladejo P, Bouaziz H, Duriez M, et al. (1994) Angiotensin converting enzyme inhibition prevents the increase in aortic collagen in rats. *Hypertension* **23**, 74–82.

Anderson S, Rennke HG and Brenner BM (1986) Therapeutic advantage of converting enzyme inhibitors in arresting progressive renal disease associated with systemic hypertension in the rat. *Journal of Clinical Investigation* **77**, 1993–2000.

Anon (1991) Effect of enalapril on survival in patients with reduced left ventricular ejection fractions and congestive heart failure. The SOLVD Investigators. *New England Journal of Medicine* **325**, 293–302.

Anon (1992) Effect of enalapril on mortality and the development of heart failure in asymptomatic patients with reduced left ventricular ejection fractions. The SOLVD Investigators. *New England Journal of Medicine* **327**, 685–691.

Anversa P, Leri A, Li B, et al. (2000) Ischemic cardiomyopathy and the cellular renin–angiotensin system. *Journal of Heart and Lung Transplantation* **19**, S1–S11.

Atalar E, Tokgozoglu SL, Alikasifoglu M, et al. (2003) Angiotensin-converting enzyme genotype predicts valve damage in acute rheumatic fever. *Journal of Heart Valve Diseases* **12**, 7–10.

Baicu CF, Stroud JD, Livesay VA, et al. (2003) Changes in extracellular collagen matrix alter myocardial systolic performance. *American Journal of Physiology* **284**, H122–H132.

Bélichard P, Savard P, Cardinal R, et al. (1994) Markedly different effects on ventricular remodeling result in a decrease in inducibility of ventricular arrhythmias. *Journal of the American College of Cardiology* **23**, 505–513.

van Belle E, Bauters C, Wernert N, et al. (1995) Neointimal thickening after balloon denudation is enhanced by aldosterone and inhibited by spironolactone, and aldosterone antagonist. *Cardiovascular Research* **29**, 27–32.

Benetos A, Lacolley P and Safar ME (1997a) Prevention of aortic fibrosis by spironolactone in spontaneously hypertensive rats. *Arteriosclerosis, Thrombosis and Vascular Biology* **17**, 1152–1156.

Benetos A, Lacolley P and Safar ME (1997b) Prevention of aortic fibrosis by spironolactone in spontaneously hypertensive rats. *Arteriosclerosis, Thrombosis and Vascular Biology* **17**, 1152–1156.

Benjamin IJ, Jalil JE, Tan LB, et al. (1989) Isoproterenol-induced myocardial fibrosis in relation to myocyte necrosis. *Circulation Research* **65**, 657–670.

Brilla CG, Pick R, Tan LB, et al. (1990) Remodeling of the rat right and left ventricle in experimental hypertension. *Circulation Research* **67**, 1355–1364.

Burdmann EA, Andoh TF, Nast CC, et al. (1995) Prevention of experimental cyclosporin-induced interstitial fibrosis by losartan and enalapril. *American Journal of Physiology* **269**, F491–F499.

Campbell SE and Katwa LC (1997) Angiotensin II stimulated expression of transforming growth factor-β1 in cardiac fibroblasts and myofibroblasts. *Journal of Molecular and Cellular Cardiology* **29**, 1947–1958.

Campbell SE, Janicki JS, Matsubara BB and Weber KT (1993) Myocardial fibrosis in the rat with mineralocorticoid excess: prevention of scarring by amiloride. *American Journal of Hypertension* **6**, 487–495.

Campbell SE, Janicki JS and Weber KT (1995) Temporal differences in fibroblast proliferation and phenotype expression in response to chronic administration of angiotensin II or aldosterone. *Journal of Molecular and Cellular Cardiology* **27**, 1545–1560.

Chappell MC, Tallant EA, Diz DI and Ferrario CM (2000) The renin–angiotensin system and cardiovascular homeostasis. In *Drugs, Enzymes and Receptors of the Renin–Angiotensin System: Celebrating a Century of Discovery*, Husain A and Graham RM (eds), Harwood, Amsterdam, pp. 3–22.

Chester AH, Misfeld M and Yacoub MH (2000) Receptor-mediated contraction of aortic valve leaflets. *Journal of Heart Valve Disease* **9**, 250–254.

Cleutjens JPM, Verluyten MJA, Smits JFM and Daemen MJAP (1995) Collagen remodeling after myocardial infarction in the rat heart. *American Journal of Pathology* **147**, 325–338.

Cohen EP, Moulder JE, Fish BL and Hill P (1994) Prophylaxis of experimental bone marrow transplant nephropathy. *Journal of Laboratory and Clinical Medicine* **124**, 371–380.

Darrow DC and Miller HC (1942) The production of cardiac lesions by repeated injections of desoxycorticosterone acetate. *Journal of Clinical Investigation* **21**, 601–611.

Delcayre C and Swynghedauw B (2002) Molecular mechanisms of myocardial remodeling. The role of aldosterone. *Journal of Molecular and Cellular Cardiology* **34**, 1577–1584.

Delcayre C, Silvestre JS, Garnier A, et al. (2000) Cardiac aldosterone production and ventricular remodeling. *Kidney International* **57**, 1346–1351.

Delyani JA, Robinson EL and Rudolph AE (2001) Effect of a selective aldosterone receptor antagonist in myocardial infarction. *American Journal of Physiology* **281**, H647–H654.

Desmouliére A, Redard M, Darby I and Gabbiani G (1995) Apoptosis mediates the decrease in cellularity during the transition between granulation tissue and scar. *American Journal of Pathology* **146**, 56–66.

Diamond JR and Anderson S (1990) Irreversible tubulointerstitial damage associated with chronic aminonucleoside nephrosis. *American Journal of Pathology* **137**, 1323–1332.

Dixon IMC, Ju H, Jassal DS and Peterson DJ (1996) Effect of ramipril and losartan on collagen expression in right and left heart after myocardial infarction. *Molecular and Cellular Biochemistry* **165**, 31–45.

El-Adawi H, Deng L, Tramontano A, et al. (2003) The functional role of the Jak-STAT pathway in post-infarction remodeling. *Cardiovascular Research* **57**, 129–138.

Erdös EG (2001) Perspectives on the early history of angiotensin-converting enzyme (ACE) – recent follow-ups. In *Angiotensin-Converting Enzyme (ACE): Clinical and Experimental Insights*, Giles TD (ed), Health Care Communications, Fort Lee, NJ, pp. 3–16.

Falkenhahn M, Franke F, Bohle RM, et al. (1995) Cellular distribution of angiotensin-converting enzyme after myocardial infarction. *Hypertension* **25**, 219–226.

Fiebeler A, Schmidt F, Müller DN, et al. (2001) Mineralocorticoid receptor affects AP_1 and nuclear factor-κB activation in angiotensin II-induced cardiac injury. *Hypertension* **37**, 787–793.

Filip DA, Radu A and Simionescu M (1986) Interstitial cells of the heart valves possess characteristics similar to smooth muscle cells. *Circulation Research* **59**, 310–320.

Francis GS, Benedict C, Johnstone DE, et al. (1990) Comparison of neuroendocrine activation in patients with left ventricular dysfunction with and without congestive heart failure: a substudy of the Studies of Left Ventricular Dysfunction (SOLVD). *Circulation* **82**, 1724–1729.

Frimm CdC, Sun Y and Weber KT (1997) Angiotensin II receptor blockade and myocardial fibrosis of the infarcted rat heart. *Journal of Laboratory and Clinical Medicine* **129**, 439–446.

Goumenos DS, Brown CB, Shortland J and El Nahas AM (1994) Myofibroblasts, predictors of progression of mesangial IgA nephropathy. *Nephrology Dialysis Transplantation* **9**, 1418–1425.

Hall CE and Hall O (1965) Hypertension and hypersalimentation. I. Aldosterone hypertension. *Laboratory Investigation* **14**, 285–294.

Hanatani A, Yoshiyama M, Kim S, et al. (1995) Inhibition by angiotensin II type 1 receptor antagonist of cardiac phenotypic modulation after myocardial infarction. *Journal of Molecular and Cellular Cardiology* **27**, 1905–1914.

Hashimoto K, Hirose M, Furukawa K, et al. (1977) Changes in hemodynamics and bradykinin concentration in coronary sinus blood in experimental coronary artery occlusion. *Japanese Heart Journal* **18**, 679–689.

Hatakeyama H, Miyamori I, Fujita T, et al. (1994) Vascular aldosterone. Biosynthesis and a link to angiotensin II-induced hypertrophy of vascular smooth muscle cells. *Journal of Biological Chemistry* **269**, 24316–24320.

Hayashi M, Tsutamoto T, Wada A, et al. (2001) Relationship between transcardiac extraction of aldosterone and left ventricular remodeling in patients with first acute myocardial infarction: extracting aldosterone through the heart promotes ventricular remodeling after acute myocardial infarction. *Journal of the American College of Cardiology* **38**, 1375–1382.

Hein S, Arnon E, Kostin S, et al. (2003) Progression from compensated hypertrophy to failure in the pressure-overloaded human heart: structural deterioration and compensatory mechanisms. *Circulation* **107**, 984–991.

Henney AM, Parker DJ and Davies MJ (1982) Collagen biosynthesis in normal and abnormal human heart valves. *Cardiovascular Research* **16**, 624–630.

Hirsch AT, Talsness CE, Schunkert H, et al. (1991) Tissue-specific activation of cardiac angiotensin converting enzyme in experimental heart failure. *Circulation Research* **69**, 475–482.

Hokimoto S, Yasue H, Fujimoto K, et al. (1995) Increased angiotensin converting enzyme activity in left ventricular aneurysm of patients after myocardial infarction. *Cardiovascular Research* **29**, 664–669.

Ihara M, Urata H, Shirai K, et al. (2000) High cardiac angiotensin-II-forming activity in infarcted and non-infarcted human myocardium. *Cardiology* **94**, 247–253.

Ikoma M, Kawamura T, Kakinuma Y, et al. (1991) Cause of variable therapeutic efficiency of angiotensin converting enzyme inhibitor on glomerular lesions. *Kidney International* **40**, 195–202.

Ishidoya S, Morrissey J, McCracken R, et al. (1995) Angiotensin II receptor antagonist ameliorates renal tubulointerstitial fibrosis caused by unilateral ureteral obstruction. *Kidney International* **47**, 1285–1294.

Ishidoya S, Morrissey J, McCracken R and Klahr S (1996) Delayed treatment with enalapril halts tubulointerstitial fibrosis in rats with obstructive nephropathy. *Kidney International* **49**, 1110–1119.

Jugdutt BI (1995) Effect of captopril and enalapril on left ventricular geometry, function and collagen during healing after anterior and inferior myocardial infarction in a dog model. *Journal of the American College of Cardiology* **25**, 1718–1725.

Jugdutt BI, Schwarz-Michorowski BL and Khan MI (1992) Effect of long-term captopril therapy on left ventricular remodeling and function during healing of canine myocardial infarction. *Journal of the American College of Cardiology* **19**, 713–721.

Jugdutt BI, Khan MI, Jugdutt SJ and Blinston GE (1995) Effect of enalapril on ventricular remodeling and function during healing after anterior myocardial infarction in the dog. *Circulation* **91**, 802–812.

Juncos LI, Carrasco Dueñas S, et al. (1993) Long-term enalapril and hydrochlorothiazide in radiation nephritis. *Nephron* **64**, 249–255.

Kaneto H, Morrissey J, McCracken R, et al. (1994) Enalapril reduces collagen type IV synthesis and expansion of the interstitium in the obstructed rat kidney. *Kidney International* **45**, 1637–1647.

van Kats JP, Duncker DJ, Haitsma DB, et al. (2000) Angiotensin-converting enzyme inhibition and angiotensin II type 1 receptor blockade prevent cardiac remodeling in pigs after myocardial infarction: role of tissue angiotensin II. *Circulation* **102**, 1556–1563.

Katwa LC, Ratajska A, Cleutjens JPM, et al. (1995) Angiotensin converting enzyme and kininase-II-like activities in cultured valvular interstitial cells of the rat heart. *Cardiovascular Research* **29**, 57–64.

Katwa LC, Tyagi SC, Campbell SE, et al. (1996) Valvular interstitial cells express angiotensinogen, cathepsin D, and generate angiotensin peptides. *International Journal of Biochemistry and Cell Biology* **28**, 807–821.

Katwa LC, Campbell SE, Tyagi SC, et al. (1997) Cultured myofibroblasts generate angiotensin peptides *de novo*. *Journal of Molecular and Cellular Cardiology* **29**, 1375–1386.

Keeley FW, Elmoselhi A and Leenen FHH (1992) Enalapril suppresses normal accumulation of elastin and collagen in cardiovascular tissues of growing rats. *American Journal of Physiology* **262**, H1013–H1021.

Kim S, Ohta K, Hamaguchi A, et al. (1994) Contribution of renal angiotensin II type I receptor to gene expressions in hypertension-induced renal injury. *Kidney International* **46**, 1346–1358.

Kim S, Ohta K, Hamaguchi A, et al. (1995) Angiotensin II type I receptor antagonist inhibits the gene expression of transforming growth factor-β1 and extracellular matrix in cardiac and vascular tissues of hypertensive rats. *Journal of Pharmacology and Experimental Therapeutics* **273**, 509–515.

van Krimpen C, Schoemaker RG, Cleutjens JPM, et al. (1991a) Angiotensin I converting enzyme inhibitors and cardiac remodeling. *Basic Research in Cardiology* **86**, 149–155.

van Krimpen C, Smits JFM, Cleutjens JPM, et al. (1991b) DNA synthesis in the non-infarcted cardiac interstitium after left coronary artery ligation in the rat heart: effects of captopril. *Journal of Molecular and Cellular Cardiology* **23**, 1245–1253.

Lacolley P, Safar ME, Lucet B, et al. (2001) Prevention of aortic and cardiac fibrosis by spironolactone in old normotensive rats. *Journal of the American College of Cardiology* **37**, 662–667.

Lacolley P, Labat C, Pujol A, et al. (2002) Increased carotid wall elastic modulus and fibronectin in aldosterone-salt-treated rats: effects of eplerenone. *Circulation* **106**, 2848–2853.

Lafayette RA, Mayer G and Meyer TW (1993) The effects of blood pressure reduction on cyclosporine nephrotoxicity in the rat. *Journal of the American Society of Nephrology* **3**, 1892–1899.

Lefroy DC, Wharton J, Crake T, et al. (1996) Regional changes in angiotensin II receptor density after experimental myocardial infarction. *Journal of Molecular and Cellular Cardiology* **28**, 429–440.

Litwin SE, Litwin CM, Raya TE, et al. (1991) Contractility and stiffness of noninfarcted myocardium after coronary ligation in rats. Effects of chronic angiotensin converting enzyme inhibition. *Circulation* **83**, 1028–1037.

Majno G, Gabbiani G, Hirschel BJ, et al. (1971) Contraction of granulation tissue *in vitro*: similarity to smooth muscle. *Science* **173**, 548–550.

Makino N, Matsui H, Masutomo K, et al. (1993) Effect of angiotensin converting enzyme inhibitor on regression in cardiac hypertrophy. *Molecular and Cellular Biochemistry* **119**, 23–28.

Martinez DV, Rocha R, Matsumura M, et al. (2002) Cardiac damage prevention by eplerenone: comparison with low sodium diet or potassium loading. *Hypertension* **39**, 614–618.

Mavroidis M and Capetanaki Y (2002) Extensive induction of important mediators of fibrosis and dystrophic calcification in desmin-deficient cardiomyopathy. *American Journal of Pathology* **160**, 943–952.

Messier RH, Bass BL, Aly HM, et al. (1994) Dual structural and functional phenotypes of the porcine aortic valve interstitial population: characteristics of the leaflet myofibroblast. *Journal of Surgical Research* **57**, 1–21.

Michel J-B, Lattion A-L, Salzmann J-L, et al. (1988) Hormonal and cardiac effects of converting enzyme inhibition in rat myocardial infarction. *Circulation Research* **62**, 641–650.

Mizuno Y, Yoshimura M, Yasue H, et al. (2001) Aldosterone production is activated in failing ventricle in humans. *Circulation* **103**, 72–77.

Molteni A, Ward WF, Ts'ao C, et al. (1985) Monocrotaline-induced pulmonary fibrosis in rats: amelioration by captopril and penicillamine. *Proceedings of the Society for Experimental Biology and Medicine* **180**, 112–120.

Morrissey JJ, Ishidoya S, McCracken R and Klahr S (1996) The effect of ACE inhibitors on the expression of matrix genes and the role of p53 and p21 (WAF1) in experimental renal fibrosis. *Kidney International* **49**, S83–S87.

Nakamura T, Honma H, Ikeda Y, et al. (1994) Renal protective effects of angiotensin II receptor I antagonist CV-11974 in spontaneously hypertensive stroke-prone rats (SHR-sp). *Blood Pressure* **3**, 61–66.

Nakamura T, Obata J, Kuroyanagi R, et al. (1996) Involvement of angiotensin II in glomerulosclerosis of stroke-prone spontaneously hypertensive rats. *Kidney International* **49**, S109–S112.

Nakamura Y, Yoshiyama M, Omura T, et al. (2003) Beneficial effects of combination of ACE inhibitor and angiotensin II type 1 receptor blocker on cardiac remodeling in rat myocardial infarction. *Cardiovascular Research* **57**, 48–54.

Needleman P, Marshall GR and Sobel BE (1975) Hormone interactions in the isolated rabbit heart. Synthesis and coronary vasomotor effects of prostaglandins, angiotensin, and bradykinin. *Circulation Research* **37**, 802–808.

Nicoletti A, Mandet C, Challah M, et al. (1996) Mediators of perivascular inflammation in the left ventricle of renovascular hypertensive rats. *Cardiovascular Research* **31**, 585–595.

Nio Y, Matsubara H, Murasawa S, et al. (1995) Regulation of gene transcription of angiotensin II receptor subtypes in myocardial infarction. *Journal of Clinical Investigation* **95**, 46–54.

Noda K, Sasaguri M, Ideishi M, et al. (1993) Role of locally formed angiotensin II and bradykinin in the reduction of myocardial infarct size in dogs. *Cardiovascular Research* **27**, 334–340.

O'Brien KD, Shavelle DM, Caulfield MT, et al. (2002) Association of angiotensin-converting enzyme with low-density lipoprotein in aortic valvular lesions and in human plasma. *Circulation* **106**, 2224–2230.

Park HK, Park SJ, Kim CS, et al. (2001) Enhanced gene expression of renin–angiotensin system, TGF-beta1, endothelin-1 and nitric oxide synthase in right-ventricular hypertrophy. *Pharmacology Research* **43**, 265–273.

Passier RC, Smits JF, Verluyten MJ and Daemen MJ (1996) Expression and localization of renin and angiotensinogen in rat heart after myocardial infarction. *American Journal of Physiology* **271**, H1040–H1048.

Petrov VV, Fagard RH and Lijnen PJ (2000) Transforming growth factor-beta(1) induces angiotensin-converting enzyme synthesis in rat cardiac fibroblasts during their differentiation to myofibroblasts. *Journal of the Renin Angiotensin Aldosterone System* **1**, 342–352.

Pimentel JL, Jr, Martinez-Maldonado M, Wilcox JN, et al. (1993) Regulation of renin–angiotensin system in unilateral ureteral obstruction. *Kidney International* **44**, 390–400.

Pimentel JL, Jr, Sundell CL, Wang S, et al. (1995) Role of angiotensin II in the expression and regulation of transforming growth factor-β in obstructive nephropathy. *Kidney International* **48**, 1233–1246.

Pinto JE, Viglione P and Saavedra JM (1991) Autoradiographic localization and quantification of rat heart angiotensin converting enzyme. *American Journal of Hypertension* **4**, 321–326.

Pitt B, Zannad F, Remme WJ, et al. (1999) The effect of spironolactone on morbidity and mortality in patients with severe heart failure. Randomized Aldactone Evaluation Study Investigators. *New England Journal of Medicine* **341**, 709–717.

Pitt B, Remme W, Zannad F, et al. (2003) Eplerenone, a selective aldosterone blocker, in patients with left ventricular dysfunction after myocardial infarction. *New England Journal of Medicine* **348**, 1309–1321.

Ratajska A, Campbell SE, Sun Y and Weber KT (1994) Angiotensin II associated cardiac myocyte necrosis: role of adrenal catecholamines. *Cardiovascular Research* **28**, 684–690.

Robert V, Van Thiem N, Cheav SL, et al. (1994) Increased cardiac types I and III collagen mRNAs in aldosterone-salt hypertension. *Hypertension* **24**, 30–36.

Roberts ISD, Burrows C, Shanks JH, et al. (1997) Interstitial myofibroblasts: predictors of progression in membranous nephropathy. *Journal of Clinical Pathology* **50**, 123–127.

Rocha R, Chander PN, Khanna K, et al. (1998) Mineralocorticoid blockade reduces vascular injury in stroke-prone hypertensive rats. *Hypertension* **31**, 451–458.

Rocha R, Chander PN, Zuckerman A and Stier CT, Jr (1999) Role of aldosterone in renal vascular injury in stroke-prone hypertensive rats. *Hypertension* **33**, 232–237.

Rocha R, Stier CT, Jr, Kifor I, et al. (2000) Aldosterone: a mediator of myocardial necrosis and renal arteriopathy. *Endocrinology* **141**, 3871–3878.

Rocha R, Rudolph AE, Frierdich GE, et al. (2002) Aldosterone induces a vascular inflammatory phenotype in the rat heart. *American Journal of Physiology* **283**, H1802–H1810.

Rouleau JL, de Champlain J, Klein M, et al. (1993) Activation of neurohormonal systems in postinfarction left ventricular hypertrophy. *Journal of the American College of Cardiology* **22**, 390–398.

Sappino AP, Skalli O, Jackson B, et al. (1988) Smooth-muscle differentiation in stromal cells of malignant and non-malignant breast tissues. *International Journal of Cancer* **41**, 707–712.

Schieffer B, Wirger A, Meybrunn M, et al. (1994) Comparative effects of chronic angiotensin-converting enzyme inhibition and angiotensin II type 1 receptor blockade on cardiac remodeling after myocardial infarction in the rat. *Circulation* **89**, 2273–2282.

Selye H (1960) Protection by a steroid-spironolactone against certain types of cardiac necroses. *Proceedings of the Society of Experimental Biology and Medicine* **104**, 212–213.

Serneri GG, Boddi M, Cecioni I, et al. (2001) Cardiac angiotensin II formation in the clinical course of heart failure and its relationship with left ventricular function. *Circulation Research* **88**, 961–968.

Shibouta Y, Chatani F, Ishimura Y, et al. (1996) TCV-116 inhibits renal interstitial and glomerular injury in glomerulosclerotic rats. *Kidney International* **49**, S115–S118.

Silvestre J-S, Robert V, Heymes C, et al. (1998) Myocardial production of aldosterone and corticosterone in the rat. *Journal of Biological Chemistry* **273**, 4883–4891.

Silvestre J-S, Heymes C, Oubénaïssa A, et al. (1999) Activation of cardiac aldosterone production in rat myocardial infarction. Effect of angiotensin II receptor blockade and role in cardiac fibrosis. *Circulation* **99**, 2694–2701.

Skalli O, Schürch W, Seemayer T, et al. (1989) Myofibroblasts from diverse pathologic settings are heterogeneous in their content of actin isoforms and intermediate filament proteins. *Laboratory Investigation* **60**, 275–285.

Slight SH, Ganjam VK, Gómez-Sánchez CE, et al. (1996) High affinity NAD^+-dependent 11β-hydroxysteroid dehydrogenase in the human heart. *Journal of Molecular and Cellular Cardiology* **28**, 781–787.

Slight SH, Chilakamarri VK, Nasr S, et al. (1998) Inhibition of tissue repair by spironolactone: role of mineralocorticoids in fibrous tissue formation. *Molecular and Cellular Biochemistry* **189**, 47–54.

Smits JFM, van Krimpen C, Schoemaker RG, et al. (1992) Angiotensin II receptor blockade after myocardial infarction in rats: effects on hemodynamics, myocardial DNA synthesis, and interstitial collagen content. *Journal of Cardiovascular Pharmacology* **20**, 772–778.

Studer R, Reinecke H, Müller B, et al. (1994) Increased angiotensin-I converting enzyme gene expression in the failing human heart. Quantification by competitive RNA polymerase chain reaction. *Journal of Clinical Investigation* **94**, 301–310.

Sun Y and Weber KT (1994) Angiotensin II receptor binding following myocardial infarction in the rat. *Cardiovascular Research* **28**, 1623–1628.

Sun Y and Weber KT (1996a) Cells expressing angiotensin II receptors in fibrous tissue of rat heart. *Cardiovascular Research* **31**, 518–525.

Sun Y and Weber KT (1996b) Angiotensin-converting enzyme and wound healing in diverse tissues of the rat. *Journal of Laboratory and Clinical Medicine* **127**, 94–101.

Sun Y and Weber KT (1996c) Angiotensin converting enzyme and myofibroblasts during tissue repair in the rat heart. *Journal of Molecular and Cellular Cardiology* **28**, 851–858.

Sun Y, Ratajska A, Zhou G and Weber KT (1993) Angiotensin converting enzyme and myocardial fibrosis in the rat receiving angiotensin II or aldosterone. *Journal of Laboratory and Clinical Medicine* **122**, 395–403.

Sun Y, Diaz-Arias AA and Weber KT (1994a) Angiotensin-converting enzyme, bradykinin and angiotensin II receptor binding in rat skin, tendon and heart valves: an *in vitro* quantitative autoradiographic study. *Journal of Laboratory and Clinical Medicine* **123**, 372–377.

Sun Y, Cleutjens JPM, Diaz-Arias AA and Weber KT (1994b) Cardiac angiotensin converting enzyme and myocardial fibrosis in the rat. *Cardiovascular Research* **28**, 1423–1432.

Sun Y, Ramires FJA and Weber KT (1997a) Fibrosis of atria and great vessels in response to angiotensin II or aldosterone infusion. *Cardiovascular Research* **35**, 138–147.

Sun Y, Ramires FJA, Zhou G, et al. (1997b) Fibrous tissue and angiotensin II. *Journal of Molecular and Cellular Cardiology* **29**, 2001–2012.

Sun Y, Zhang JQ, Zhang J and Ramires FJA (1998) Angiotensin II, transforming growth factor-β1 and repair in the infarcted heart. *Journal of Molecular and Cellular Cardiology* **30**, 1559–1569.

Sun Y, Zhang J, Zhang JQ and Weber KT (2001) Renin expression at sites of repair in the infarcted rat heart. *Journal of Molecular and Cellular Cardiology* **33**, 995–1003.

Swedberg K, Eneroth P, Kjekshus J and Wilhelmsen L (1990) Hormones regulating cardiovascular function in patients with severe congestive heart failure and their relation to mortality. CONSENSUS Trial Study Group. *Circulation* **82**, 1730–1736.

Takeda Y, Miyamori I, Yoneda T, et al. (1995) Production of aldosterone in isolated rat blood vessels. *Hypertension* **25**, 170–173.

Takeda Y, Miyamori I, Yoneda T, et al. (1996) Regulation of aldosterone synthase in human vascular endothelial cells by angiotensin II and adrenocorticotropin. *Journal of Clinical Endocrinology and Metabolism* **81**, 2797–2800.

Tanaka R, Sugihara K, Tatematsu A and Fogo A (1995) Internephron heterogeneity of growth factors and sclerosis – modulation of platelet-derived growth factor by angiotensin II. *Kidney International* **47**, 131–139.

Taylor PM, Allen SP and Yacoub MH (2000) Phenotypic and functional characterization of interstitial cells from human heart valves, pericardium and skin. *Journal of Heart Valve Disease* **9**, 150–158.

Thompson JS, Palmieri GM, Eliel LP and Crawford RL (1972) The effect of porcine calcitonin on osteoporosis induced by adrenal cortical steroids. *Journal of Bone and Joint Surgery. American Volume* **54**, 1490–1500.

Tsutamoto T, Wada A, Maeda K, et al. (2000) Spironolactone inhibits the transcardiac extraction of aldosterone in patients with congestive heart failure. *Journal of the American College of Cardiology* **36**, 838–844.

Volders PGA, Willems IEMG, Cleutjens JPM, et al. (1993) Interstitial collagen is increased in the non-infarcted human myocardium after myocardial infarction. *Journal of Molecular and Cellular Cardiology* **25**, 1317–1323.

Ward WF, Molteni A and Ts'ao C (1989) Radiation-induced endothelial dysfunction and fibrosis in rat lung: modification by the angiotensin converting enzyme inhibitor CL242817. *Radiation Research* **117**, 342–350.

Ward WF, Molteni A, Ts'ao C-H and Hinz JM (1990) Captopril reduces collagen and mast cell accumulation in irradiated rat lung. *International Journal of Radiation Oncology, Biology, Physics* **19**, 1405–1409.

Ward WF, Molteni A, Ts'ao C, et al. (1992) Radiation pneumotoxicity in rats: modification by inhibitors of angiotensin converting enzyme. *International Journal of Radiation Oncology, Biology, Physics* **22**, 623–625.

Weber KT (1989) Cardiac interstitium in health and disease: the fibrillar collagen network. *Journal of the American College of Cardiology* **13**, 1637–1652.

Weber KT (1997a) Fibrosis, a common pathway to organ failure: angiotensin II and tissue repair. *Seminars in Nephrology* **17**, 467–491.

Weber KT (1997b) Extracellular matrix remodeling in heart failure. A role for *de novo* angiotensin II generation. *Circulation* **96**, 4065–4082.

Weber KT (2001) Aldosterone in congestive heart failure. *New England Journal of Medicine* **345**, 1689–1697.

Weber KT, Brilla CG and Janicki JS (1993) Myocardial fibrosis: functional significance and regulatory factors. *Cardiovascular Research* **27**, 341–348.

Weber KT, Sun Y, Katwa LC and Cleutjens JPM (1995) Connective tissue: a metabolic entity? *Journal of Molecular and Cellular Cardiology* **27**, 107–120.

Willems IEMG, Havenith MG, De Mey JGR and Daemen MJAP (1994) The α-smooth muscle actin-positive cells in healing human myocardial scars. *American Journal of Pathology* **145**, 868–875.

Wollert KC, Studer R, Doerfer K, et al. (1997) Differential effects of kinins on cardiomyocyte hypertrophy and interstitial collagen matrix in the surviving myocardium after myocardial infarction in the rat. *Circulation* **95**, 1910–1917.

Yamada H, Fabris B, Allen AM, et al. (1991) Localization of angiotensin converting enzyme in rat heart. *Circulation Research* **68**, 141–149.

Yamagishi H, Kim S, Nishikimi T, et al. (1993) Contribution of cardiac renin–angiotensin system to ventricular remodelling in myocardial-infarcted rats. *Journal of Molecular and Cellular Cardiology* **25**, 1369–1380.

Yanagisawa H, Morrissey J, Morrison AR and Klahr S (1990) Eicosanoid production by isolated glomeruli of rats with unilateral ureteral obstruction. *Kidney International* **37**, 1528–1535.

Yoshimura M, Nakamura S, Ito T, et al. (2002) Expression of aldosterone synthase gene in failing human heart: quantitative analysis using modified real-time polymerase chain reaction. *Journal of Clinical Endocrinology and Metabolism* **87**, 3936–3940.

Young M, Head G and Funder J (1995) Determinants of cardiac fibrosis in experimental hypermineralocorticoid states. *American Journal of Physiology* **269**, E657–E662.

Zannad F, Alla F, Dousset B, et al. (2000) Limitation of excessive extracellular matrix turnover may contribute to survival benefit of spironolactone therapy in patients with congestive heart failure: insights from the randomized aldactone evaluation study (RALES). Rales Investigators. *Circulation* **102**, 2700–2706.

Zhang G, Moorhead PJ and el Nahas AM (1995) Myofibroblasts and the progression of experimental glomerulonephritis. *Experimental Nephrology* **3**, 308–318.

11

Trophic Effects of Aldosterone

Claude Delcayre, Christophe Heymes,
Paul Milliez and Bernard Swynghedauw

Introduction

Cardiac remodeling is a complex issue which results from combined effects of mechanical overload, susceptibility factors, etiologies, and the neurohormonal reaction, including the adrenal and myocardial secretion of aldosterone. Aldosterone production plays an important role in cardiac remodeling.

There is experimental evidence that aldosterone induces fibrosis in the cardiovascular system in the presence of a high sodium diet. However, the pathways of aldosterone-induced fibrosis are still unclear. The aldosterone receptor is a transcription factor whose cardiovascular target genes are largely unknown. The RALES trial has recently evidenced a significant beneficial effect of spironolactone on both mortality and morbidity in heart failure, and a substudy has shown that these improvements are linked to a reduction of cardiac fibrosis.

An intracardiac production of aldosterone and corticosterone has been shown in the rat. Aldosterone production is regulated by low sodium/high potassium diets and by angiotensin II (Ang II) and is evidenced in both atria and ventricles. Cardiac production is low as compared to the adrenal production, nevertheless it results in high local concentrations, just like Ang II. In rats, myocardial infarction activates aldosterone production and this activation is prevented by losartan. Heart failure, in humans, activates aldosterone production and is accompanied by a significant increase of the arteriovenous difference in aldosterone by the myocardium.

Thus, in both myocardial infarction and heart failure increased adrenal (as part of the neurohormonal reaction) and cardiovascular productions of aldosterone have detrimental consequences on cardiac function. Aldosterone effects on coronary function and pericoronary structure, and on the induction of tissular fibrosis are key factors to explain these detrimental consequences.

Renal effects of aldosterone

Aldosterone was first isolated 50 years ago (Simpson and Tait, 1953), and is now identified as the main determinant of sodium reabsorption and potassium release by the epithelial cells of the kidneys, intestine, and sweat and salivary glands. Aldosterone prevents sodium and water loss during the periods of dietary salt deprivation. It also prevents hyperkalemia after consumption of potassium-rich food or after intense exercise. From an evolutionary perspective, the aldosterone system has confered a highly selective advantage to living organisms which became able to regulate their internal sodium homeostasis in the absence of external sea water. Cells in the cortical collecting duct of the distal nephron have been considered for a long time as the unique cellular targets of aldosterone, and the activation of sodium reabsorption and potassium excretion as its unique physiological function (Weber, 2001). However, it is now clear that other cell types in nonepithelial tissues are also potential targets for aldosterone, but the functions that this hormone controls in nonepithelial tissues are still a matter of debate. Aldosterone production is a end-component of the renin angiotensin system, and both renin and Ang II secretion are obligatory links between salt and water homeostasis and glomerular filtration. Indeed, the pivotal role of aldosterone in control of sodium homeostasis designates this hormone as a key actor in the control of blood pressure.

In heart failure, the primary afferent signal that initiates salt and water retention, and edema, is likely to be a threat to blood pressure (Anand, 1997). This induces a baroreceptor-mediated activation of both the autonomous system (towards a high sympathetic activity and a low vagal drive (Malliani, 2000) and the renin angiotensin aldosterone system (RAAS). As far as aldosterone metabolism is concerned, the net result is an increased plasma aldosterone concentration (from 100–400 pmol/l in control subjects up to 8000 pmol/l in patients with heart failure). Increased aldosterone is likely the main determinant of the extravascular volume expansion which helps to maintain blood pressure. This increased aldosterone production may be even exacerbated by a reduced hepatic metabolic clearance during the end-stage of heart failure. Such an extravascular expansion, in turn, is controlled by several negative feedback mechanisms, such as the atrial natriuretic factors, vasopressin and adrenomedullin. As a consequence, patients with systolic dysfunction may have a compensated heart failure for a long time, with symptoms occurring only during heavy exercise. A good index of how these opposite systems are in fact playing their role is the urinary sodium:potassium ratio, which is above 1 in compensatory heart failure (Weber, 2001).

Trophic effects of aldosterone

Mechanisms of action

The aldosterone receptor, the so-called mineraloreceptor, is basically different from Ang II receptors. The latter are plasma membrane receptors and they belong to the R7G family that bind G proteins and possess seven hydrophobic spanning regions in their molecular structure. The R7G family also includes the adrenergic receptors. By contrast, the aldosterone receptor is an intracellular nuclear hormone receptor that possesses together with its C-terminal steroid recognition region, a central highly conserved DNA binding site, and a finger-like structure. This broad receptor family also includes thyroxine, glucocorticoids, androgen, estrogen and progesterone receptors. They all act as transcription factors, which is likely the basis of the complexity of their physiologic function. This is a major issue for understanding some of the adverse effects of blocking aldosterone therapy.

A crucial issue for understanding the effects of aldosterone in heart is that the aldosterone receptor is a transcription factor, and that the ligand-binding domain and the DNA-binding site of both the aldosterone and glucocorticoid receptors are highly homologous. The specificity of both the ligand binding and the regulation of transcription makes these systems complex, and it is essential to mention that the interaction with several pleiotropic genes and pleiotropic signaling systems is certainly a major point that deserves further studies. Our current knowledge of the corticosteroid systems mode of action raises namely the question of aldosterone binding to its mineraloreceptor in heart. In epithelial cells glucocorticoids (that are 100- to 1000-fold higher in plasma than aldosterone) are inactivated by the type 2 11-β-hydroxysteroid-dehydrogenase (Funder *et al.*, 1988). This enzyme has been evidenced in the human and rat heart but its enzymatic activity is far too low to protect the cardiac mineraloreceptor from glucocorticoids (review in Farman and Rafestin-Oblin, 2001). Thus, other mechanisms are required to explain the aldosterone specific binding (Farman and Refestin-Oblin, 2001) or one must admit that the cardiac mineraloreceptor is predominantly occupied by glucocorticoids (Funder, 1997). This fascinating question is still open. There is another important feature that distinguishes epithelial from nonepithelial tissues. Indeed, nonepithelial cells are not polarized, which means that aldosterone does not induce any transcellular ionic transport there (if we hypothesize that aldosterone controls ionic movements in cardiac cells as it does in kidney cells). Thus, the major consequence of aldosterone action in nonepithelial cells is a modification of their intracellular ionic composition. This may have fundamental consequences for the cell's metabolism and survival.

Cell hypertrophy

The trophic effects of aldosterone were first identified on the kidneys. The compensatory hypertrophy of the kidney that follows uninephrectomy is accompanied by an enlargement of distal and collecting tubule cells, which is very alike that observed after dietary manipulations that are known to stimulate aldosterone excretion. Aldosterone itself induces morphological changes in the renal structure with intensive hypertrophy of the epithelial cells and increased expression of the Na^+, K^+-ATPase (Horisberger and Rossier, 1992; Weber, 2001).

Collagen metabolism

Chronic infusion of aldosterone in rats that have undergone uninephrectomy and are supplemented in dietary salt induces systemic hypertension, left ventricular hypertrophy, nephrosclerosis and perivascular fibrosis in atria, the two ventricles, aorta and systemic organs including kidneys (Brilla *et al.*, 1990; Robert *et al.*, 1994, 1995; Young *et al.*, 1995). Aldosterone-induced fibrosis is not linked to cardiac hypertrophy *per se*, or to hypertensive cardiopathy, and there are many models of cardiac hypertrophy (with or without pressure overload) without fibrosis (reviewed in Swynghedauw, 2000). Fibrosis is a general process that may involve sodium changes in fibroblasts (see above). Fibrosis in the experimental hyperaldosteronism model is observed in organs which are not hemodynamically overloaded, as the right ventricle. Subhypotensive doses of spironolactone prevent fibrosis and the intracerebroventricular infusion of RU28318, an aldosterone-receptor antagonist that abolishes the central mineralocorticoid effects of aldosterone, normalizes blood pressure, while it does not prevent fibrosis. Fibrosis does not occur if sodium supplementation is omitted (Young et al., 1995).

Aldosterone-induced fibrosis is likely to be both reparative and reactive. Collagen accumulation is preceded by myocardial fibrinoid necrosis (Robert et al., 1995), intramacrophagic iron deposit and increase of inflammation markers (Nicoletti and Michel, 1999; Rocha and Funder, 2002). Microscopic scaring and reparative fibrosis are, in part, prevented by the potassium sparing diuretic amiloride and by potassium supplementation suggesting that hypokalemia may play an additional role as a determinant of necrosis (Weber, 2001). The increased collagen concentration is pretranslationally regulated, and is preceded

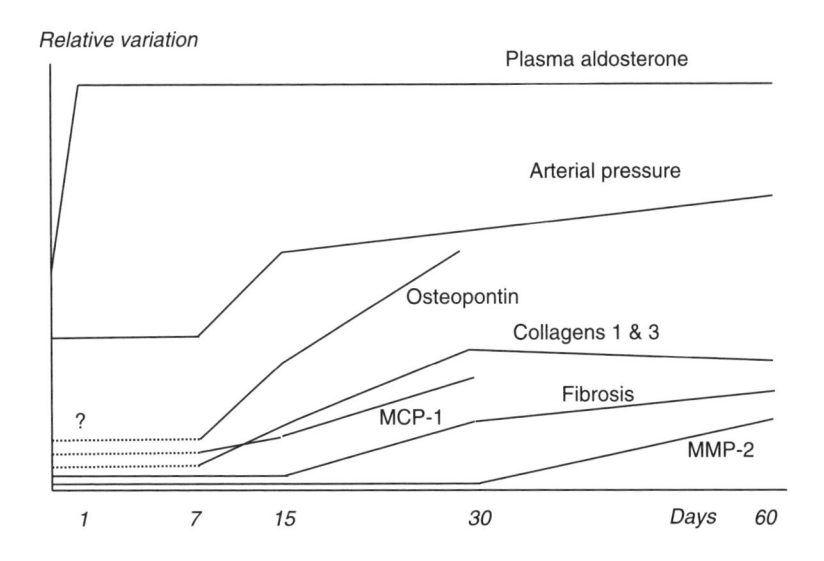

Figure 11.1 Time course of events related to remodeling in the heart of a rat treated with aldosterone-salt. Aldosterone (0.75 µg/h infused by osmotic minipumps) increases in plasma on the first day. '?' indicates that early aldosterone-driven events are still unknown. Then, the first evidences of perivascular inflammation are seen at 7 days (MCP-1 and osteopontin mRNAs as markers). Related or not, the collagens mRNAs increase at 15 days and perivascular and interstitial fibrosis are histologically obvious at 30 days. Anti-aldosterone treatment (20 mg/kg/day spironolactone or 100 mg/kg/day eplerenone) attenuates these modifications despite blood pressure remains elevated (combined results from Robert et al., 1995, 1999; Rocha et al., 2002)

by an enhanced tissue mRNA concentrations in collagen. The increase in cardiac collagen is not immediate and needs a few weeks to be observed, at least 2 weeks for the mRNA, reinforcing the idea that the fibrotic effect is not direct (Horisberger and Rossier, 1992; Robert et al., 1995). Aldosterone-induced fibrosis is not due to a reduction in collagenase activity, as during senescence, but it is associated with a reactive increase in cardiac total matrix metalloprotease activity (Robert et al., 1997). As compared to Ang II, aldosterone is unlikely to have any direct effect on collagen synthesis in the fibroblasts, and to cause fibrosis through an ischemic mechanism. The mechanism of aldosterone-induced fibrosis is multifactorial and may involve the renin angiotensin system and early inflammatory events (see below). Indeed, aldosterone infusion upregulates the Ang II receptor type 1 (Robert et al., 1999), endothelin and bradykinin receptors, the angiotensin-converting enzyme (ACE), and is attenuated by specific blockers of these components (reviewed in Delcayre and Swynghedauw, 2002) (Figure 11.1).

Other effects

The increased plasma levels of aldosterone result in a paradoxical upregulation of the aldosterone receptors. Nevertheless, such an upregulation is restricted to the overloaded part of the heart (i.e. the left ventricle), and is likely to have a hemodynamic origin. In contrast, aldosterone infusion is also associated with reduced plasma levels of corticosterone and a homologous upregulation of the glucocorticoid receptors in the two parts of the heart and in the kidneys (Silvestre et al., 2000).

The activated aldosterone receptors have several well-documented effects on transcription that explain aldosterone late renal effects (Horisberger and Rossier, 1992). In kidney, the hormone induces the expression of the genes encoding the Na^+/K^+-ATPase. Nevertheless, in the heart, *in vivo*, but not *in vitro*, aldosterone does not modify levels of the sodium pump subunits (Robert et al., 1995). There are also suggestions that, at least *in vitro*, aldosterone raises the activities of both the Cl/HCO_3 exchanger and the Na^+/H^+ antiport. For the moment, the only well documented finding is the evidence made by Vassort's group that aldosterone induces the expression of the calcium channels and augments the corresponding current which is potentially arrhythmogenic (Benitah and Vassort, 1999). This increase in inward calcium current is likely involved in the effect of Ang II which increases the action potential duration in rat heart (De Mello, 2002). Recently, it was suggested that there are other aldosterone receptors than those we know since years. This was supported by the discovery that aldosterone has cellular effects on protein kinase C which are not inhibited by spironolactone (Sato et al., 1997).

Results from clinical trials

Two trials with aldosterone blockade

In heart failure, several clinical reports have evidenced that under ACEI treatment the plasma levels of aldosterone usually 'escape' after 3 months and return to elevated values (Pitt, 1995). Such an escape phenomenon may be due to incomplete RAAS blockade (Ang II escape), to Ang II synthesis by pathways other than the converting enzyme pathways (the chymase pathway for example (Urata et al., 1993) or to a decrease in aldosterone hepatic catabolism (see above). Such observations have stimulated researches towards an effect of aldosterone blockade in heart failure.

The Randomized Aldactone Evaluation Study (RALES), has been conducted in patients with severe heart failure (NYHA class III/IV) and has evaluated the effect of spironolactone in addition to an optimal treatment (Pitt et al., 1999). This study was ended before its scheduled term since the primary end point – decrease in mortality – had been reached. The trial has demonstrated that the addition of 26 mg/day of spironolactone to the conventional treatment of heart failure reduced mortality from all causes by 30 percent, and mortality of cardiovascular origin by 31 percent. In addition, spironolactone has a beneficial effect on cardiac function since some patients who were initially in class IV have been assigned to class III at the end of the study.

More recently, another randomized, double-blind, placebo-controlled trial, EPHESUS, using eplerenone, a novel aldosterone inhibitor with greater selectivity for the mineralocorticoid receptor at the dose of 42 mg/day was conducted in patients with acute myocardial infarction complicated by left ventricular dysfunction (Pitt et al., 2003). The EPHESUS study is quite different from the RALES trial. Patients were eligible for randomization 3–14 days after acute myocardial infarction. The mean follow-up was 16 months. Again, aldosterone blockade was beneficial in patients who received optimal therapy, and significantly reduced the overall and cardiovascular mortality rate and hospitalization for cardiovascular events. Interestingly, the reduction in cardiovascular mortality was in large part due to a 21 percent reduction in the rate of sudden death from cardiac causes. In addition, the incidence of gynecomastia, a known adverse effect of spironolactone, was not greater than that in the placebo group.

Aldosterone blockade mechanisms of action

The reasons that explain this effect of aldosterone blockade are likely complex. Effects of aldosterone blockers on plasma volume and electrolyte excretion have been recognized for many years, and up to now aldosterone blockers are the only diuretic agents that significantly improve cardiovascular mortality in heart failure (reviewed in Swynghedauw, 2000).

At the myocardial level, the low dose of spironolactone used in RALES, or of eplerenone in the 2003 study, had no influence on blood pressure, thus suggesting that aldosterone blockade acts through mechanisms that were unrelated to loading conditions. (i) An inhibitory effect of cardiac fibrosis did certainly play a role. For example, in a substudy of RALES, Zannad and colleagues using a plasma assay of the N-terminal fragment of collagen III have observed a relationship between mortality and the initial degree of cardiac fibrosis and has shown that spironolactone reduced fibrosis with a higher efficiency in patients who had initially the highest degree of cardiac fibrosis (Zannad et al., 2000). (ii) One of the main determinants of re-entry arrhythmia is myocardial fibrosis. A pro-arrythmic role of aldosterone, which could act through such a mechanism, has been suggested by Ramires et al., on the basis of a 74 percent decrease of ventricular premature complexes and a 80 percent decrease of nonsustained episodes of ventricular tachycardia in patients under spironolactone therapy (Ramires et al., 2000).

At the level of large vessels:

(i) Aldosterone-induced fibrosis can be prevented by spironolactone treatment which, at least in ageing normotensive rats, prevents the increase of aortic stiffness and the increase of aortic collagen (Lacolley et al., 2001).

(ii) Aldosterone-salt treatment in rats increases arterial stiffness and induces an aortic accumulation of fibronectin EIIIa, which can be prevented by eplerenone, suggesting a role of aldosterone as a determinant in the structural alterations of the large vessels in hyperaldosteronism (Lacolley et al., 2002).

(iii) In heart failure, spironolactone improves the endothelial dysfunction (Farquharson and Struthers, 2000).

(iv) Aldosterone synthesis has been demonstrated in the human pulmonary artery and in the rat mesenteric artery, and this synthesis is increased in the spontaneously hypertensive rat (Takeda et al., 1997). These authors have suggested that the locally produced aldosterone could potentiate the trophic effect of Ang II on cultured vascular smooth muscle cells (Hatakeyama et al., 1994).

(v) Recent data have highlighted the deleterious role of aldosterone on coronary vessels (reviewed in Rocha and Funder, 2002), and two lines of evidence have suggested that the role of aldosterone in vascular injury is independent of Ang II. Aldosterone produced vascular injury in the presence of ACE inhibition, and aldosterone antagonism result in marked vascular protection, even in the presence of Ang II infusions (Rocha and Stier, 2001).

Two laboratories have recently observed the induction of a pericoronary inflammatory phenotype in the heart of aldosterone-salt treated rats (Rocha et al., 2002; Sun et al., 2002). Several markers of inflammatory cells, such as osteopontin, Cox-2 and MCP-1, are expressed in the first week of aldosterone challenge. Thus, proliferation of inflammatory cells around the coronary arteries may be one of the early events that ultimately result in cardiac fibrosis. The causative role of oxidative stress in this aldosterone-mediated vascular alterations is strongly suggested by the fact that spironolactone or antioxidants independently prevent these changes in either coronary (Sun et al., 2002) or peripheral (Virdis et al., 2002) vessels. Young and colleagues have shown that vascular smooth muscle cells, that express the aldosterone receptor and 11-β-HSD1/2 with 11-β-HSD1 showing uncharacteristic oxidase activity, are targets for mineralocorticoids (Young et al., 2002). They also have observed that both deoxycorticosterone or carbenoxolone may induce the expression of inflammation markers in rat heart, suggesting that local glucocorticoid excess may mimic mineralocorticoid excess, thus being a determinant of coronary vascular inflammatory responses under circumstances of a high salt intake. Preliminary results from our laboratory showing that cardiac aldosterone overproduction induces coronary dysfunction (detailed in the 'Transgenic models' section) reinforce the idea that vascular injury is probably one of the early events that may be harmful to cardiac function, and help to explain the beneficial effect of anti-aldosterone treatment in heart failure.

Cardiac aldosterone production

Normal heart

The mitochondrial P-450 aldosterone-synthase (AS) catalyzes the synthesis of aldosterone from deoxycorticosterone in the adrenal cortex. This synthesis is regulated by the plasma levels of both Ang II and potassium, and also although more weakly, by adrenocorticotrophic hormone (ACTH) and sodium. This is the 'classic' view of aldosterone synthesis.

Extra-adrenal sites for aldosterone production have been identified in the aorta (Hatakeyama et al., 1994) and in the brain (Gomez-Sanchez et al., 1997) of rodents, and in the pulmonary artery in humans (Hatakeyama et al., 1994). In the rat heart, aldosterone production was first evidenced in our group in 1998 (Silvestre et al., 1998).

(i) Quantitative RT–PCR is able to detect significant levels of 11-β-hydroxylase and AS mRNAs, the terminal enzymes of corticosterone and aldosterone synthesis, respectively. In the heart, 11-β-hydroxylase is seven-fold more abundant than AS, and this ratio is identical in the adrenal gland. The total amount of both mRNAs in the whole heart is approximately 100-fold lower than in adrenals, and there are no significant differences between the right and left parts of the heart. This makes this category of cytochrome P450 enzymes different from cytochromes 2D6 (the enzymes that metabolizes several drugs, as beta-blockers for example), which are concentrated in the right ventricle.

(ii) Production of aldosterone, corticosterone and deoxycorticosterone has been detected by celite column chromatography coupled to radioimmunoassay in the perfusate of isolated Langendorff perfused hearts. The production is increased acutely by Ang II, and more weakly by ACTH.

(iii) *In vivo*, 1 week's treatment with low sodium or high potassium diets or with Ang II increases myocardial aldosterone synthase mRNA concentration, showing that the cardiac aldosterone production is also regulated on a long-term basis.

(iv) In normal conditions, the cardiac aldosterone concentration is 17-fold higher than that of the plasma. Interestingly, concentrations far higher in tissue than in plasma are also observed for Ang II in the normal dog heart (Dell'Italia et al., 1997).

Despite the mechanisms that result in such high levels of active hormones in cardiac tissue are unknown, these observations suggest that these local hormonal systems may have up to now unexpected significant effects (De Mello and Danser, 2000).

Work from our laboratory, and in collaboration with Capponi's group has identified two key factors for aldosterone synthesis in the rat heart, namely the steroidogenic acute regulatory (StAR) protein that plays a pivotal role in the rate-limiting step of steroidogenesis, i.e. intramitochondrial cholesterol transfer, and the AS (Silvestre et al., 1998; Casal et al., 2003). The level of expression of these factors is low in normal conditions, which indeed corresponds to a low level of cardiac aldosterone synthesis. This could be considered as unsignificant, but it should be realized that the hormone produced in cardiac tissue will act in conditions very different from the circulating hormones (i.e., on a very limited area and with a short time response). Thus, it is quite possible that instantaneous high concentrations of aldosterone may be reached locally despite a low production (Figure 11.2). Interestingly,

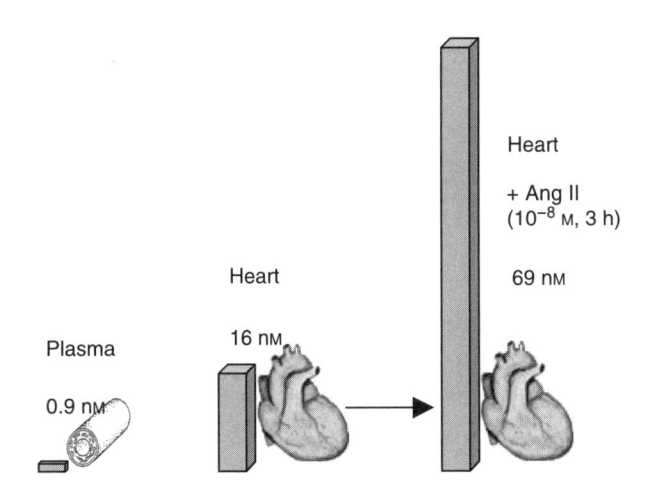

Figure 11.2 The tissue concentration of aldosterone is likely much higher in the cardiac tissue than that measured in the plasma. In normal rat heart (middle) aldosterone concentration is 17 times higher than in the same rat's plasma (left). The right column shows that aldosterone concentration rises to very high levels in an isolated rat heart perfused for 3 h with 10^{-8} M Ang II. These experimental conditions are obviously far from physiological conditions. Nevertheless, this observation suggests that a long-lasting increase of circulating or intracardiac synthesis of Ang II (as is the case in myocardial infarction or in heart failure) may well result in a sustained synthesis of cardiac aldosterone. Therefore, one cannot rule out the possibility that in severe pathological conditions the cardiac level of aldosterone may reach values high enough to induce the detrimental cardiac remodeling observed in experimental hyperaldosteronism (data taken from Silvestre et al., 1999)

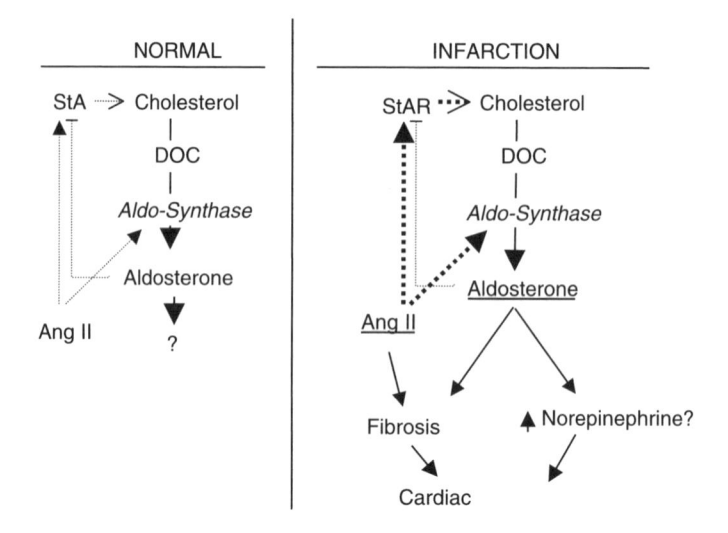

Figure 11.3 Consequences of myocardial infarction on synthesis of cardiac aldosterone. One month after an experimental myocardial infarction in rat, the level of Ang II is two-fold increased in the noninfarcted zone of left ventricle. This induces an increased expression of the StAR protein and of aldosterone synthase, which results in an increased aldosterone synthesis in the infarcted heart. Both Ang II and aldosterone participate in the development of fibrosis in the ventricle (data taken from Silvestre et al., 1999)

this local synthesis is stimulated one month after myocardial infarction in parallel to the local synthesis of Ang II (Silvestre et al., 1999). The expression level of both StAR and AS is increased after myocardial infarction (Casal et al., 2003). The ventricular fibrosis observed in the noninfarcted part of the left ventricle is totally or partly prevented by losartan or spironolactone, respectively. Since the circulating level of these hormones is normal, cardiac fibrosis has been linked to the local production of these two hormones (Figure 11.3). The aldosterone concentration, already 15 times higher in normal rat heart than in plasma, still rises by a factor of three in the noninfarcted part of left ventricle. On the other hand, the role of sodium is critical since a diet with a moderate increase of sodium intake induces a decrease of plasma aldosterone, a stimulation of cardiac aldosterone synthesis and a moderate cardiac hypertrophy in normotensive rats (Takeda et al., 2000). A tissue RAAS thus exists in heart, and according to the local conditions that may be quite different from those estimated from the plasma assays, its role in cardiovascular pathology may be important and requires further study.

Transgenic models

It has been described above that the myocardial infarction-associated ventricular fibrosis is partly dependent on aldosterone. Several questions still remain as to regards the mechanisms since the partial inactivation of the cardiac mineraloreceptor by an inducible antimineraloreceptor antisens RNA in mice induces a syndrome of congestive heart failure associated with a major cardiac fibrosis (Beggah et al., 2002). This observation suggests that the action of aldosterone in heart may involves an equilibrium between glucoreceptor and mineraloreceptor, and that some of the effects of aldosterone may be mediated by other receptors than the mineraloreceptor, as the glucoreceptor for example. The study of the local aldosterone system is complicated by its low level of expression and also by the difficulty to identify the effects of aldosterone from tissular or from circulating origin. To resolve this issue, a transgenic strain of mice has been generated in our laboratory that overexpress AS in heart by targeting the AS gene with the alpha-myosin heavy chain promoter. Preliminary results obtained from these transgenic mice indicate that increased cardiac aldosterone induces no significant change of cardiac function, but a major coronary dysfunction. This may have harmful consequences on coronary adaptation to increased flow demand. Interestingly, this dysfunction was more severe in males. Despite explanation of this observation deserve further studies, it is in agreement with a greater incidence of cardiovascular events in males than in females.

Aldosterone production in heart failure

Experimental myocardial infarction in rats activates the myocardial production of aldosterone and doubles the myocardial content in aldosterone synthase (Silvestre et al., 1999). The myocardial renin angiotensin system is equally activated (Dell'Italia et al., 1997; van Kats et al., 2000), and the cardiac level of Ang II is doubled (Silvestre et al., 1999). In contrast, the myocardial production of corticosterone is reduced and the 11-β-hydroxylase level is downregulated. Such findings make contrast with the circulating systems, since at the same time the plasma levels of aldosterone, corticosterone, Ang II and renin remain unchanged. In this condition, the activation of the myocardial aldosterone system is mediated primarily by the renin angiotensin system, and is abolished by the simultaneous prescription of losartan. The activation of the two systems have fibrogenic consequences, myocardial infarction induces collagen deposition and the deposition is prevented by spironolactone and also by losartan. In conclusion, myocardial infarction produces a shift of the myocardial corticoid pathways through an activation of the renin angiotensin system, the shift results in an activation of the mineralocorticoid production and a reduction in glucocorticoid secretion.

In human heart failure, the cardiac aldosterone production is increased and there is a relationship between this increase and the level of ventricular dysfunction (Mizuno et al., 2001). Recently, two laboratories have described an increased AS gene expression, with a relationship to cardiac fibrosis and left ventricle dysfunction, in freshly obtained ventricular biopsies from patients with heart failure (Satoh et al., 2002; Yoshimura et al., 2002). If the cellular types of synthesis are still undetermined, recent works detailed below indicate that vascular cells may be one of the primary targets of this aldosterone generated 'from the inside'.

An interesting hypothesis from Weber (2000) is to propose the existence of two different forms of ACE: a constitutive ACE bound to endothelial cells to regulate circulating concentrations of Ang II that normally contribute to circulatory homeostasis, and a recruitable form of ACE bound to myofibroblasts and macrophages that regulates local concentrations of Ang II and is involved in tissue repair. According to this hypothesis, recruitable ACE appears in the infarcted area and is responsible for elevated concentrations of Ang II and aldosterone that, in turn, would lead to fibrotic tissue. Then, recruitable Ang II and aldosterone would be linked together, as also shown by Silvestre (Silvestre et al., 1999) and would be major determinants of both scar and fibrosis of the noninfarcted area, which could be a reasonable explanation for the results of EPHESUS (Pitt et al., 2003).

The activation of aldosterone production during heart failure may have multiple origins. The first hypothesis is that such a reexpression belongs to the fetal program, in parallel to the ventricular expression of natriuretic peptides. Nevertheless, the capacity of the fetal myocardium to produce aldosterone is not documented now. Information concerning development does not support this hypothesis: (i) in mouse, the concentration of plasma aldosterone rises progressively from E17 till birth and then falls (Mitani et al., 1997); (ii) in rat, the development of the adrenal zona glomerulosa and the expression of both AS and 11-β-hydroxylase occurs in two different phases, one before E17, and another after E19 with a continuum until birth (Mitani et al., 1997; Wotus et al., 1998). The regulation of the myocardial system is the same as that of the adrenal system, the myocardial production of aldosterone being indeed sensitive to low sodium/high potassium and to Ang II, and the other hypothesis is that the activation of the myocardial aldosterone production is just a new component of the neurohormonal reaction.

References

Anand IS (1997) Pathogenesis of salt and water retention in the congestive heart failure syndrome. In *Heart Failure. Scientific Principles and Clinical Practice*, Poole-Wilson PA, Colucci WS, Massie BM, *et al.* (eds), Churchill Livingstone, New York, pp. 155–171.

Beggah AT, Escoubet B, Puttini S, *et al.* (2002) Reversible cardiac fibrosis and heart failure induced by conditional expression of an antisense mRNA of the mineralocorticoid receptor in cardiomyocytes. *Proceedings of the National Academy of Sciences of the United States of America* **99**, 7160–7165.

Benitah JP and Vassort G (1999) Aldosterone upregulates Ca^{2+} current in adult rat cardiomyocytes. *Circulation Research* **85**, 1139–1145.

Brilla CG, Pick R, Tan LB, *et al.* (1990) Remodeling of the rat right and left ventricles in experimental hypertension. *Circulation Research* **67**, 1355–1364.

Casal AJ, Silvestre JS, Delcayre C and Capponi AM (2003) Expression and modulation of the steroidogenic acute regulatory (StAR) protein mRNA in rat cardiocytes and after myocardial infarction. *Endocrinology* **144**, 1861–1868.

Delcayre C and Swynghedauw B (2002) Molecular mechanisms of myocardial remodeling. The role of aldosterone. *Journal of Molecular and Cellular Cardiology* **34**, 1577–1584.

Dell'Italia LI, Meng QC, Balcells E, *et al.* (1997) Compartimentalization of angiotensin II generation in the dog heart. Evidence for independent mechanisms in intravascular and interstitial spaces. *Journal of Clinical Investigation* **100**, 253–258.

De Mello WC (2002) Aldosterone modulates the effect of angiotensin II on the electrical properties of rat heart. *Journal of Cardiovascular Pharmacology* **40**, 90–95.

De Mello WC and Danser AH (2000) Angiotensin II and the heart: on the intracrine renin–angiotensin system. *Hypertension* **35**, 1183–1188.

Farman N and Rafestin-Oblin ME (2001) Multiple aspects of mineralocorticoid selectivity. *American Journal of Physiology. Renal Physiology* **280**, F181–F192.

Farquharson CAJ and Struthers AD (2000) Spironolactone increases nitric oxide bioactivity, improves endothelial vasodilator dysfunction, and supresses vascular angiotensin I/angiotensin II conversion in patients with chronic heart failure. *Circulation* **101**, 594–597.

Funder JW (1997) Glucocorticoid and mineralocorticoid receptors. Biology and clinical relevance. *Annual Reviews of Medicine* **448**, 231–240.

Funder JW, Pearce PT, Smith R and Smith AI (1988) Mineralocorticoid action: target tissue specificity is enzyme, not receptor, mediated. *Science* **242**, 583–585.

Gomez-Sanchez CE, Zhou MY, Cozza EN, *et al.* (1997) Aldosterone biosynthesis in the rat brain. *Endocrinology* **138**, 3369–3373.

Hatakeyama H, Miyamori I, Fujita T, *et al.* (1994) Vascular aldosterone: biosynthesis and a link to angiotensin II-induced hypertrophy of vascular smooth muscle cells. *Journal of Biology Chemistry* **269**, 24316–24320.

Horisberger JD and Rossier BC (1992) Aldosterone regulation of gene transcription leading to control of ion transport. *Hypertension* **19**, 221–227.

van Kats JP, Duncker DJ, Haitsma DB, *et al.* (2000) Angiotensin-converting enzyme inhibition and angiotensin II type 1 receptor blockade prevent cardiac remodeling in pigs after myocardial infarction: role of tissue angiotensin II. *Circulation* **102**, 1556–1563.

Lacolley P, Safar ME, Lucet B, *et al.* (2001) Prevention of aortic and cardiac fibrosis by spironolactone in old normotensive rats. *Journal of the American College of Cardiology* **37**, 662–667.

Lacolley P, Labat C, Pujol A, *et al.* (2002) Increased carotid wall elastic modulus and fibronectin in aldosterone-salt treated rats. Effects of Eplerenone. *Circulation* **106**, 2848–2853.

Malliani A (2000) *Principle of Cardiovascular Neural Regulation in Health and Disease*. Kluwer Academic Publishers, Boston.

Mitani F, Mukai K, Ogawa T, *et al.* (1997) Expression of cytochromes P450ado and P45011beta in rat adrenal gland during late gestational and neonatal stages. *Steroids* **62**, 57–61.

Mizuno Y, Yoshimura M, Yasue H, *et al.* (2001) Aldosterone production is activated in failing ventricle in humans. *Circulation* **103**, 72–77.

Nicoletti A and Michel JB (1999) Cardiac fibrosis and inflammation: interaction with hemodynamic and hormonal factors. *Cardiovascular Research* **41**, 532–543.

Pitt B (1995) 'Escape' of aldosterone production in patients with left ventricular dysfunction treated with an angiotensin converting enzyme inhibitor: implications for therapy. *Cardiovascular Drugs Therapy* **9**, 145–149.

Pitt B, Remme W, Zannad F, *et al.* (2003) Eplerenone, a selective aldosterone blocker, in patients with left ventricular dysfunction after myocardial infarction. *New England Journal of Medicine* **348**, 1309–1321.

Pitt B, Zannad F, Remme WJ, *et al.* for the Randomized Aldactone Evaluation Study Investigators (1999) The effect of spironolactone on morbidity and mortality in patients with severe heart failure. *New England Journal of Medicine* **341**, 709–717.

Ramires FJA, Mansur A, Coelho O, *et al.* (2000) Effect of spironolactone on ventricular arrythmias in congestive heart failure secondary to idiopathic dilated or to ischemic cardiomyopathy. *American Journal of Cardiology* **85**, 1207–1211.

Robert V, Thiem NV, Cheav SL, *et al.* (1994) Increased cardiac collagens (I) and (III) mRNAs in aldosterone-salt hypertension. *Hypertension* **24**, 30–36.

Robert V, Silvestre JS, Charlemagne D, *et al.* (1995) Biological determinants of aldosterone-induced cardiac fibrosis in rat. *Hypertension* **26**, 971–978.

Robert V, Besse S, Sabri A, *et al.* (1997) Differential regulation of matrix metalloproteinases associated with aging and hypertension in the rat heart. *Laboratory Investigation* **76**, 729–738.

Robert V, Heymes C, Silvestre JS, *et al.* (1999) Angiotensin AT1 receptor subtype as a cardiac target of aldosterone; role in aldosterone-salt induced fibrosis. *Hypertension* **33**, 981–986.

Rocha R and Stier CT (2001) Pathophysiological effects of aldosterone in cardiovascular tissues. *Trends in Endocrinology and Metabolism* **12**, 308–314.

Rocha R and Funder JW (2002) The pathophysiology of aldosterone in the cardiovascular system. *Annals of the New York Academy Science* **970**, 89–100.

Rocha R, Rudolph AE, Frierdich GE, et al. (2002) Aldosterone induces a vascular inflammatory phenotype in the rat heart. *American Journal of Physiology. Heart and Circulatory Physiology* **283**, H1802–H1810.

Sato A, Liu JP and Funder JW (1997) Aldosterone rapidly represses protein kinase C activity in neonatal rat cardiomyocytes *in vitro*. *Endocrinology* **138**, 3410–3416.

Satoh M, Nakamura M, Saitoh H, et al. (2002) Aldosterone synthase (CYP11B2) expression and myocardial fibrosis in the failing human heart. *Clinical Science (London)* **102**, 381–386.

Silvestre J, Heymes C, Oubenaissa A, et al. (1999) Activation of cardiac aldosterone production in rat myocardial infarction. Effect of angiotensin II receptor blockade and role in cardiac fibrosis. *Circulation* **99**, 2694–2701.

Silvestre JS, Robert V, Heymes C, et al. (1998) Myocardial production of aldosterone and corticosterone in the rat. Physiological Regulations. *Journal of Biological Chemistry* **273**, 4883–4891.

Silvestre JS, Robert V, Escoubet E, et al. (2000) Different regulation of cardiac and renal corticosteroid receptors in aldosterone-salt treated rats; effect of hypertension and glucocorticoids. *Journal of Molecular and Cellular Cardiology* **32**, 1249–1253.

Simpson SAS and Tait JF (1953) Physicochemical methods of detection of a previously unidentified adrenal hormone. *Memoirs of the Society of Endocrinologist* **2**, 9–24.

Sun Y, Zhang J, Lu L, et al. (2002) Aldosterone-induced inflammation in the rat heart. *American Journal of Pathology* **161**, 1773–1781.

Swynghedauw B (2000) Myocardial remodelling: pharmacological targets. *Expert Opinion on Investigative Drugs* **11**, 661–674.

Takeda Y, Miyamori I, Inaba S, et al. (1997) Vascular aldosterone in genetically hypertensive rats. *Hypertension* **29**, 45–48.

Takeda Y, Yoneda T, Demura M, et al. (2000) Sodium-induced cardiac aldosterone synthesis causes cardiac hypertrophy. *Endocrinology* **141**, 1901–1904.

Urata H, Boehm KD, Philip A, et al. (1993) Cellular localization and regional distribution of an angiotensin II-forming chymase in the heart. *Journal of Clinical Investigation* **91**, 1269–1281.

Virdis A, Neves MF, Amiri F, et al. (2002) Spironolactone improves angiotensin-induced vascular changes and oxidative stress. *Hypertension* **40**, 504–510.

Weber KT (2000) Recruitable ACE and tissue repair in the infarcted heart. *Journal of the Renin Angiotensin Aldosterone System* **1**, 295–303.

Weber KT (2001) Aldosterone in congestive heart failure. *New England Journal of Medicine* **345**, 1689–1697.

Wotus C, Levay-Young BK, Rogers LM, et al. (1998) Development of adrenal zonation in fetal rats defined by expression of aldosterone synthase and 11beta-hydroxylase. *Endocrinology* **139**, 4397–4403.

Young M, Head G and Funder J (1995) Determinants of cardiac fibrosis in experimental hypermineralocorticoid states. *American Journal of Physiology* **269**, E657–E662.

Zannad F, Alla F, Dousset B, et al. (2000) Limitation of excessive extracellular matrix turnover may contribute to survival benefit of spironolactone therapy in patients with congestive heart failure: insights from the Randomized Aldactone Evaluation Study (RALES). *Circulation* **102**, 2700–2706.

12

Intracellular Angiotensin and the Actions of Intracrine Hormones

Richard N. Re

Introduction

The renin angiotensin aldosterone system is an important regulator of intravascular volume and blood pressure. Over the last three decades increasing evidence has accumulated to indicate that in fact there exist angiotensin generating systems in nonrenal tissues and in cells (Re, 2001). In the early 1980s we reported the synthesis of renin in arterial smooth muscle cells and soon thereafter we and our colleagues reported, for the first time, the presence of renin in cardiac myocytes (Re et al., 1982; Dzau and Re, 1987). In 1984, based on our studies of intracellular angiotensin action, we coined the term *intracrine* for the action of a peptide or growth factor hormone within its cell of synthesis and then extended the definition to include internalized peptide hormones as well (Re and Bryan, 1984; Re, 1989). In the ensuing two decades, the notion of intracellular angiotensin action has commanded more interest and considerable investigation is ongoing to further define that action (Harris, 1999; Re, 1999). Even more impressive is the enormous growth in understanding of intracrine hormone action in general and the growing appreciation of the widely varying nature of such factors. The study of intracrine action has expanded from the study of established growth factors and hormones such as neural growth factor, platelet-derived growth factor (PDGF), epidermal growth factor, insulin and angiotensin to include homeodomain transcription factors and even metabolic enzymes (Bouche et al., 1987; Rakowicz-Szulczynska and Koprowski, 1989; Re, 1989, 2002a, b, 2003a, b; Morel, 1994; Rakowicz-Szulczynska, 1994). This expanded view of intracrine action provides new insights into the nature and functions of signaling molecules.

Intracrine angiotensin

As early as 1971 it had been shown that when injected into the circulation of the rat tritiated angiotensin localized to the nuclei and mitochondria of cardiac cells (Robertson and Khairallah, 1971; Re, 2003a). It was similarly shown that isolated mitochondria possessed angiotensin receptors. Our group later demonstrated high affinity, specific angiotensin II receptors on hepatic nuclei and further demonstrated angiotensin binding to chromatin. In addition we showed an up-regulation of transcription following angiotensin binding to isolated nuclei and demonstrated that this binding was also associated with enhanced susceptibility of chromatin to nuclease as would be expected if angiotensin binding produced altered chromatin conformation in advance of the stimulation of transcription. Angiotensin was shown to enhance the solubility to nuclease of its own chromatin receptor and a DNP particle which specifically bound angiotensin was isolated from solubilized chromatin (Re, 1999, 2000, 2002a, b, 2003a, b). Collectively, these observations strongly suggested an intracellular physiologic role for Ang II on gene transcription. Subsequently, others demonstrated that nuclear angiotensin receptors were AT_1-like in that they were blocked by losartan (Re, 2003a). Several years later the existence of both nuclear membrane and chromatin angiotensin binding sites was confirmed in studies of isolated nuclei and binding of angiotensin to those receptors was associated with up-regulation of renin, angiotensinogen and PDGF gene expression (Eggena et al., 1996). Others performed electron microscopic studies using colloidal gold-tagged anti-angiotensin antibody to demonstrate angiotensin associated with transcriptionally active euchromatin in the nuclei of hepatic, adrenal and cerebellar cells (Erdmann et al., 1996). Recently, confocal microscopy has revealed the trafficking of AT_1 receptor green fluorescent protein fusions from cell membrane to nucleus following exposure of cells to angiotensin thereby supporting the notion that angiotensin traffics from the cell surface to nucleus (Chen et al., 2000).

In addition to trafficking to nucleus and regulating transcription, other actions have been suggested for intracellular Ang II. For example, instillation of renin or angiotensin in cardiac cells alters intracellular calcium concentrations, ion fluxes, and intercellular conduction, suggesting action at intracellular calcium channels (De Mello, 1995, 2001; Haller et al., 1999; De Mello and Danser, 2000; Eto et al., 2002). It is also likely that angiotensin acts at the mitochondrion. Following nephrectomy, renin immunoreactivity accumulates in mitochondria, and angiotensin receptors have been reported to be present on isolated mitochondria. In rodents this mitochondrial renin increases after nephrectomy and appears to support the synthesis of aldosterone in these animals (Peters et al., 1999). Of note is the fact that several groups have recently reported the existence of a renin transcript that does not encode a secretory signal peptide (Lee-Kirsch et al., 1999; Clausmeyer et al., 2000; Sinn and Sigmund, 2000). This renin, known as renin exon 1A, is therefore expected to not be secreted but rather to remain in the cell. Based on the expected sequence of renin 1A it is also expected to be synthesized as an active renin rather than as a prorenin. Finally, there is evidence to suggest that renin exon 1A can traffick to mitochondria (Clausmeyer et al., 2000). Thus the adrenal appears to synthesize both full-length secreted prorenin as well as renin exon 1A which likely is retained in the cell where it regulates steroidogenesis. Interestingly, renin 1A is the only renin transcript detected in rodent left ventricle and it, rather than secreted renin, is up-regulated following infarction (Clausmeyer et al., 2000).

In nephrectomized rats maintained on dialysis, adrenal renin is up-regulated and renin granules appear in mitochondria. Aldosterone secretion is maintained. Of note, however, the administration of angiotensin to the animals actually results in a diminution of aldosterone production, likely because the action of angiotensin to suppress adrenal renin synthesis is greater than its direct stimulation of aldosterone. In addition, the angiotensin AT_1 receptor blocker losartan suppresses aldosterone secretion in this model, raising the possibility that it blocks the intracellular action of angiotensin (Peters et al., 1999). Taken with studies demonstrating that the introduction of renin into cardiac myocytes can alter junctional conductance through a mechanism inhibitable by angiotensin converting enzyme inhibition, this observation supports the contention that intracellular renin angiotensin systems exist in some cells (Re and Bryan, 1984). To be sure there is good evidence to suggest such intracellular angiotensin synthesis in the juxtaglomerular cells of the kidney, but the generation of the peptide in other cell types has been questioned (Mercure et al., 1998). The preponderance of evidence, however, supports both the internalization and the intracellular synthesis of angiotensin in specific cases

(De Mello, 1995; Pierzchalski et al., 1997; Peters et al., 1999, 2002; Re, 2001).

Recently, our group addressed the issue of intracellular angiotensin action by stably transfecting rat hepatoma cells with an angiotensinogen gene construct lacking the sequence which encodes the secretion signal sequence (Cook et al., 2001, 2002). The angiotensinogen produced in this way was expected to remain intracellular. Indeed, we were able to show in subsequent studies employing angiotensinogen–green fluorescent protein fusion constructs, that while native angiotensinogen is rapidly secreted from the cell, the protein synthesized from the experimental construct remains intracellular (Cook et al., 2002). Because the cells expressed renin and angiotensin-converting enzyme, we suspected the cells would produce intracellular Ang II driven by the expression of the angiotensinogen construct. Indeed, we could show that the cellular content of angiotensin was elevated in transfected cells (Cook et al., 2002). Moreover, the cells proliferated more rapidly than did untransfected cells or cells transfected with a scrambled control construct. In order to assess the locus of angiotensin action transfected cells were treated with the angiotensin AT_1 blocker losartan. Unexpectedly, losartan reduced the proliferation of the cells to control levels, suggesting that the angiotensin produced by the cells was working at extracellular receptors rather than at an intracellular site. However, in reviewing the literature we were impressed that in spite of assertions to the effect that nonpeptide angiotensin receptor blockers are not internalized, the data were also consistent with a low but definite rate of losartan internalization. We therefore tested the insurmountable AT_1 receptor blocker candesartan CV11971. Not only did candesartan not reduce the proliferation of transfected cells, pretreatment of the cells with candesartan eliminated the ability of losartan to inhibit proliferation, consistent with the idea that losartan is acting in the cells after internalization via the AT_1 receptor (which once bound to candesartan could not internalize and was not available for losartan internalization). In order to further investigate this possibility we treated the cells with phenylarsine oxide, an agent known to inhibit receptor internalization. This agent also blocked the inhibitory effect of losartan (Cook et al., 2001). This again was consistent with an intracellular locus of losartan action and is consistent with the data supporting an intracellular action of losartan in the rodent adrenal (Peters et al., 1999).

Also of note was the observation that PDGF A was up-regulated in transfected cells and in particular, expression of the long form of PDGF was increased. This is consistent with earlier studies demonstrating that angiotensin up-regulates PDGF transcription in isolated nuclei. In addition, although the administration of excess anti-angiotensin antibodies (in a concentration adequate to block the proliferative action of extracellular angiotensin on control cells) did not inhibit the growth of transfected cells, the administration of anti-PDGF antibodies did reduce proliferation by about 30 percent, suggesting that PDGF up-regulated by intracellular angiotensin acts at least in part in the extracellular space to stimulate proliferation (Cook et al., 2001). Evidence was also developed which suggested that the long form of PDGF was activated by an amidation reaction. Finally, losartan but not candesartan blocked the up-regulation of PDGF transcription (Cook et al., 2002).

Of note was the finding that antirenin antisense oligonucleotides inhibited the proliferation of transfected cells, confirming that the proliferation resulted from an activation of a renin angiotensin sytem. Moreover, we demonstrated that the renin transcript produced by these cells was the renin exon 1A transcript (Cook et al., 2001).

Collectively, these studies indicate that the transfected cells produced angiotensin which acted in the cell to stimulate PDGF transcription and proliferation. They further indicate that losartan enters cells and acts within the cellular interior whereas candesartan does not. In is noteworthy that a recent study demonstrates the robust internalization of AT_1 receptor-fluorescent fusion proteins after exposure to losartan, confirming our assumption that losartan can be internalized via an AT_1 mechanism (Merian et al., 2001).

Intracrine renin

Although somewhat controversial still, there is accumulating evidence to indicate the synthesis of renin in extrarenal tissues in health and disease (Re, 2001). In general, the quantity of locally synthesized renin is small, raising the possibility that it acts in a paracrine, autocrine or intracrine mode. In addition, receptors for renin and prorenin of various sorts have been reported. Prorenin binds to the mannose/IGF-II receptor and is internalized and activated, although it now appears likely that this represents a clearance pathway. Recently a prorenin/renin receptor has been reported that generates intracellular second messengers following prorenin binding. In addition, prorenin/renin bound to the receptor demonstrates enhanced angiotensinogen cleavage so that binding potentially results in the augmentation of angiotensin generation in the near environment of the cell surface angiotensin receptor (Nguyen et al., 1996, 2002). In addition, there is evidence from transgenic models that prorenin/renin can be internalized by a mechanism different from the mannose/IGF-II receptor and act within cardiac myocytes with the generation of angiotensin and the production of pathological changes (Peters *et al.*, 2002). These findings, coupled with earlier studies showing a biological effect associated with the intracellular intraduction of renin in cardiac myocytes, again supports the possibility that complete intracellular renin angiotensin systems exist and are functional.

Clinical implications

The clinical implications of intracrine renin and angiotensin are multiple. Clearly, if intracellular angiotensin can produce pathology or enhanced proliferation, the intracrine renin angiotensin system becomes a potential therapeutic target. If renin exon 1A is up-regulated following myocardial infarction in man, the suppression of its intracellular generation of angiotensin or the interruption of the action of that angiotensin could be clinically relevant in preventing the sequelae of infarction. Potentially important in this regard is the possibility that various angiotensin converting enzyme inhibitors and angiotensin AT_1 blockers have differential access to the intracellular sites of angiotensin generation or action. If so, tailoring therapy toward the intracrine renin angiotensin system could already be possible and further studies will be needed to test the potential clinical utility of such directed pharmaceutical intervention.

Intracrine physiology

Given the emerging evidence that angiotensin can act within cells either after internalization or retention in its cell of synthesis, one can ask if such intracrine action is common among signaling proteins and if so, whether there are any general principles of intracrine action. In approaching this issue it is helpful to precisely define *intracrine*. Here, the term will be used to mean the intracellular action of a peptide hormone or factor either after internalization or retention in its cell of synthesis. Because too little work has in general been done on the intracellular action of potential intracrines, it will, however, also here be assumed that the trafficking of a candidate intracrine to a cellular organelle not associated with secretion or degradation is *prima facie* evidence of intracellular action – that is, it is assumed that any such organelle-associated factor is biologically active. Thus even though angiotensin has been shown to exert some of its activity in the endocytic vesical after cell surface receptor binding and internalization, the endosomal localization of the peptide would not satisfy the criteria for intracrine action because the interior of the endosome is topologically extracellular space and the endosome itself can be considered part of the degratory pathway (Harris, 1999). Rather, the nuclear and mitochondrial trafficking of the hormone meet the criteria here being used. In recent years the term intracrine has been applied to a wide variety of factors other than peptides and in particular to steroid hormones. However, here the term will be used in its original meaning and applied only to peptide hormones and factors (Re and Bryan, 1984; Re, 1989). Some use intracrine to refer only to the case of a hormone acting in the cell that synthesized it – that is, the intracellular action of internalized hormone would not be included in the definition (Schuijt and Danser, 2002). However, we will again hold to the original definition, which has the advantage of allowing the term to be used in the case of a hormone that is secreted and immediately taken up to act in the cell that synthesized it. In addition, many intracrines act in both modes and it is problematic as to whether enough investigation has been done on any peptide that acts after internalization to exclude the possibility that it also is retained in cells which synthesize. But most important, many intracrines operate in both modes and there are reasons to believe this may be an important part of their biology (see below). For these reasons, the original definition of the term will be used in the following analysis (Re and Bryan, 1984; Re, 1989, 1999, 2002a, b).

Using the definition of intracrine above, a wide variety of hormones and growth factors can be considered to be intracrines (Table 12.1). The vast majority of these factors have been shown to localize in nucleus or nucleolus, although trafficking to mitochondria and other cytoplasmic sites also is seen (Re, 2002a, b). It is immediately apparent that, as defined, the intracrines differ widely in structure (except that they are all by definition peptide) and known function. Some such as insulin and prolactin are easily recognized hormones. Some like nerve growth factor and epidermal growth factor are growth factors. Some like interleukin are cytokines. Others, however, are not usually appreciated to be signaling molecules. For example, amphoterin, also known as high mobility group protein B1 (HMGB1), is a nontranscription factor nuclear protein which is secreted and then regulates target cell growth and maturation (Re, 2003a). Engrailed and HOXA5 are homeobox transcription factors and yet appear capable of being secreted, taken up by nearby cells and acting within those cells (Prochiantz and Theodore, 1995; Prochiantz, 1999, 2000; Re, 2003a). Even more surprising is the fact that several enzymes qualify for intracrine designation. For example,

Table 12.1 Selected intracrines

Insulin	Heregulin/neuregulins	
Leukemia inhibitory factor		
Angiotensin	Homeoproteins	Dynorphin B
FGF 1 (aFGF)	Lactoferrin	Thyrotropin releasing hormone
FGF 2 (bFGF)	Vasoactive intestinal peptide	Maspin*
FGF 3	IFN-γ, IFN-β	Renin/prorenin
Epidermal growth factor	Vascular endothelial growth factor	Leptin
Midkine	Pleiotrophin (HB-GAM)	
Neural growth factor	Parathyroid hormone-related hormone	Amphoterin (HMGB1)
Platelet-derived growth factor	Angiogenin (an RNase)	PD-ECGF
Growth hormone	Somatostatin	Transforming growth factor-α
Prolactin	Proenkephalin	IGFBP 3, 5
Interleukins	Defensins	Granzyme A, B
Insulin-like growth factor I	Factor J	Hepatopoietin
Pigmented epithelium-derived factor*	Tat	ESkine/CCL 27
Brain-derived neurotrophic factor	Schwannoma-derived growth factor	
Gonadotropin	Phospholipase A2-I	Thioredoxin
Gonadotropin releasing hormone	Macrophage colony-stimulating factor	
Hepatoma-derived growth factor	Chorionic gonadotropin	
Neuroleukin/autocrine motility factor/phosphoglucose isomerase		

FGF, Fibroblast growth factor; IFN, interferon; PD-ECGF, platelet-derived endothelial cell growth factor (thymidine phosphorylase); IGFBP, insulin-like growth factor binding proteins 3 and 5.
*A member of the serine protease inhibitor family (serpin).
From Re, 2002a, b, 2003a, b; Haga, 2000; Morel, 1994.

the tumor angiogenic factor angiogenin is an RNase and that enzymatic activity is essential for angiogenin's angiogenic action (Moroianu and Riordan, 1994; Re, 2003a, b). Phosphoglucose isomerase, also known as neuroleukin, is an important enzyme in the glycolysis pathway, but also induces differentiation in neurons. Moreover, it has also been identified as autocrine motility factor, a factor which induces motility in tumor cells (Haga et al., 2000). Thus the intracrines are structurally and functionally diverse. They frequently combine intracellular regulatory processes with extracellular signaling.

The analysis above also leads to the surprising conclusion that renin and prorenin should properly be considered intracrines. Although neither has been reported in association with nucleus, renin trafficking to mitochondria – where it presumably acts to stimulate aldosterone synthesis – has been reported (Peters *et al.*, 1999; Re, 1999). Renin and prorenin clearly are secreted by the kidney, salivary glands and likely to a lesser extent by other tissues as well (Re, 2001). Recent data indicate that renin binding to a cell-surface receptor can generate second messengers and renin internalization is associated with physiologic action (Nguyen *et al.*, 2002; Peters *et al.*, 2002). Thus renin/prorenin satisfies the criteria for intracrine functionality. It is also of note that, like many intracrines, renin appears to be synthesized in both a form destined to be retained in the cell (renin exon 1A) and a form destined for secretion (prorenin). Renin synthesis also utilizes alternative transcription start sites, alternative message processing, and the use of an internal AUG start codon, features of the action of other intracrines (Re, 2003a). Finally, like other intracrines, renin participates in intracellular interactions with other intracrines in that it appears capable in at least some cells of synthesizing the intracrine angiotensin in the cell (De Mello, 1995; Mercure *et al.*, 1998; Peters *et al.*, 2002). The realization that renin is a signaling molecule and an intracrine, along with the accumulating evidence of intracrine functionality associated with peptides and proteins not traditionally thought of as growth factors or hormones, must be considered in any attempt to develop a theory of intracrine action.

This point is further emphasized by the reports of intracrine action associated with homeodomain transcription factors and other DNA binding proteins. In the early 1990s it was found that the homeodomain transcription factor antennopedia could be internalized by target cells. It was soon shown that the homeodomain region of other homeotranscription factors was also taken up by cells. Indeed, evidence was developed to indicate that the homeotranscription factor Engrailed could be secreted via an atypical mechanism and then be taken up by cells in coculture (Prochiantz, 1999, 2000; Re, 2003a). The homeodomain transcription factor HOXA5 was similarly shown to be internalized by target cells. Moreover, a portion of the third helix of the homeodomain of antennopedia was used to form fusion proteins with other proteins of interest and was shown to transfer these fusion proteins to cytoplasm or nucleus. This then raised the possibility that homeodomain sequences could prove to be useful research tools or effective pharmaceuticals by virtue of their ability to convey active peptides into the cell. Recently it has been suggested that the internalization of homeodomain transcription factors and other DNA proteins results from membrane holes produced artifactually during fixation which permit cell surface bound factors to traffick to nucleus by virtue of their positive charge. While this phenomenon may occur, it does not explain the functional activities transferred into cells by homeodomain transcription factor fusion proteins or by fusion proteins made from other DNA or RNA binding proteins such as the herpes virus protein VP 22, the Tat protein of human immunodeficiency virus, or others (Re, 2003). Thus the preponderance of the evidence indicates that homeodomain transcription factors can be secreted by cells, be taken up by nearby cells, and then act in those cells.

Although the idea that transcription factors can act as intracrines may seem startling, this activity is mirrored in the action of plant transcription factors and of bacterial virulence factors. Plant homeotranscription factors like KNOTTED or other plant transcription factors such as LEAFY can leave one plant cell, traffick to distant cells where they are taken up, and then move to nucleus where they function. Virulence factors such as AvrXa7 are in effect injected by bacteria via the type three secretory mechanism into plant cells where they traffick to nucleus and alter host cell transcription (Re, 2002a, b, 2003a, b). This activity is similar to that of the human intracrines granzyme A and B which are secreted by T cells, enter target cells aided by perforin and then traffick to nucleolus to induce apoptosis (Jans et al., 1998; Re, 2003).

Yet another feature of intracrine action broadly defined is the fact that a large minority of known intracrines traffick not only to nucleus but also to nucleolus. Remarkably, virtually all intracrines which traffick to nucleolus are either angiogenic or anti angiogenic either directly or indirectly through the regulation of another intracrine (Re, 2003a, b). The relationship between nuclear binding and angiogenesis was first suggested by Moroianu and Riordan and remains an interesting clue to the nature and origin of intracrine action on the one hand and to the nature/regulation of angiogenesis on the other (Moroianu and Riordan, 1994). The relationship between intracrine biology and the nucleolus goes even farther. For example, the major nucleolar protein nucleolin participates in rDNA transcriptional regulation, in ribosomal synthesis, in tRNA maturation and in a variety of other functions. It also is a membrane protein which has been shown to shuttle the angiogenic intracrines midkine, pleitrophin and factor J from the external cell surface to the nucleolus. In addition, some intracrines directly interact with rRNA (Re, 2002a, b, 2003a, b). Thus, there is a close relationship between intracrine action and nucleolar function.

A theory of intracrine action

Based on the totality of the available information we proposed two hypotheses regarding the etiology and nature of intracrine functionality.

The first, the *intracrine memory hypothesis*, was based on the observation that intracellular feedback loops by which intracrines up-regulated their own synthesis, that of their signaling apparatus, or that of other intracrines are seen among intracrine hormones (Re, 1999, 2000, 2002a, b, 2003a, b). The hypothesis states that such action permits the establishment of long-lived, active feedback loops which have the effect of producing a memory in the cell of an external stimulus such as exposure to an extracellular intracrine which after internalization resets the intracellular autoregulatory feedback loop. Such loops could produce forms of memory, differentiation, or altered hormonal responsiveness. The second hypothesis, the *intracrine origin hypothesis*, states that intracrine action had its origins in mechanisms for coupling cellular trophic activities with ribosomal synthesis and function. The simultaneous establishment of self-supporting feedback loops then preserves a memory of the initial stimulus. With the advent of the metazoan organism, such intracellular regulatory factors developed the capacity to spread to nearby cells thereby permitting a wave of differentiation to spread across a tissue (Re, 2002a, b, 2003a, b). The implications of this view include the suggestion that some factors currently recognized as intracellular transcription factors also have the capacity to traffick between cells as signaling molecules – that is, some transcription factors are in fact intracrines. The observation that transcription factors, including intracrine transcription factors, form feedback loops is also consistent with the intracrine memory hypothesis, as are the important roles played by intracrines in tissue differentiation and stem cell biology (Re, 2003a). These notions and their possible implications/applications are further explored elsewhere. However, the theory of intracrine action which these hypotheses comprise suggests tests of its validity, clinical applications and new avenues for research and therapeutics.

Finally, the diversity of intracrine functions and structures suggests that metabolic/genetic regulation, cellular memory/differentiation, and intercellular signaling often evolved simultaneously in metazoans, utilizing the product of a single gene, or alternative isoforms of a single gene product, in all three roles. The co-ordinated evolution of all three functions in the same molecule could then have occurred as an intrinsic part of the evolution of intracrine genes, thus relieving the organism of the need to develop parallel mechanisms to transmit information to other sites regarding developmental or adaptive gene expression in a particular tissue. Once this view is adopted, the intracrine signaling activity of enzymes and transcription factors becomes explicable, as do the intracellular regulatory actions of signaling molecules such as peptide hormones.

References

Bouche G, Gas N, Prats H, et al. (1987) Basic fibroblast growth factor enters the nucleolus and stimulates the transcription of ribosomal genes in ABAE cells undergoing G0–G1 transition. *Proceedings of the National Academy of Science of the United States of America* **84**, 6770–6774.

Chen R, Mukhin YV, Garnovskaya MN, et al. (2000) A functional angiotensin II receptor-GFP fusion protein: evidence for agonist-dependent nuclear translocation. *American Journal of Physiology Renal Physiology* **279**, F440–F448.

Clausmeyer S, Reinecke A, Farrenkopf R, et al. (2000) Tissue-specific expression of a rat renin transcript lacking the coding sequence for the prefragment and its stimulation by myocardial infarction. *Endocrinology* **141**, 2963–2970.

Cook JL, Zhang Z and Re RN (2001) *In vitro* evidence for an intracellular site of angiotensin action. *Circulation Research* **89**, 1138–1146.

Cook JL, Giardina JF, Zhang Z and Re RN (2002) Intracellular angiotensin II increases the long isoform of PDGF in rat hepatoma cells. *Journal of Molecular and Cellular Cardiology* **34**, 1525–1537.

De Mello WC (1995) Influence of intracellular renin on heart cell communication. *Hypertension* **25**, 1172–1177.

De Mello WC (2001) Cardiac arrhythmias: the possible role of the renin angiotensin system. *Journal of Molecular Medicine* **79**, 103–108.

De Mello WC and Danser AHJ (2000) Angiotensin II and the heart: on the intracrine renin angiotensin system. *Hypertension* **35**, 1183–1188.

Dzau VJ and Re RN (1987) Evidence for the existence of renin in the heart. *Circulation* **75** (Suppl I), 1134–1136.

Eggena P, Zhu JH, Sereevinyayut S, et al. (1996) Hepatic angiotensin II nuclear receptors and transcription of growth-related factors. *Journal of Hypertension* **14**, 961–968.

Erdmann B, Fuxe K and Ganten D (1996) Subcellular localization of angiotensin II immunoreactivity in the rat cerebellar cortex. *Hypertension* **28**, 818–824.

Eto K, Ohya Y, Nakamura Y, et al. (2002) Intracellular angiotensin II stimulates voltage-operated Ca channels in arterial myocytes. *Hypertension* **39**, 474–478.

Gerber H-P, Malik AK, Solar GP, et al. (2002) VEGF regulates haematopoietic stem cell survival by an internal autocrine loop mechanism. *Nature* **417**, 954–958.

Haga A, Niinaka Y and Raz A (2000) Phosphohexose isomerase/autocrine motility factor/neuroleukin/maturation factor is a multifunctional phosphoprotein. *Biochimica et Biophysica Acta* **1480**(1–2), 235–244.

Haller H, Lidschau C, Quass P and Luft FC (1999) Intracellular actions of angiotensin II in vascular smooth muscle cells. *Journal of the American Society of Nephrology* **10** (Suppl 11), S75–S83.

Harris RC (1999) Potential mechanisms and physiologic actions of intracellular angiotensin II. *American Journal of Medical Science* **318**, 374–379.

Jans DA, Briggs LJ, Jans P, et al. (1998) Nuclear targeting of the serine protease granzyme A (fragmentin-1). *Journal of Cell Science* **111**, 2645–2654.

Lee-Kirsch MA, Gaudet F, Cardoso MC and Lindpaintner K (1999) Distinct renin isoforms generated by tissue-specific transcription initiation and alternative splicing. *Circulation Research* **84**, 240–246.

Mercure C, Ramla D, Garcia R, et al. (1998) Evidence for intracellular generation of angiotensin II in rat juxtaglomerular cells. *FEBS Letters* **422**, 395–399.

Merian AJ, Kanashiro CA, Krieger JE and Paiva ACM (2001) Ligand-induced endocytosis and nuclear localization of angiotensin II receptors expressed in CHO cells. *Brazilian Journal of Medical and Biological Research* **34**, 1175–1183.

Morel G (1994) Internalization and nuclear localization of peptide hormones. *Biochemical Pharmacology* **47**, 63–76.

Moroianu J and Riordan JF (1994) Nuclear translocation of angiogenic proteins in endothelial cells: an essential step in angiogenesis. *Biochemistry* **33**, 12535–12539.

Nguyen G, Delarue F, Berrou J, et al. (1996) Specific receptor binding of renin on human mesangial cells in culture increases plasminogen activator inhibitor-1 antigen. *Kidney International* **50**, 1897–1903.

Nguyen G, Delarue F, Burckle C, et al. (2002) Pivotal role of the renin/prorenin receptor in angiotensin II production and cellular responses to renin. *Journal of Clinical Investigation* **109**, 1417–1427.

Peters J, Obermüller N, Alexander Woyth A, et al. (1999) Losartan and angiotensin II inhibit aldosterone production in anephric rats via different actions on the intraadrenal renin–angiotensin system. *Endocrinology* **140**, 675–682.

Peters J, Farrenkopf R, Clausmeyer S, et al. (2002) Functional significance of prorenin internalization in the rat heart. *Circulation Research* **90**, 1135–1141.

Pierzchalski P, Reiss K, Cheng W, et al. (1997) p53 induces myocyte apoptosis via the activation of the renin–angiotensin system. *Experimental Cell Research* **234**, 57–65.

Prochiantz A (1999) Homeodomain-derived peptides in and out of the cells. *Annals of the New York Academy of Science* **886**, 172–179.

Prochiantz A (2000) Proteines messageres. *Journal de la Societé de Biologie* **194**, 119–123.

Prochiantz A and Theodore L (1995) Nuclear/growth factors. *Bioessays* **17**, 39–43.

Rakowicz-Szulczynska EM (1994) Chromatin receptors for growth fractors. In *Nuclear Localization of Growth Factors and of Monoclonal Antibodies*, Rakowicz-Szulcynska EM (ed), CRC Press, Boca Raton, pp. 3–102.

Rakowicz-Szulczynska EM and Koprowski H (1989) Antagonistic effect of PDGF and NGF on transcription of ribosomal DNA and tumor cell proliferation. *Biochemical and Biophysical Research Communications* **163**, 649–656.

Re RN (1982) The nature of intracrine peptide hormone action. *Hypertension* **34**, 534–538.

Re RN (1989) The cellular biology of angiotensin: paracrine, autocrine and intracrine actions in cardiovascular tissues. *Journal of Molecular and Cellular Cardiology* **21** (Suppl 5), 63–69.

Re RN (1999) The nature of intracrine peptide hormone action. *Hypertension* **34**, 534–538.

Re RN (2000) On the biological actions of intracellular angiotensin. *Hypertension* **35**, 1189–1190.

Re RN (2001) The clinical implication of tissue renin angiotensin systems. *Current Opinion in Cardiology* **16**, 317–327.

Re RN (2002a) The origins of intracrine hormone action. *American Journal of Medical Science*, **323**, 43–48.

Re RN (2002b) Toward a theory of intracrine hormone action. *Regulatory Peptides* **106**, 1–6.

Re RN (2003a) The intracrine hypothesis and intracellular peptide hormone action. *Bioessays* **25**, 401–409.

Re RN (2003b) The implications of intracrine hormone action for physiology and medicine. *American Journal of Physiology* **284**, H751–H757.

Re RN and Bryan SE (1984) Functional intracellular renin–angiotensin systems may exist in multiple tissues. *Clinical and Experimental Hypertension, Part A, Theory and Practice* **A6** (Suppl 10 & 11), 1739–1742.

Re RN, Fallon TJ, Dzau VS, *et al.* (1982) Renin synthesis by cultured arterial smooth muscle cells. *Life Sciences* **30**, 99–106.

Robertson AL and Khairallah PA (1971) Angiotensin: rapid localization in nuclei of smooth and cardiac muscle. *Science* **172**, 1138–1140.

Sinn PL and Sigmund CD (2000) Identification of three human renin mRNA isoforms from alternative tissue-specific transcriptional initiation. *Physiological Genomics* **3**, 25–31.

Schuijt MP and Danser AH (2002) Cardiac angiotensin II: and intracrine hormone? *American Journal of Hypertension* **15**, 1109–1116.

13

Angiotensin II and Myocardial Fibrosis, Clinical Implications

Begoña López, Arantxa González and Javier Díez

Introduction

In response to mechanical and/or metabolic stress the heart undergoes structural remodeling involving cardiomyocyte hypertrophy and myocardial fibrosis. Cardiomyocyte hypertrophy includes an increase in contractile and embryonic protein content, which appears largely on the activation of transcription of the corresponding cardiac genes that encode these proteins (Hunter *et al.*, 1999). Myocardial fibrosis is the result of the exaggerated deposition of collagen types I and III fibers as a consequence of the predominance of the synthesis over the degradation of collagen types I and III molecules (Weber, 1997a). Cardiac remodeling is accompanied by a progressive decline in cardiac function over time, which underlies the pathogenesis of heart failure in patients with chronic cardiac conditions (Cohn *et al.*, 2000).

It is now accepted that a number of systemic and locally expressed factors have key roles in the process of cardiac remodeling (Swynghedauw, 1999). One of these factors is angiotensin II (Ang II). Whereas the role of Ang II in cardiomyocyte hypertrophy is well established and has been recently reviewed (Lijnen and Petrov, 1999; Yamazaki *et al.*, 1999), emerging evidence is providing support for the notion that this peptide induces myocardial fibrosis. Thus, this chapter will focus on the review of the available information supporting the fibrotic role of Ang II in the

Renin Angiotensin System and the Heart Edited by Walmor De Mello
© 2004 by John Wiley & Sons Ltd. ISBN 0 470 86292 0

heart, mostly in the hypertensive left ventricle, as well as the potential cellular and molecular mechanisms involved. In addition, the clinical impact of myocardial fibrosis will be also considered.

General aspects of myocardial fibrosis

Collagen types I and III are the major fibrillar collagens produced by fibroblasts in the adult heart. They exhibit the characteristic triple helical conformation formed by three polypeptide chains (α chains). Fibrillar collagen of the heart provides the structural scaffolding for cardiomyocytes and coronary vessels and imparts cardiac tissue with physical properties that include stiffness and resistance to deformation (Weber, 1989). In addition, fibrillar collagen may also act as a link between contractile element of adjacent cardiomyocytes and as a conduit of information that is necessary for cell function.

As in other organs, collagen turnover of normal adult heart results from the equilibrium between the synthesis and degradation of collagen types I and III molecules (Burlew and Weber, 2000). The synthesis of collagen molecules follows the normal pattern of protein synthesis, but it differs from the synthesis of many proteins in that the newly formed α chains undergo a number of postranslational modifications. On the other hand, extracellular degradation of collagen fibers is mediated by collagenase and other members of the matrix metalloproteinase (MMP) family of zinc-containing endoproteinases. The active form of collagenase can be inhibited by interaction with naturally occurring specific tissue inhibitors of MMPs (TIMPs).

A number of factors have been described that may alter the balance of fibrillar collagen in favor of either the synthesis or the degradation (Table 13.1) (Burlew and Weber, 2000). Predominance of synthesis over degradation leads to increased interstitial and perivascular deposition of collagen types I and III or fibrosis that accompanies cardiac diseases such as hypertensive heart disease (Figure 13.1), ischemic cardiomyopathy, diabetic cardiomyopathy, and hypertrophic cardiomyopathy.

Several arguments support the concept that myocardial fibrosis has a particularly important influence in the process of heart failure associated with cardiac remodeling, namely in hypertensive heart disease (HHD) (Diez et al., 2001b). First, interstitial fibrosis contributes to ventricular wall stiffness and consequently impairs cardiac compliance, contributing to impaired diastolic function. Second, because neither the collagen network nor the fibroblasts contribute to systolic contraction, increased collagen deposition and fibroblast volume means that

Table 13.1 Factors involved in myocardial fibrosis

Profibrotic factors
Vasoactive substances
  Ang II, endothelin-1, catecholamines
Growth factors
  Transforming growth factor-β1, platelet-derived growth factor, basic fibroblast growth factor, insulin-like growth factor-1
Hormones
  Aldosterone, deoxycorticosterone
Cytokines
  Interleukin-1
Adhesion molecules
  Osteopontin

Antifibrotic factors
Vasoactive substances
  Bradykinin, prostaglandins, nitric oxide, natriuretic peptides
Growth factors
  Hepatocyte growth factor
Hormones
  Glucocorticoids
Cytokines
  Tumor necrosis factor-α, interferon-γ
Endogenous peptides
  N-Acetyl-seryl-aspartyl-lysyl-proline (Ac-SDKP)

systolic work is being performed by a smaller proportion of the cardiac mass, contributing to systolic dysfunction. Third, perivascular fibrosis leads to increased distance that oxygen must diffuse and therefore potentially lowers PaO_2 for the working cardiomyocytes. Finally, electrical coupling on the cardiomyocytes may be impaired by the accumulation of collagen proteins and fibroblasts since such accumulation causes morphologic separation of cardiomyocytes.

Role of Ang II in myocardial fibrosis

The observation that myocardial fibrosis is present not only in the left ventricle but also in the right ventricle and the interventricular septum of animals and patients with arterial hypertension suggests that besides hypertension, some systemically and/or locally produced humoral factor may also contribute to hypertensive myocardial fibrosis. Various lines of evidence support a role for Ang II as one potential candidate factor (González et al., 2002).

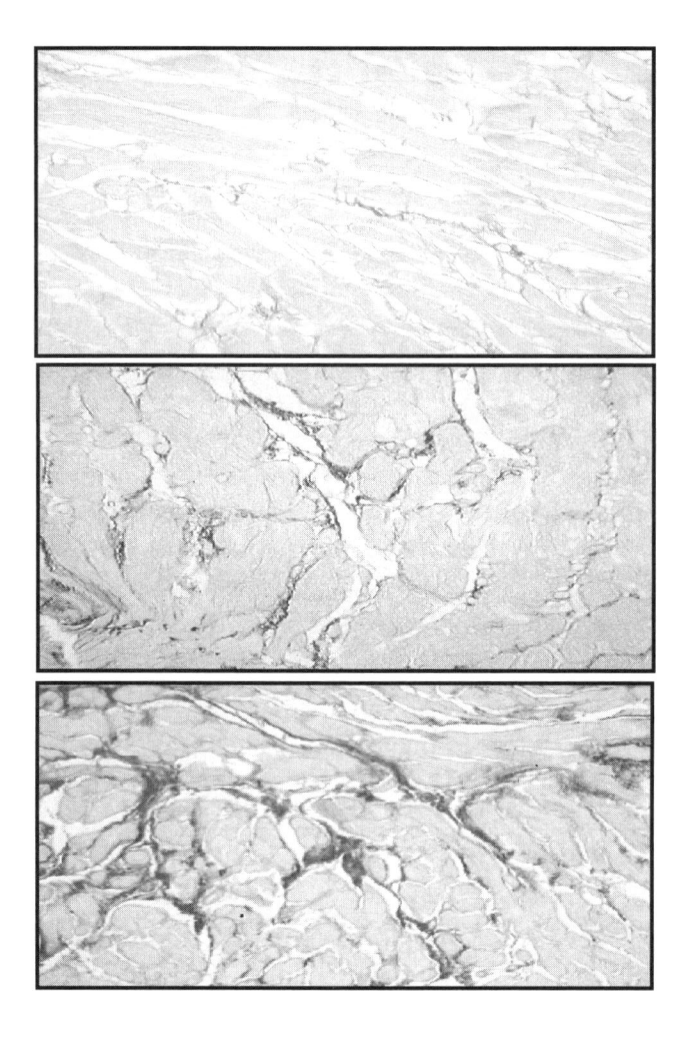

Figure 13.1 Histological sections of interventricular septal specimen biopsies from a normotensive subject (upper panel), a hypertensive patient with left ventricular hypertrophy (middle panel) and a hypertensive patient with heart failure (lower panel). Sections were stained with picrosirius red, and the interstitial collagen was identified in red. (Magnification ×20.) A colour reproduction of this figure can be found in the color plate section

In vivo evidence

Animal models

Endogenous elevations in circulating Ang II that accompany unilateral renal artery stenosis (Sun *et al.*, 1997) or the infusion of exogenous

Ang II (Jalil et al., 1991) are associated with increased blood pressure and fibrosis. The appearance of such fibrous tissue formation is preceded by increased expression of Ang II type 1 (AT$_1$) receptors, transforming growth factor-β1 (TGF-β1), and mRNA for collagen types I and III (Everett et al., 1994). In addition, development of fibrosis involves proliferating fibroblasts and cell differentiation into myofibroblasts (Campbell et al., 1995). Two observations suggest that the ability of Ang II to induce cardiac fibrosis in these models is independent of its hypertensive action. First, fibrosis in the renal artery stenosis model develops in both low-pressure right and left atria and right ventricle and high-pressure left ventricle (Brilla et al., 1993). Second, cardiac fibrosis in the Ang II infusion model can be prevented by either angiotensin-converting enzyme (ACE) inhibitors or AT$_1$ receptor antagonists, but not hydralazine or prazosin, despite a similar antihypertensive efficacy of these compounds (Crawford et al., 1994; Kim et al., 1995). The critical role of Ang II in hypertension-associated cardiac fibrosis is further supported by the observation that experimental infrarenal aortic binding, which does not induce Ang II, causes blood pressure elevation and cardiomyocyte hypertrophy but not cardiac fibrosis (Brilla et al., 1993).

The hypertensive ren2 rat provides a well-established model of Ang II-dependent cardiac hypertrophy (Lee et al., 1996). Several studies have revealed that interstitial and perivascular fibrosis, along with extensive collagen types I and III deposition are present in ren2 rats (Bishop et al., 2000; Pinto et al., 2000; Rothermund et al., 2002). Increased cardiac renin and Ang II levels have been described in this transgenic rat model (Lee et al., 1996). In addition, cardiac lesions are very sensitive to ACE inhibition and AT$_1$ receptor antagonism in ren2 rats (Teisman et al., 1998). As a result, the development of hypertrophy and fibrosis in the heart of these animals has been attributed, at least partially, to a local activation of the cardiac renin angiotensin system.

Pharmacological studies

Experimental findings

Pharmacological interventions with ACE inhibitors or AT$_1$ receptor antagonists have underscored the potential importance of Ang II in the mediation of cardiac fibrosis in pathologic conditions such as primary hypertension. In rats with spontaneous hypertension (SHR) and left ventricular hypertrophy myocardial fibrosis has been shown to regress by treatment with the ACE inhibitor lisinopril (Brilla et al., 1991). This effect occurred independently of the drug's antihypertensive effect (Brilla et al., 1991). On the other hand, it has been found that chronic AT_1 receptor antagonism with losartan resulted in reversal of fibrosis (as assessed by the measurement of myocardial collagen volume fraction or CVF), inhibition of the post-transcriptional synthesis of procollagen type I, inhibition of TIMP-1 expression and stimulation of collagenase activity in the left ventricle of adult SHR (Varo et al., 1999, 2000). Analysis of the individual data showed that the intensity of these myocardial changes was independent of the antihypertensive efficacy of the drug SHR (Varo et al., 1999, 2000).

Clinical findings

The fibrogenic role of Ang II in humans has been investigated in three recent prospective trials of limited size using biopsy-proven myocardial fibrosis in patients with essential hypertension and HHD. Schwartzkopff et al. (2000) studied 14 patients before and after 1 year of treatment with the ACE inhibitor perindopril. Structural analysis revealed diminution of perivascular and interstitial fibrosis with treatment. The observed regression of fibrosis on ACE inhibitor treatment was observed in the nonpressure-overloaded right ventricle, indicating that the antifibrotic effect was not accounted for by left ventricular pressure reduction alone. Brilla et al. (2000) randomized 35 previously treated patients with controlled blood pressure to receive either the ACE inhibitor lisinopril or the diuretic hydrochlorothiazide for 6 months. Only patients randomized to lisinopril had a significant reduction in myocardial fibrosis. Blood pressure reduction was similar in patients treated with either lisinopril or hydrochlorothiazide. Finally, López et al. (2001a) studied 37 treated patients with uncontrolled blood pressure. After randomization, 21 patients were assigned to the AT_1 receptor antagonist losartan and 16 to the calcium channel blocker amlodipine for 12 months. Whereas myocardial fibrosis decreased significantly in losartan-treated patients, this parameter remained unchanged in amlodipine-treated patients. A similar reduction of blood pressure in losartan-treated patients than in amlodipine-treated patients was reported in this study. Collectively, these observations support the concept that in addition to pressure overload, Ang II induces myocardial fibrosis in essential hypertension.

Cellular and molecular mechanisms

Increasing evidence strongly indicates that Ang II exerts multiple profibrotic effects within the heart including induction of fibroblast hyperplasia, activation of collagen biosynthetic pathways and inhibition of collagen degradative pathways. In addition, available data indicates that these effects may result from either the direct action of Ang II or a synergistic co-operation between this peptide and other profibrotic factors (Figure 13.2).

Stimulation of fibroblast proliferation

In vitro studies of rat and human cardiac fibroblasts have shown that Ang II stimulates cell proliferation via the AT_1 receptor (Sadoshima and Izumo, 1993). Results in the literature indicate that the proliferative response of fibroblasts to Ang II might well be mediated by stimulation of the synthesis of growth or inflammatory substances like platelet-derived growth factor (PDGF) and cytokines, by integrin activation due to adhesion proteins or by a combination of these mechanisms (Schnee and Hsueh, 2000; Bouzegrhane and Thibault, 2002).

For instance, Ang II strongly upregulates the expression of osteopontin and its ligand αVβ3 integrin in rat and human cardiac fibroblasts (Ashizawa *et al.*, 1996; Graf *et al.*, 2000). Interestingly, elevated left ventricular osteopontin expression has been reported in the ren2 rat model characterized by high myocardial Ang II concentrations (Rothermund *et al.*, 2002). Monoclonal antibodies directed against either osteopontin or αVβ3 completely blocked the mitogenic effect of Ang II on cultured rat

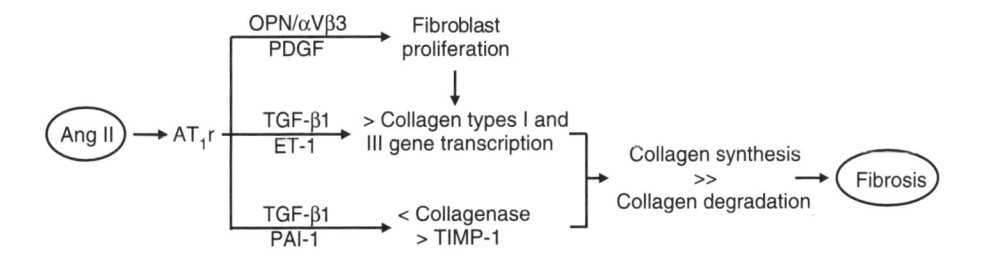

Figure 13.2 Angiotensin II (Ang II) type 1 receptor (AT_1r)-mediated effects of Ang II on fibrillar collagen metabolism in cardiac fibroblasts. Cofactors of these effects are: OPN, osteopontin; αVβ3, integrin αVβ3; TGF-β1, transforming growth factor-β1; ET-1, endothelin-1; PAI-1, plasminogen activator inhibitor-1. (TIMP-1, tissue inhibitor of matrix metalloproteinase-1.)

cardiac fibroblasts (Ashizawa et al., 1996), thus suggesting that osteopontin mediates Ang II-induced fibroblast proliferation acting via an integrin-dependent pathway.

Stimulation of collagen synthesis

Although different signaling pathways of the AT_1 receptor may subserve direct Ang II-induced collagen synthesis in cardiac fibroblasts (Dostal et al., 1996), recent data suggest that the MAP/ER kinase pathway appears to play a major role (Tharaux et al., 2000). The end result of signaling mechanisms is activation of transcription factors which bind to various 'cis-acting' elements in the regulatory sequences of $\alpha 1$ and $\alpha 2$ collagen type I and $\alpha 1$ collagen type III genes (Ghiggeri et al., 2000; Tharaux et al., 2000). This, in turn, will couple with gene expression and the synthesis of collagen types I and III precursor molecules (Villarreal et al., 1993; Crabos et al., 1994).

On the other hand, a number of studies provide strong evidence that Ang II indirectly regulates collagen synthesis by cardiac fibroblasts via specific growth factors (Dostal, 2001). The principal candidates include TGF-β1 and endothelin-1.

In fact, Ang II has been shown to induce collagen type I gene expression via activation of TGF-β1 signaling pathways (e.g., connective tissue growth factor – CTGF – and Smad proteins) and these effects were blocked by the AT_1 receptor antagonist losartan (Hao et al., 2000). Ang II has been also shown to increase the expression of TGF-β1 in cultured cardiac fibroblasts via stimulation of the AT_1 receptor (Sadoshima and Izumo, 1993). Recent data suggest that a Krüppel-like zinc-finger transcription factor 5 (KLF5; also known as BTEB2 and IKLF) is critically involved in Ang II-induced TGF-β1 expression, collagen synthesis and development of cardiac fibrosis (Shindo et al., 2002). Besides upregulation of cardiac gene TGF-β1 expression, Ang II has been reported to convert latent TGF-β1 to the active protein *in vivo* in the heart (Tomita et al., 1998).

Endothelin-1 is synthesized and released by cardiac fibroblasts in response to the interaction of Ang II with the AT_1 receptor (Gray et al., 1998) and has been shown to stimulate the synthesis of collagen types I and III in these cells (Guarda et al., 1993). In several rat models of arterial hypertension, blockade of endothelin receptors is associated with decrease in left ventricular collagen accumulation (Ammarguellat et al., 2001; Yamamoto et al., 2002).

There is some *in vivo* evidence that Ang II also influences post-translational processing of cardiac fibrillar collagen. It has been shown that

Ang II infusion is associated with stimulation of prolyl-4-hydroxylase (an enzyme that mediates hydroxylation of procollagen α-chains in the endoplasmic reticulum of cardiac fibroblasts) in the rat left ventricle (Leipala et al., 1988). In addition, it has been reported that immunoreactive prolyl-4-hydroxylase concentration decreases significantly in the ventricle of post-myocardial infarction rats treated with the AT_1 receptor antagonist losartan (Ju et al., 1997).

Inhibition of collagen degradation

In addition to collagen synthesis, Ang II stimulation of the AT_1 receptor has been shown to regulate collagen degradation by attenuating interstitial collagenase activity in adult rat (Sadoshima and Izumo, 1993) and human (Funck et al., 1997) cardiac fibroblasts and by enhancing TIMP-1 production in rat heart endothelial cells (Chua et al., 1996).

A number of factors may mediate the inhibitory effect of Ang II on cardiac collagen degradation (e.g., TGF-β1 and plasminogen activator inhibitor-1, PAI-1). Cell culture studies on human fibroblasts show that exposure of these cells to TGF-β1 in the presence of other growth factors (e.g., epidermal growth factor and basic fibroblastic growth factor) resulted in downregulation of collagenase and upregulation of TIMP-1 (Edwards et al., 1987; Chua et al., 1991). Similar findings have been reported in the fibrotic myocardium of TGF-β1 transgenic mice (Seeland et al., 2002).

Activation of the AT_1 receptor in human cardiac fibroblasts has been shown to promote stimulation of PAI-1 expression (Kawano et al., 2000). This stimulatory effect has been confirmed in the left ventricle of Ang II-induced hypertensive rats (Kobayashi et al., 2002). PAI-1 inhibits the activation of collagenase and other matrix metalloproteinases and thereby collagen degradation (Dollery et al., 1995; Yamamoto and Saito, 1998).

Alteration of collagen type I turnover

Fibrillar collagen type I is synthesized in the fibroblasts as procollagen type I containing an amino-terminal and a carboxy-terminal propeptide (Nimmi, 1993). After procollagen type I has been secreted into the extracellular space, the propeptides are removed by specific proteinases, allowing integration of the rigid collagen triple helix into the growing fibril (Nimmi, 1993).

The 100-kDa procollagen type I carboxy-terminal propeptide (PIP) is cleaved from procollagen type I during the synthesis of fibril-forming collagen type I and is released into the bloodstream (Smedsrod et al., 1990). A stoichiometric ratio of 1:1 exists between the number of collagen type I molecules produced and that of PIP released. Circulating PIP is cleared from the blood by the liver (Smedsrod et al., 1990). Several clinical observations have demonstrated that high serum levels of the propeptide measured by specific radioimmunoassay reflect continuous tissue fibrosis (Risteli and Risteli, 1990). Therefore, the serum concentration of PIP can be considered as a useful marker of collagen type I synthesis in conditions of preserved liver function.

The rate-limiting step in the degradation of collagen type I fibrils is catalytic cleavage by interstitial collagenase (Janicki, 1995). The resulting 36-kDa and 12-kDa telopeptides maintain their helical structure and are resistant to further proteolytic degradation. The small 12-kDa pyridoline cross-linked C-terminal telopeptide resulting from the cleavage of collagen type I (CITP) is found in an immunochemically intact form in blood, where it appears to be derived from tissues with a stoichiometric ratio of 1:1 between the number of collagen molecules degraded and that of CITP released (Risteli et al., 1993). CITP appears to be cleared from the circulation via glomerular filtration (Risteli et al., 1993). In recent clinical studies, serum concentrations of CITP measured by radioimmunoassay were found to be related to the intensity of the degradation of collagen type I fibrils (Risteli and Risteli, 1990). Therefore, the serum concentration of this peptide can be considered as a useful marker of collagen type I degradation in conditions of normal renal function.

In accordance with that we have proposed that the measurement of serum PIP and CITP may provide indirect information on the potential influence of a number of factors (e.g., Ang II) on collagen type I turnover *in vivo* (López et al., 2001b). In this regard, we have reported that serum PIP and CITP concentrations are abnormally increased and decreased, respectively in SHR (Díez et al., 1996; Varo et al., 1999, 2000) and hypertensive patients (Díez et al., 1995; Laviades et al., 1998, 2000; Querejeta et al., 2000) with HHD. These findings have been confirmed recently by other groups (Camilión de Hurtado et al., 2002; Lindsay et al., 2002; Cingolani et al., 2003; Muiesan et al., 2003). In addition, we found that serum PIP concentrations correlated directly with CVF in SHR (Díez et al., 1996) and patients (Querejeta et al., 2000) with HHD.

In a number of recent studies we observed that a strong association exists between treatment-induced changes in myocardial fibrosis and the balance between PIP and CITP in SHR (Díez et al., 1996; Varo et al., 1999, 2000) and hypertensive patients (López et al., 2001; Díez et al., 2002). In fact, chronic administration of either lisinopril or losartan was accompanied by a simultaneous decrease in CVF and the ratio PIP:CITP in treated SHR and hypertensive patients. Interestingly, this association was independent of the antihypertensive efficacy of the two drugs. Thus, Ang II may play a major role in alterations of collagen type I turnover leading to myocardial fibrosis in arterial hypertension.

Clinical consequences

As mentioned before, myocardial fibrosis predisposes to ventricular dysfunction, diminished coronary reserve and ventricular arrhythmias, which, in turn, confer increased risk of adverse cardiovascular events to patients with HHD (Figure 13.3). Some observations suggest that the fibrogenic role of Ang II may possess clinical impact in HHD.

Ventricular dysfunction

Myocardial tissue exhibits a resistance to stretch (i.e., stiffness) during diastole. It includes postcontraction relengthening of tissue during the

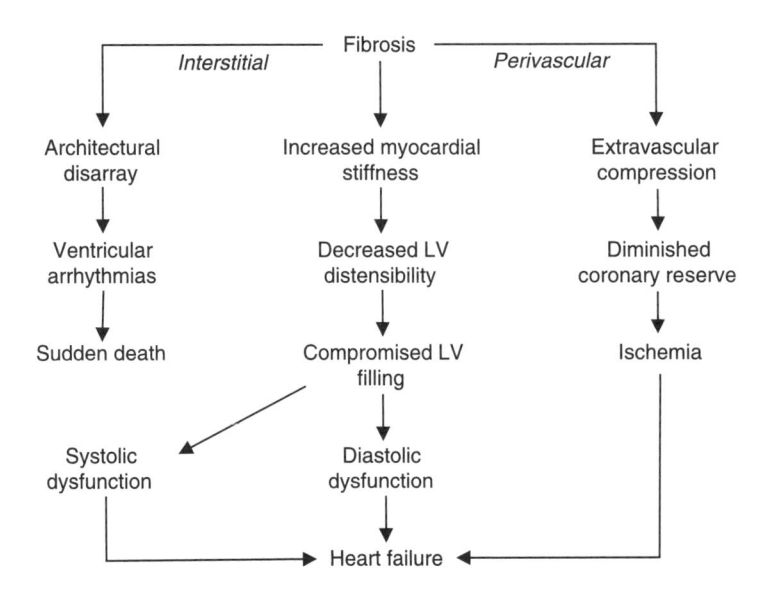

Figure 13.3 Proposed detrimental consequences of myocardial fibrosis on the heart of patients with arterial hypertension. (LV, left ventricle.)

isovolumic relaxation period and stretching of tissue during rapid filling and following atrial contraction (Weber, 1997b). Furthermore, dynamic elastance of tissue is present during contraction (Weber, 1997b).

Various clinical and experimental studies have demonstrated the importance of fibrosis on tissue stiffness. As reviewed elsewhere (Weber et al., 1993), these studies addressed: (i) the presence of fibrosis in the hypertrophied ventricle with abnormal stiffness; (ii) the importance of fibrosis to abnormal myocardial stiffness, with or without cardiomyocyte hypertrophy; (iii) the prevention of fibrosis to preserve normal tissue stiffness; and (iv) regression of fibrosis, which would normalize tissue stiffness in either hypertrophied or nonhypertrophied ventricles. Thus, the following broad statements have been made (Weber, 2000): a two- to threefold increase in CVF adversely influences diastolic stiffness (or diastolic dysfunction) whereas systolic stiffness is preserved, and a fourfold or more rise in CVF is associated with a further rise in diastolic stiffness and a decline in systolic stiffness (or systolic dysfunction).

This statement is supported by several clinical findings. Sugihara et al. (1988) and Ohsato et al. (1992) reported that CVF was the most significant factor related to diastolic dysfunction, as assessed by Doppler echocardiography measurements, in hypertensive patients. Furthermore, López et al. (2001) found that an inverse correlation exists between CVF and Doppler mitral A wave deceleration time (DT), an index of left ventricular distensibility (European Study Group on Diastolic Heart Failure, 1998), in hypertensives. Finally, an inverse relation has been found between left ventricular ejection fraction and CVF in hypertensive patients (McLenachan and Dargie, 1990). Furthermore, in the same study systolic function was reported to be preserved when moderate amounts of fibrosis (CVF of 5 to 10 percent) was present, but declined when fibrosis became more severe (McLenachan and Dargie, 1990).

Some epidemiological and clinical considerations strength the potential relevance of these relationships. Diastolic heart failure accounts for 30 to 50 percent of congestive heart failure in clinical practice, and HHD is the major cause of this type of heart failure (Vasan et al., 1999). Exercise-induced systolic dysfunction in hypertensive patients with HHD has been found to arise predominantly from impaired diastolic filling, leading to inadequate augmentation of end-diastolic filling during exercise to maintain systolic function (Cuocolo et al., 1990). Recent findings in patients with hypertensive pulmonary edema and a normal left ventricular ejection fraction after treatment indicate a high probability that the pulmonary congestion was due to isolated, transient diastolic dysfunction with increases in both left ventricular end-diastolic pressure and left atrial pressure (Ghandi et al., 2001).

Recently, Brilla et al. (2000) reported that diminution of CVF after chronic treatment with the ACE inhibitor lisinopril was accompanied by improved left ventricular diastolic dysfunction in patients with essential hypertension. On the other hand, Díez et al. (2002) have reported that chronic AT_1 blockade with losartan is associated with diminution of both myocardial collagen content and left ventricular chamber stiffness in patients with essential hypertension. Interestingly, in the two studies was found that the ability of either lisinopril or losartan to improve both mechanics and diastolic performance of the left ventricle was independent of LVH regression and the efficacy of lowering blood pressure. Therefore, these findings point out to the potential relevance of Ang II in fibrosis-related diastolic dysfunction associated with arterial hypertension.

Diminished coronary reserve

It is increasingly recognized that patients with HHD have symptoms and signs of myocardial ischemia despite angiographically normal coronary arteries, and this was found to be related to impaired coronary flow reserve (Houghton et al., 1990). The impairment of coronary vasodilator reserve is likely to initiate a process of myocardial malperfusion and malnutrition, which can provoke functional depression of the myocardial performance, a loss of contractile proteins and an overall decrease in contractile function in long-standing HHD (Vogt and Strauer, 1995).

Functional and structural abnormalities of the coronary microcirculation have been described in HHD that may be related to impaired coronary reserve including endothelial dysfunction, thickening of the media wall with reduced lumen size and accumulation of collagen fibers in the periarteriolar region (Schwartzkopff et al., 1993). The importance of periarteriolar collagen for coronary reserve was further elucidated by Isoyama et al. (1992) in experimental hypertension. In the rat, the normalization of blood pressure after debanding of the aorta induced regression of media hypertrophy, but the normalization of coronary reserve was achieved only after the additional inhibition and reversal of collagen accumulation in the adventitia with β-aminopropionitrile. Thus, it can be assumed that the overall amount of perivascular fibrosis is a limiting factor for vascular distensibility also in patients with HHD.

Schwartzkopff et al. (1993) have demonstrated that total and perivascular CVF correlated with the increased minimal coronary resistance in hypertensives with reduced coronary flow reserve. Furthermore, the same group has demonstrated that long-term therapy with the ACE inhibitor perindopril induced a decrease of coronary resistance and improvement of coronary reserve in hypertensive patients that was associated with significant regression of periarteriolar fibrosis and slight but not significant reduction of media hypertrophy (Schwartzkopff et al., 2000). These findings emphasize the potential relevance of the profibrotic actions of Ang II in alterations of coronary reserve present in hypertensive patients.

Ventricular arrhythmias

Epidemiological surveys, such as the Framingham study (Levy et al., 1987), have shown a high incidence of ventricular arrhythmias in patients with HHD. In addition, asymptomatic arrhythmias are associated with a higher mortality rate in these patients, including sudden death.

McLenachan and Dargie (1990) analyzed possible correlates of left ventricular arrhythmias in patients with HHD. They found that patients with arrhythmias exhibited higher values of left ventricular mass and CVF than patients without arrhythmias. Ejection fraction and the frequency of coronary vessels with significant (>50 percent) stenosis were similar in the two groups of patients. Thus, the high incidence of arrhythmias in patients with HHD cannot be entirely attributed to coexistent coronary artery disease, nor to left ventricular dysfunction, but may be related to fibrosis and the adaptational phenotypic changes in membrane proteins associated with cardiomyocyte hypertrophy.

Fibrosis would create arrhythmias both by anatomical uncoupling due to myocardial heterogeneity and by a re-entry mechanism generated by the zig-zag propagation of the transverse waveform (Assayag et al., 1997). Triggered activity and automaticity would depend on the membrane phenotype of the cardiomyocyte (Assayag et al., 1997).

Some years ago we reported that treatment with the ACE inhibitor lisinopril is associated with diminution in the number of daily ventricular extrasystoles and decrease in the concentrations of PIP in hypertensive patients with HHD (Díez et al., 1995). Whether this means that the blockade of the profibrotic actions of Ang II is involved in the antiarrhytmic properties of ACE inhibitors in hypertensive patients (Díez et al., 2001a) deserves further studies.

Therapeutic implications

Reparation of pathological remodeling in cardiac diseases is a concept based on specifically targeting such remodeling with a pharmacological intervention that will intend to promote the regression of, and perhaps even normalize, abnormalities in tissue structure, thereby improving or even correcting associated functional derangements (Weber, 2000).

In HHD, this concept focuses on a regression of fibrosis and reduction of the associated risk of cardiovascular events. A cardioreparative agent should counteract the disproportionate balance that exists between factors that stimulate and factors that inhibit turnover of collagen types I and type III molecules. In accordance with this, those antihypertensive agents with cardioreparative properties include ACE inhibitors, AT_1 receptor antagonists, antagonists of endothelin receptors, and aldosterone antagonists (Weber, 2000).

The cardioreparative concept has been proven clinically in four recent prospective trials performed in patients with essential hypertension receiving either an ACE inhibitor (Brilla et al., 2000; Schwartzkopff et al., 2000) or an AT_1 receptor anatgonist (López et al., 2001; Díez et al., 2002) as treatment. The main findings of these studies can be summarized as follows: (1) the ability of ACE inhibitors and AT_1 receptor antagonists to reduce myocardial fibrosis is not exclusively linked to their capacity to reduce blood pressure but may be also related to their efficacy in interfering with nonhemodynamic fibrogenic factors (i.e., Ang II and TGF-β1); and (2) the ability of these drugs to induce regression of myocardial fibrosis is associated with improvement of left ventricular function.

Conclusions and perspectives

Structural homogeneity of cardiac tissue is governed by mechanical and humoral factors that regulate cell growth, apoptosis, phenotype, and extracellular matrix turnover. Ang II has endocrine, autocrine and paracrine properties that influence the behavior of cardiac cells and matrix via AT_1 receptor binding. Thus various paradigms have been suggested, including Ang II-mediated upregulation of collagen types I and III formation and deposition in cardiac conditions such as HHD. A number of data indicate that myocardial fibrosis predisposes to an enhanced risk of diastolic and/or systolic ventricular dysfunction, symptomatic heart failure, ischemic heart disease, and arrhythmias in patients with HHD. Thus, management of these patients must be aimed to detect and target hypertensive myocardial fibrosis. Preliminary data suggest that the goal of reducing myocardial fibrosis is achievable in patients with HHD treated with agents interfering with either ACE or AT_1 receptor. Furthermore, the beneficial effects of these drugs in patients with HHD may be related to their capacity to repair myocardial fibrosis.

References

Ammarguellat F, Larouche II and Schiffrin EL (2001) Myocardial fibrosis in DOCA-salt hypertensive rats: effect of endothelin (ETA) receptor antagonism. *Circulation* **103**, 319–324.

Ashizawa N, Graf K, Do YS, et al. (1996) Osteopontin is produced by rat cardiac fibroblasts and mediates AII-induced DNA synthesis and collagen gel contraction. *Journal of Clinical Investigation* **98**, 2218–2227.

Assayag P, Carré F, Chevalier B, et al. (1997) Compensated cardiac hypertrophy: arrhythmogenicity and the new myocardial phenotype. I. Fibrosis. *Cardiovascular Research* **34**, 439–444.

Bishop JE, Kiernan LA, Montgomery HE, et al. (2000) Raised blood pressure, not renin–angiotensin system, causes cardiac fibrosis in TGRm(ren2)27 rats. *Cardiovascular Research* **47**, 57–67.

Bouzegrhane F and Thibault G (2002) Is angiotensin II a proliferative factor of cardiac fibroblasts? *Cardiovascular Research* **53**, 304–312.

Brilla CG, Janicki JS and Weber KT (1991) Impaired diastolic function and coronary reserve in genetic hypertension: role of interstitial fibrosis and medial thickening of intramyocardial coronary arteries. *Circulation Research* **69**, 107–115.

Brilla CG, Matsubara LS and Weber KT (1993) Anti-aldosterone treatment and the prevention of myocardial fibrosis in primary and secondary aldosteronism. *Journal of Molecular and Cellular Cardiology* **25**, 563–575.

Brilla CG, Funck RC and Rupp RH (2000) Lisinopril-mediated regression of myocardial fibrosis in patients with hypertensive heart disease. *Circulation* **102**, 1388–1393.

Burlew BS and Weber KT (2000) Connective tissue and the heart. Functional significance and regulatory mechanisms. *Cardiology Clinics* **18**, 435–442.

Camilión de Hurtado MC, Portiansky EL, Pérez NG, et al. (2002) Regression of cardiomyocyte hypertrophy in SHR following chronic inhibition of Na^+/H^+ exchanger. *Cardiovascular Research* **53**, 862–868.

Campbell JE, Janicki JS and Weber KT (1995) Temporal differences in fibroblast proliferation and phenotype expression in response to chronic administration of angiotensin II or aldosterone. *Journal of Molecular and Cellular Cardiology* **27**, 1545–1560.

Chua CC, Chua BH, Zhao ZY, et al. (1991) Effect of growth factors on collagen metabolism in cultured human heart fibroblasts. *Connective Tissue Research* **26**, 271–281.

Chua CH, Hamdy RC and Chua BH (1996) Angiotensin II induces TIMP-1 production in rat heart endothelial cells. *Biochimica et Biophysica Acta* **1311**, 175–180.

Cingolani HE, Rebolledo OR, Portiansky EL, et al. (2003) Regression of hypertensive myocardial fibrosis by Na$^+$/H$^+$ exchange inhibition. *Hypertension* **41**, 373–377.

Cohn JN, Ferrari R and Sharpe N, on behalf of an International Forum on Cardiac Remodeling (2000) Cardiac remodeling-concepts and clinical implications: a consensus paper from an international forum on cardiac remodeling. *Journal of the American College of Cardiology* **35**, 569–582.

Crabos M, Roth M, Hahn AW and Erne P (1994) Characterization of angiotensin II receptors in cultured adult rat cardiac fibroblasts. Coupling to signaling systems and gene expression. *Journal of Clinical Investigation* **93**, 2372–2378.

Crawford DC, Chobanian AV and Brecher P (1994) Angiotensin II induces fibronectin expression associated with cardiac fibrosis in the rat. *Circulation Research* **74**, 727–739.

Cuocolo A, Sax FL, Brush JE, et al. (1990) Left ventricular hypertrophy and impaired diastolic filling in essential hypertension. Diastolic mechanisms for systolic dysfunction during exercise. *Circulation* **81**, 978–986.

Díez J, Laviades C, Mayor G, et al. (1995) Increased serum concentrations of procollagen peptides in essential hypertension. Relation to cardiac alterations. *Circulation* **91**, 1450–1456.

Díez J, Panizo A, Gil MJ, et al. (1996) Serum markers of collagen type I metabolism in spontaneously hypertensive rats: relation to myocardial fibrosis. *Circulation* **93**, 1026–1032.

Díez J, González A, López B, et al. (2001a) Effects of antihypertensive agents on the left ventricle. Clinical implications. *American Journal of Cardiovascular Drugs* **1**, 263–279.

Díez J, Lopez B, Gonzalez B and Querejeta R (2001b) Clinical aspects of hypertensive myocardial fibrosis. *Current Opinion in Cardiology* **16**, 328–335.

Díez J, Querejeta R, López B, et al. (2002) Losartan-dependent regression of myocardial fibrosis is associated with reduction of left ventricular chamber stiffness in hypertensive patients. *Circulation* **105**, 2512–2517.

Dollery CM, McEwan JR and Henney AM (1995) Matrix metalloproteinases and cardiovascular diseases. *Circulation Research* **77**, 863–868.

Dostal DE (2001) Regulation of cardiac collagen. Angiotensin and cross-talk with local growth factors. *Hypertension* **37**, 841–844.

Dostal DE, Booz GW and Baker KM (1996) Angiotensin II signaling pathways in cardiac fibroblasts: conventional versus novel mechanisms in mediating cardiac growth and function. *Molecular and Cellular Biochemistry* **157**, 15–21.

Edwards DR, Murphy G, Reynolds JJ, et al. (1987) Transforming growth factor beta modulates the expression of collagenase and metalloproteinase inhibitor. *EMBO Journal* **6**, 1899–1904.

European Study Group on Diastolic Heart Failure (1998) How to diagnose diastolic heart failure. *European Heart Journal* **19**, 990–1003.

Everett AD, Tufro-McReddie A, Fisher A and Gomez RA (1994) Angiotensin receptor regulates cardiac hypertrophy and transforming growth factor-β1 expression. *Hypertension* **23**, 587–592.

Funck RC, Wilke A, Rupp H and Brilla CG (1997) Regulation and role of myocardial matrix remodeling in hypertensive heart disease. *Advances in Experimental Medicine and Biology* **432**, 35–44.

Ghandi SK, Powers JC, Nomeir AM, et al. (2001) The pathogenesis of acute pulmonary edema associated with hypertension. *New England Journal of Medicine* **344**, 17–22.

Ghiggeri GM, Oleggini R, Musante L, *et al.* (2000) A DNA element in the α1 type III collagen promoter mediates a stimulatory response by angiotensin II. *Kidney International* **58**, 537–548.

González A, López B, Querejeta R and Díez J (2002) Regulation of myocardial fibrillar collagen by angiotensin II. A role in hypertensive heart disease? *Journal of Molecular and Cellular Cardiology* **34**, 1585–1593.

Graf K, Neuss M, Stawowy P, *et al.* (2000) Angiotensin II and alpha(V)beta(3) integrin expression in rat neonatal cardiac fibroblasts. *Hypertension* **35**, 978–984.

Gray MO, Long CS, Kalinyak JE, *et al.* (1998) Angiotensin II stimulates cardiac myocyte hypertrophy via paracrine release of TGF-beta1 and endothelin-1 from fibroblasts. *Cardiovascular Research* **40**, 352–363.

Guarda E, Katwa LC, Myers PR, *et al.* (1993) Effects of endothelins on collagen turnover in cardiac fibroblasts. *Cardiovascular Research* **27**, 2130–2134.

Hao J, Wang B, Jones SC, *et al.* (2000) Interaction between angiotensin II and Smad proteins in fibroblasts in failing heart and *in vitro*. *American Journal of Physiology* **279**, H3020–H3030.

Houghton JL, Frank MJ, Carr AA, *et al.* (1990) Relations among impaired coronary flow reserve, left ventricular hypertrophy and thallium perfusion defects in hypertensive patients without obstructive artery disease. *Journal of the American College of Cardiology* **15**, 43–51.

Hunter JJ, Grace A and Chien KR (1999) Molecular and cellular biology of cardiac hypertrophy and failure. In *Molecular Basis of Cardiovascular Disease*, Chien KR (ed), WB Saunders, Philadelphia, pp. 211–250.

Isoyama S, Ito N, Satoh K and Takishima T (1992) Collagen deposition and the reversal of coronary reserve in cardiac hypertrophy. *Hypertension* **20**, 491–500.

Jalil JE, Janicki JS, Pick R and Weber KT (1991) Coronary vascular remodeling and myocardial fibrosis in the rat with renovascular hypertension: response to captopril. *American Journal of Hypertension* **4**, 51–55.

Janicki JS (1995) Collagen degradation in the heart. In *Molecular Biology of Collagen Matrix in the Heart*, Eghbali-Webb M (ed), RG Landes, Austin, pp. 61–76.

Ju H, Zhao S, Jassal DS and Dixon IM (1997) Effect of AT_1 receptor blockade on cardiac collagen remodeling after myocardial infarction. *Cardiovascular Research* **35**, 223–232.

Kawano H, Do YS, Kawano Y, *et al.* (2000) Angiotensin II has multiple profibrotic effects in human cardiac fibroblasts. *Circulation* **101**, 1130–1137.

Kim S, Ohta K, Hamaguchi A, *et al.* (1995) Angiotensin II-induced cardiac phenotypic modulation and remodeling *in vivo* in rats. *Hypertension* **25**, 1252–1259.

Kobayashi N, Nakano S, Mita S, *et al.* (2002) Involvement of Rho-kinase pathway for angiotensin II-induced plasminogen activator inhibitor-1 gene expression and cardiovascular remodeling in hypertensive rats. *Journal of Pharmacology and Experimental Therapeutics* **301**, 459–466.

Laviades C, Varo N, Fernández J, *et al.* (1998) Abnormalities of the extracellular degradation of collagen type I in essential hypertension. *Circulation* **98**, 535–540.

Laviades C, Varo N and Díez J (2000) Transforming growth factor-β in hypertensives with cardiorenal damage. *Hypertension* **36**, 517–522.

Lee MA, Bohm M, Paul M, *et al.* (1996) Physiological characterization of the hypertensive transgenic rat TGR(mren2)27. *American Journal of Physiology* **270**, E919–E929.

REFERENCES

Leipala JA, Takala TE, Ruskoaho H, et al. (1988) Transmural distribution of biochemical markers of total protein and collagen synthesis, myocardial contraction speed and capillary density in the rat left ventricle in angiotensin II-induced hypertension. *Acta Physiologica Scandavica* **133**, 325–333.

Levy D, Anderson K, Savage DD, et al. (1987) Risk of ventricular arrhythmias in left ventricular hypertrophy: the Framingham heart study. *American Journal of Cardiology* **60**, 560–565.

Lijnen P and Petrov V (1999) Renin–angiotensin system, hypertrophy and gene expression in cardiac myocytes. *Journal of Molecular and Cellular Cardiology* **31**, 949–970.

Lindsey MM, Maxwell P and Dunn FG (2002) TIMP-1. A marker of left ventricular diastolic dysfunction and fibrosis in hypertension. *Hypertension* **40**, 136–141.

López B, González A, Varo N, et al. (2001a) Biochemical assessment of myocardial fibrosis in hypertensive heart disease. *Hypertension* **38**, 1222–1226.

López B, Querejeta R, Varo N, et al. (2001b) Usefulness of serum carboxy-terminal propeptide of procollagen type I in assessment of the cardioreparative ability of antihypertensive treatment in hypertensive patients. *Circulation* **104**, 286–291.

McLenachan JM and Dargie HJ (1990) Ventricular arrhythmias in hypertensive left ventricular hypertrophy. Relationship to coronary artery disease, left ventricular dysfunction, and myocardial fibrosis. *American Journal of Hypertension* **3**, 735–740.

Muiesan ML, Rizzoni D, Salvetti M, et al. (2003) Left ventricular mass and function are related to collagen turnover markers in essential hypertension. *American Journal of Hypertension*, **16** (part 2), 4A.

Nimmi ME (1993) Fibrillar collagens: their biosynthesis, molecular structure, and mode of assembly. In *Extracellular Matrix*, Zern MA and Reid LM (eds), Marcel Dekker, New York, pp. 121–148.

Ohsato K, Shimizu M, Sugihara N, et al. (1992) Histopathological factors related to diastolic function in myocardial hypertrophy. *Japanese Circulation Journal* **56**, 325–333.

Pinto YM, Pinto-Sietsma SJ, Philipp T, et al. (2000) Reduction in left ventricular messenger RNA for transforming growth factor beta (1) attenuates left ventricular fibrosis and improves survival without lowering blood pressure in the hypertensive TGR(mren2)27 rat. *Hypertension* **36**, 747–754.

Querejeta R, Varo N, López B, et al. (2000) Serum carboxy-terminal propeptide of procollagen type I is a marker of myocardial fibrosis in hypertensive heart disease. *Circulation* **101**, 1729–1735.

Risteli L and Risteli J (1990) Noninvasive methods for detection of organ fibrosis. In *Focus on Connective Tissue in Health and Disease*, Rojkind M (ed), CRC Press, Boca Raton, pp. 61–68.

Risteli J, Elomaa I, Niemi S, et al. (1993) Radioimmunoassay for the pyridoline cross-linked carboxy-terminal telopeptide of type I collagen: a new serum marker of bone collagen degradation. *Clinical Chemistry* **39**, 635–640.

Rothermund L, Kreutz R, Kossmehl P, et al. (2002) Early onset of chondroitin sulfate and osteopontin expression in angiotensin II-dependent left ventricular hypertrophy. *American Journal of Hypertension* **15**, 644–652.

Sadoshima J and Izumo S (1993) Molecular characterization of angiotensin II-induced hypertrophy of cardiac myocytes and hyperplasia of cardiac fibroblasts. *Circulation Research* **73**, 413–423.

Schnee JM and Hsueh WA (2000) Angiotensin II, adhesion, and cardiac fibrosis. *Cardiovascular Research* **46**, 264–268.

Schwartzkopff B, Motz W, Frenzel H, et al. (1993) Structural and functional alterations of the intramyocardial coronary arterioles in patients with arterial hypertension. *Circulation* **88**, 993–1003.

Schwartzkopff B, Brehm M, Mundehenke M and Strauer BE (2000) Repair of coronary arterioles after treatment with perindopril in hypertensive heart disease. *Hypertension* **36**, 220–225.

Seeland U, Haeuseler C, Hinrichs R, et al. (2002) Myocardial fibrosis in transforming growth factor-β1 (TGF-β1) transgenic mice is associated with inhibition of interstitial collagenase. *European Journal of Clinical Investigation* **32**, 295–303.

Shindo T, Manabe I, Fukushima Y, et al. (2002) Krüppel-like zinc-finger transcription factor KLF5/BTEB2 is a target for angiotensin II signaling and an essential regulator of cardiovascular remodeling. *Nature Medicine* **8**, 856–863.

Smedsrod B, Melkko J, Risteli L and Risteli J (1990) Circulating C-terminal propeptide of type I procollagen is cleared mainly via a mannose receptor in the liver endothelial cells. *Biochemical Journal* **271**, 345–350.

Sugihara N, Genda A, Shimizu M, et al. (1988) Diastolic dysfunction and its relation to myocardial fibrosis in essential hypertension. *Journal of Cardiology* **18**, 353–361.

Sun Y, Ramires FJA and Weber KT (1997) Fibrosis of atria and great vessels in response to angiotensin II or aldosterone infusion. *Cardiovascular Research* **35**, 138–147.

Swynghedauw B (1999) Molecular mechanisms of myocardial remodeling. *Physiological Reviews* **79**, 215–262.

Teisman AC, Pinto YM, Buikema H, et al. (1998) Dissociation of blood pressure reduction from end-organ damage in TGR(mren2)27 transgenic hypertensive rats. *Journal of Hypertension* **16**, 1759–1765.

Tharaux PL, Chatziantoniou C, Fakhouri F and Dussaule JC (2000) Angiotensin II activates collagen I gene through a mechanism involving the MAP/ER kinase pathway. *Hypertension* **36**, 330–336.

Tomita H, Egahsira K, Ohara Y, et al. (1998) Early induction of transforming growth factor-β via angiotensin II type 1 receptors contributes to cardiac fibrosis induced by long-term blockade of nitric oxide synthesis in rats. *Hypertension* **32**, 273–279.

Varo N, Etayo JC, Zalba G, et al. (1999) Losartan inhibits the posttranscriptional synthesis of collagen type I and reverses left ventricular fibrosis in spontaneously hypertensive rats. *Journal of Hypertension* **17**, 101–114.

Varo N, Iraburu M, Varela M, et al. (2000) Chronic AT_1 blockade stimulates extracellular collagen type I degradation and reverses myocardial fibrosis in spontaneously hypertensive rats. *Hypertension* **35**, 1197–1202.

Vasan RS, Larson MG, Benjamin EJ, et al. (1999) Congestive heart failure in subjects with normal versus reduced left ventricular ejection fraction: prevalence and mortality in a population-based cohort. *Journal of the American College of Cardiology* **33**, 1948–1955.

Villarreal FJ, Kim NN, Ungab GD, et al. (1993) Identification of functional angiotensin II receptors on cardiac fibroblasts. *Circulation* **88**, 2849–2861.

Vogt M and Strauer BE (1995) Systolic ventricular dysfunction and heart failure due to coronary microangiopathy in hypertensive heart disease. *American Journal of Cardiology* **76**, 48D–53D.

Weber KT (1989) Cardiac interstitium in health and disease: the fibrillar collagen network. *Journal of the American College of Cardiology* **13**, 1637–1652.

Weber KT (1997a) Extracellular matrix remodeling in heart failure. A role for *de novo* angiotensin II generation. *Circulation* **96**, 4065–4082.

Weber KT (1997b) Cardiac interstitium. In *Heart Failure. Scientific Principles and Clinical Practice*, Poole-Wilson PA, Colucci WS, Massie BM, *et al.* (eds), Churchill Livingstone, New York, pp. 13–31.

Weber KT (2000) Targeting pathological remodeling. Concepts of cardioprotection and reparation. *Circulation* **102**, 1342–1345.

Weber KT, Brilla CG and Janicki JS (1993) Myocardial fibrosis. Functional significance and regulatory factors. *Cardiovascular Research* **27**, 341–348.

Yamamoto K and Saito H (1998) A pathological role of increased expression of plasminogen activator inhibitor-1 in human or animal disorders. *International Journal of Hematology* **68**, 371–385.

Yamamoto K, Masuyama T, Sakata Y, *et al.* (2002) Prevention of diastolic heart failure by endothelin type A receptor antagonist through inhibition of ventricular structural remodeling in hypertensive heart. *Journal of Hypertension* **20**, 753–761.

Yamazaki T, Komuro I and Yazaki Y (1999) Role of the renin–angiotensin system in cardiac hypertrophy. *American Journal of Cardiology* **83** (12A), 53H–57H.

14

Hypertensive Heart Disease: Significance of the Renin Angiotensin System

Jasmina Varagic and Edward D. Frohlich

Introduction

Elevated arterial pressure is a well-established predisposing factor for the development of stroke, hypertensive heart and peripheral artery disease, as well as for cardiac and renal failure. Over the past several decades we have witnessed the great impact antihypertensive therapy has had on the incidence of stroke, coronary heart disease and other mostly pressure-dependent emergencies (Collins et al., 1990; Thijs et al., 1992). On the other hand, we remain far from preventing, postponing or improving the prognosis and mortality from congestive heart failure (CHF) (Vasan et al., 1995, 1996). According to the earliest and most recent reports from the Framingham Heart Study hypertension is the most common cause of CHF (Kannel et al., 1972; Vasan et al., 1996). Hypertension induces alterations in cardiac structure and function manifested by left ventricular hypertrophy (LVH), which is associated with impaired coronary hemodynamics and ventricular fibrosis that proceeds to altered left ventricular (LV) performance. Each of these derangements contributes to the increased cardiovascular morbidity and mortality resulting from LV failure (Vasan et al., 1996; Frohlich, 1999). Moreover, in addition to increased arterial pressure, nonhemodynamic mechanisms participate importantly in hypertension-associated cardiovascular injury. Among these factors, the renin angiotensin system

(RAS) seems to have a major role. Indeed, numerous studies have demonstrated that angiotensin II, independent of its effect on arterial pressure, is implicated in ischemia and apoptosis, as a mitogenic and growth factor, each participating importantly in the development and continuance of hypertensive heart disease (HHD) and its progression to CHF. As intriguing as this concept is, it is further compounded by the existence of a local cardiac RAS in addition to the existence of the classical endocrine RAS.

Structural and functional alterations in HHD

HHD is a clinical and pathophysiological entity linked with a sustained increase in arterial pressure and is characterized by the presence of LVH. Increased LV wall thickness and cardiac mass represent an early adaptive structural response to an increased hemodynamic load (pressure or volume) that normalizes myocardial tension and maintains cardiac performance. Thickening of the LV wall is mainly achieved by enlargement of cardiac myocytes that also undergo specific changes in the expression of different isoforms of contractile proteins, myocardial enzymes, and secretory products (Susic and Frohlich, 1993; Swynghedauw, 1999). In addition, structural and functional alterations of the coronary circulation occur besides changes in the size and number of nonmyocyte cells, excessive accumulation of collagen and apoptosis as periphenomena of LVH; and each importantly contribute to deterioration of LV performance.

Although resting coronary blood flow may be normal in clinical and experimental forms of hypertension (Marcus *et al.*, 1981; Susic *et al.*, 1998), the ability of coronary vasculature to dilate in response to certain physiological or pharmacological interventions (coronary flow reserve) diminishes with persistent elevation in arterial pressure and increase in LV mass (Frohlich *et al.*, 1992; Hamasaki *et al.*, 2000; Kozakova *et al.*, 2000). This occurs primarily because of structural alterations in coronary and other arteriolar resistance vessels (vascular remodeling), which is manifested by medial wall thickening and increased wall/lumen ratio, perivascular fibrosis, as well as decreased numbers of arterioles (rarefaction) (Folkow, 1993). Increased ventricular wall compression as well as collagen and protein deposition in extracellular matrix further alter coronary hemodynamics. Moreover, functional alterations of coronary arterioles have been also demonstrated. Among the latter, endothelial dysfunction represents a dysbalance in synthesis and degradation of the various endothelial-derived vasodilating and contracting substances, which are at least in part responsible for the impaired coronary hemodynamics in hypertension (Kelm et al., 1996; Feletou and Vanhoutte, 1999; Spieker et al., 2000). Each of these foregoing damages account for the remarkable progress in our understanding of silent ischemia or microvascular angina that occur in patients with HHD, especially when epicardial coronary arteries appear to be clinically normal (Scheler et al., 1994).

Excess accumulation of fibrilar collagen (predominantly collagen I and III) in the interstitium and perivascularly have become well accepted in HHD (Weber, 2000). The increased ventricular collagen content impairs ventricular relaxation and further compromises myocardial perfusion since coronary flow occurs primarily during diastole. Additionally, the perivacular fibrosis may also impair vasorelaxation and consequently coronary blood flow. Moreover, diffuse interstitial fibrosis is also an important determinant of myocardial stiffness (Brilla et al., 1991b) and thereby has a prominent role in decreased ventricular compliance, impairing further LV filling. Interestingly, these changes in collagen matrix do not include only quantitative, but qualitative alterations too. Indeed, the altered collagen type I:III ratio was implied to be associated with myocardial dysfunction (Mukherjee and Sen, 1990). Besides alterations in collagen network, an impaired ventricular filling during diastole engages disarray in cardiac myocytes as well. The reduction in capacity of calcium sequestration is, at least in part, accountable for prolonged isovolemic relaxation time (Rothermund et al., 2001). Thus, as diastolic dysfunction progresses, left atrial enlargement due to increased atrial contribution to the late diastolic filling precipitates the incidence of atrial fibrillation and CHF. Furthermore, with the associated LV apoptosis, there is reduced functional contractile elements adding further to CHF development (Fortuno et al., 2001, 2003).

As a result of hypertensive LVH, myocardial tension and oxygen demand are increased, and the consequent remodeling of coronary arterioles and collagen matrix aggravate further ischemia. Thus, the ischemia, myocyte necrosis and apoptosis, as well as fibrosis, accelerate CHF progression. Eventually, the LV force-generating ability declines along with marked impairment of LV filling and increased end-diastolic LV pressure. Resting systolic function is preserved in hypertensive patients for long periods of time, although altered diastolic function occurs early in the course of hypertensive disease, even in the absence of obvious LVH (De Marchi et al., 2000) so that approximately one-third of patients with CHF have normal or preserved systolic function (Senni et al., 1999). Thus, not only is diastolic dysfunction a marker of HHD, but it is also a potential cause of CHF.

Contribution of Ang II cardiac effects to HHD

The possible role of elevated ventricular load and coronary perfusion pressure in mediating structural and functional alterations in the ventricle have been extensively discussed. However, development of LVH is not only dependent on the augmented hemodynamic load, and several lines of evidence point to the important role of activated RAS as well. The active moiety of the RAS is Ang II, which exerts potent vasoconstrictor as well as mitogenic, growth promoting and apoptotic effects predominantly through activation of AT_1 receptors. In contrast to the well-established role of the AT_1 receptor, the role of AT_2 receptor still remains more controversial.

Cardiomyocyte hypertrophy

There is now general agreement that Ang II exerts powerful stimulatory effect on myocardial growth acting predominantly on AT_1 receptors. Ang II increases protein synthesis in isolated cardiac myocytes (Baker and Aceto, 1990; Miyata and Haneda, 1994). In addition, Ang II induces expression of nuclear proto-oncogenes which are importantly involved in cell growth and proliferation through activation of different protein kinases (Kudoh et al., 1997; Pan et al., 1997). On the other hand, in vivo experiments are not always straightforward in distinguishing direct from concomitant systemic hemodynamic effects of Ang II that provide clear evidence of its independent growth action. Thus, the pressor as well as nonpressor doses of Ang II increase rat LV mass, though only doses that elevate arterial pressure simultaneously induce switch in LV myosin isoform mRNA from the adult to the fetal pattern thereby increasing the β while decreasing α myosin heavy chain mRNAs (Susic et al., 1996). The shift from V1 (homodimer of the α myosin heavy chain) to the V3 (homodimer of the β myosin heavy chain) improves contractile efficiency (Alpert and Mulieri, 1982) and provides a biochemical adaptation to increased hemodynamic load. Interestingly, an important participation of Ang II is shown in mechanical stress-induced cardiomyocyte hypertrophy (Yamazaki et al., 1999). A specific AT_1 receptor antagonist, TCV 116, partly inhibited the stretch-induced activation of second messengers such as Raf-1 kinase and extracellular signal-regulated protein kinase (ERK) which are involved in reexpression of a number of genes including skeletal α-actin and β-myosin heavy chain. When it was orally administrated to spontaneously hypertensive rats (SHR), TCV 116 lowered arterial pressure, reduced LV weight, LV wall thickness, myocytic diameter, and a shift from the V1 to the V3 isoform of myosin heavy chain (Yamazaki et al., 1994). Moreover, studies from our and other laboratories clearly indicate that reduction in LV mass induced by different drugs that interfere with RAS (either angiotensin-converting enzyme (ACE) inhibitors or AT_1 receptor antagonists) may be independent of effective pressure reduction (Ando et al., 1991; Brilla et al., 1991a; Kaneko et al., 1996, 1997; Malmqvist et al., 2001; Varagic et al., 2001b). On the other hand, the role of AT_2 receptors is less understood, although some experimental findings support their antigrowth action (van Kesteren et al., 1997b; Bartunek et al., 1999).

Coronary insufficiency

In recent years, several studies have shown experimentally and clinically, that impaired coronary hemodynamic in HHD is, at least in part, related to the increased activity of RAS. Ang I and II exert a direct coronary vasoconstriction in isolated heart preparations (Britton and Di Salvo, 1973) and the human being (Whelan et al., 1969). Besides this acute modulation of coronary vascular tone, chronic vasoconstrictor and hypertrophic effects of Ang II on smooth muscle cells and fibroblasts may explain the remarkable diminished coronary vasodilator reserve in various models of experimental hypertension and in hypertensive patients. Thus, in adult SHR, we have demonstrated decreased minimal coronary vascular resistance and increased coronary flow reserve with ACE inhibitors (Kaneko et al., 1996, 1997; Nunez et al., 1997) and AT_1 receptor blockers (Nunez et al., 1997). Furthermore, in aged SHR, interruption of RAS cascade has been shown to be profoundly effective in reversing coronary hemodynamic impairment associated with hypertension and aging (Susic et al., 1999). An ACE inhibitor was more effective than a calcium antagonist in spite of their equipotency in reducing arterial pressure. Reduction of medial thickness of intramyocardial arterioles and increased capillary density are major components of the structural basis for improved coronary hemodynamics associated with ACE inhibitors (Brilla et al., 1991a), but improved endothelial function of the coronary circulation may also participate. Thus, Ang II-induced hypertension increased concentrations of aortic oxygen free radicals, which in turn inactivated nitric oxide exacerbating the balance between endothelium derived vasodilatatory and vasoconstrictor factors. Interestingly, altered endothelium-dependent vascular relaxation was not observed after the noradrenalin infusion which produced a similar increase in arterial pressure thereby indicating Ang II involvement in the endothelial dysfunction independent of its hemodynamic effects (Rajagopalan, 1996). Furthermore, we have also demonstrated that more complete blockade of the RAS with concomitant administration of an ACE inhibitor and AT_1 receptor antagonist was superior to either of these two agents used alone in equidepressor doses (Nunez *et al.*, 1997). Importantly, these valuable effects may also be attributed to bradykinin actions mediated by Ang II-dependent (Gohlke *et al.*, 1998) or independent (Linz *et al.*, 1995) mechanisms.

More recent observations, based on clinical use of ACE inhibitors has confirmed the foregoing experimental findings providing further support to the concept of activated RAS in HHD (Motz and Straur, 1996; Strauer and Schwartzkopff, 1998; Schwartzkopff *et al.*, 2000). Thus, significant reduction in minimal coronary vascular resistance after an ACE inhibitor, but not a β-adrenergic receptor blocker, likely reflected improved wall:lumen ratio and better functional response of small arteries in essential hypertension after long-term therapy with ACE inhibitor but not with beta-blockers (Schiffrin *et al.*, 1994; Thybo *et al.*, 1995). Notably, inhibition of the RAS appeared to be particularly effective in reducing myocardial fibrosis in recent clinical studies that was associated with marked improvement in coronary flow reserve (Brilla *et al.*, 2000; Schwartzkopff *et al.*, 2000).

Ventricular fibrosis

A substantial evolution in our understanding of hypertensive heart pathophysiology has led to increased recognition of RAS contribution to structural and functional disturbance of nonmyocytic compartment as well. There has been much *in vitro* evidence of direct Ang II mitogenic and growth influence on myocardial fibroblast (Brilla *et al.*, 1994). Thus, Ang II-induced excessive extracellular accumulation of fibrilar collagen has been confirmed repeatedly and independent of its hemodynamic effects in different experimental hypertensive models. For example, in those models with elevated circulating Ang II, myocardial fibrosis was found in both, hypertrophic pressure overloaded left as well as in normotensive, nonhypertrophied right ventricle (Brilla *et al.*, 1990). Moreover, RAS blockade, but not hydralazine, prevented or reduced myocardial fibrosis in these hypertensive models (Narayan et al., 1989; Pahor et al., 1991; Crawford et al., 1994; Kim et al., 1995). Most importantly, impressive clinical data comparing antifibrotic effects of drugs that interfere with RAS (either ACE inhibitor or AT_1 receptor antagonists) with diuretic or calcium channel blocker in hypertensive patients support these experimental findings confirming fibrogenic participation of Ang II in essential hypertension (Brilla et al., 2000; Schwartzkopff et al., 2000; Lopez et al., 2001). Also, Ang II not only stimulates collagen synthesis in rat cardiac fibroblast but it also concomitantly suppresses collagenase activity (Brilla et al., 1994). These findings are in accord with *in vivo* data indicating that the antifibrotic effect of AT_1 receptor antagonists is related to inhibition of collagen synthesis together with stimulation of its degradative pathways (Varo et al., 1999, 2000). Recent attention has been focused on the intriguing role of AT_2 receptors in overall cardiac Ang II influence, but debate about its involvement in collagen matrix remodeling continues (Brilla et al., 1994; Liu et al., 1997; Ohkubo et al., 1997; Varagic et al., 2001a). For example, in our recent study in adult SHR, we reported that not only blockade of AT_1 receptors but also concomitant stimulation of AT_2 receptors may account for the observed antifibrotic effect of AT_1 receptor antagonism (Varagic et al., 2001a) providing further support for direct Ang II action on cardiac fibroblast via opposite responses on AT_1 and AT_2 receptors. On the other hand, the possible role of AT_2 receptors in mediating myocardial fibrosis has been also discussed. In addition to collagen synthesis, Ang II stimulation of AT_2 receptors inhibits collagenase activity in cultured rat cardiac (Brilla et al., 1994). Clearly, additional studies are needed to further clarify AT_2 receptor involvement in Ang II-induced cardiac damage.

Diastolic dysfunction

As mentioned above, many patients with CHF have normal or preserved systolic function. Therefore, much attention has been directed to better understanding of the factors promoting diastolic failure. Additionally, diastolic function in hypertension may be impaired early in the course of disease. Much experimental evidence has been gathered indicating RAS may directly affect myocardial vasculature and connective tissue thereby affecting diastolic performance. Moreover, in recent clinical studies, decreased interstitial and perivascular fibrosis, achieved with drugs that interrupt RAS, points to the mechanism accounting for improved diastolic function and coronary hemodynamics in hypertensive patients (Brilla *et al.*, 2000; Schwartzkopff *et al.*, 2000; Lopez *et al.*, 2001). In addition, calcium movement abnormalities have been linked to the activated RAS and the abnormal relaxation properties of cardiac myocytes in the rat model of hypertension (Yamamoto *et al.*, 2000; Rothermund *et al.*, 2001). Taken together, these observations strongly support Ang II as an important contributor to impaired diastolic function in hypertension.

Cardiac RAS in development of HHD: experimental and clinical evidence

Endocrine vs. paracrine/autocrine/intracrine RAS

The RAS had been considered to be a classic endocrine system for many decades. In this traditional view, kidney-released renin acts on liver-derived angiotensinogen to produce Ang I in circulating blood, and then, through the action of ACE in pulmonary circulation, forms the active Ang II. The effector hormone is delivered via the blood stream to its target organs to exhibit physiologic and pathophysiologic actions through its binding to specific receptors (Braun-Mendez and Page, 1958). More recently, however, a rapidly growing body of evidence suggests the existence of an additional, fully operated RAS, in local tissues, or even at the cellular level (Re, 2001) emphasizing that Ang II is a paracrine, autocrine and intracrine hormone as well. Thus, in some studies utilizing sophisticated molecular biological techniques, the presence of RAS components in many cells, including cardiac and vascular myocytes as well as fibroblast has been revealed (Schunkert *et al.*, 1990; Dostal *et al.*, 1992a, b, 1994, 2000; Sawa *et al.*, 1992; Sadoshima *et al.*, 1993; Endo-Mochizuki *et al.*, 1995; Falkenhahn *et al.*, 1995; Iwai *et al.*, 1995; Pieruzzi *et al.*, 1995; Shyu *et al.*, 1995; Zhang *et al.*, 1995; Hokimoto *et al.*, 1996; Kawaguchi and Kitabatake, 1996; Lee *et al.*, 1996; Miyata *et al.*, 1996; Fischer *et al.*, 1997). In parallel, specific angiotensin receptors, AT_1 and AT_2, necessary for Ang II to mediate its effects, have been also demonstrated (Dzau *et al.*, 1993), even intracellularly in rat cardiomyocytes and fibroblasts (Fu *et al.*, 1998). In addition, several lines of evidence have demonstrated Ang II as mediator of cardiac aldosterone synthesis supporting further the existence of a complete local renin angiotensin aldosterone system within the heart (Delcayre *et al.*, 2000). However, the evidence may be interpreted that we have oversimplified the whole system in the light of recent discoveries of nonrenin and nonACE Ang II production as well. Thus, cathepsin D has been shown to cleave angiotensinogen (Katwa et al., 1997), and chymase activity may also explain Ang I–II conversion, particularly in human heart (Balcells et al., 1997). On the other hand, failure to confirm existence of renin or angiotensinogen, both at the messenger and protein level in cardiac cells was reported (Heller et al., 1998; van Kesteren et al., 1999) suggesting their active uptake from plasma (van Kesteren et al., 1997a; Admiraal et al., 1999). Nevertheless, accumulating evidence suggests that cardiac Ang II in normal hearts originates primarily from local synthesis (Danser et al., 1994; Neri Serneri et al., 1996), regardless of whether the synthesis is driven by blood-borne renin or not. This is even more important under certain pathophysiological conditions, such as hypertension, myocardial infarction or cardiac failure where local upregulation of renin, angiotensinogen, ACE mRNA as well as AT_1 and AT_2 receptors may occur (Janiak et al., 1992; Suzuki et al., 1993; Lopez et al., 1994; Diez et al., 1997; Ohkubo et al., 1997; Barlucchi et al., 2001; Serneri et al., 2001; Sun et al., 2001).

Thus, it seems that two components of the RAS may have somewhat different roles in the cardiovascular regulation (Dzau and Re, 1987; Dzau, 1988). The endocrine part, with the prompt response of kidney renin to volume or electrolyte disturbance and consequently rapid generation of circulating Ang II explains a critical short-term restoration of cardiorenal equilibrium through acute changes in vascular tone, aldosterone release and renal sodium and water reabsorption. The more subtle changes in local cardiac Ang II production necessary for its paracrine/autocrine/intracrine actions may be more responsible for the direct mitogenic and growth-promoting cellular effects, thereby contributing to long-term control of vascular resistance as well as to development of cardiac hypertrophy, fibrosis, and apoptosis in hypertension. However, in addition to the direct cardiovascular effects of Ang II, it is well accepted that changes in cardiac preload (volume expansion with sodium retention) and afterload (increased pressure) contribute significantly to Ang II-induced vascular and cardiac hypertrophy. Thus, the more general approach appears to be also more appropriate, suggesting that the endocrine and paracrine/autocrine/intracrine RAS may act in concert with development of HHD and its progression to CHF. For example, it is well accepted that increased plasma Ang II concentration significantly contributes to the clinical outcome of CHF. Moreover, activated circulatory RAS may also represent a significant source for cardiac sequestration of its components. Thus, increased cardiac Ang II generation in patients with CHF may reflect both increased cardiac sequestration of the circulating RAS components as well as increased generation through locally upregulated ACE and angiotensinogen (Serneri et al., 2001).

The complex relationships between systemic and cardiac RAS in the development of cardiac alterations associated with increased dietary salt intake deserve particular attention as well. Recent studies have proposed that salt excess not only increases arterial pressure but may also be a mediator of increased left ventricular mass and excessive myocardial collagen deposition (Du Cailar et al., 1989; Frohlich et al., 1993; Yu et al., 1998). In addition, salt-induced cardiac and vascular derangements have been disclosed as independent of arterial pressure, underlining the role of nonhemodynamic factors (Du Cailar et al., 1989; Yuan and Leenen, 1991; Yu et al., 1998). Furthermore, accumulated experimental and clinical evidence have revealed a normal plasma concentration or even increased LV Ang II or aldosterone during salt loading, an 'inappropriate' level for given dietary salt intake (Schmieder et al., 1996; Leenen and Yuan, 1998; Takeda et al., 2001; Hodge et al., 2002). However, high dietary salt intake affects left, but not right ventricular weight and collagen content in SHR (Yu et al., 1998), making involvement of circulatory factors less likely. Thus, upregulation of cardiac ACE mRNA and protein found after salt-loading in genetic (Kreutz et al., 1995) and salt-sensitive types of hypertension (Zhao et al., 2000) provides support to the concept that the activated cardiac RAS system may contribute, at least in part, to the detrimental effects of salt overload. In the former study dietary salt excess increased levels of cardiac ACE mRNA and activity in normotensive Wistar–Kyoto rats as well, without affecting arterial pressure or LV mass, though ACE expression was more pronounced in SHR. The increased salt sensitivity of SHR cardiac ACE may be one explanation along with its higher turnover. Additionally, the salt induced increase in cardiac ACE expression and activity may very well act in accordance with increased afterload leading to the further LV enlargement in this hypertensive experimental model. Surprisingly, salt excess did not increase cardiac Ang II in either salt sensitive strain (SHR and Dahl S rats). Therefore, the possibility that upregulated ACE message and activity may be pertinent for other ACE dependent nonangiotensinergic pathways (i.e., bradykinin pathways) involved in cardiac hypertrophy can be also raised.

Transgenic models

The pathophysiological relevance of local cardiac RAS has also been confirmed in the experiment utilizing transgenic animals overexpressing the genes responsible for particular components of the system. Thus, transgenic rats overexpressing mouse renin, develop hypertension with associated and, in part, pressure-independent LV hypertrophy and dysfunction (Rothermund et al., 2001). The overexpression of angiotensinogen gene in the cardiac myocyte did not affect arterial pressure but produced both right and left ventricular hypertrophy (Mazzolai et al., 2000). Increased cardiac production of Ang II without concomitant changes in circulation Ang II level in this experimental model provides strong verification for a functional role of local RAS in HHD.

Pharmacological blockade of cardiac RAS

Whenever it has been shown that ACE inhibitors successfully control arterial pressure and ameliorate complex structural and functional alterations associated with HHD independent of the systemic plasma ACE inhibition, the role of locally synthesized Ang II as a mediator of these alterations has received substantial attention. Almost two decades ago the antihypertensive effect of ACE inhibitors were shown to persist 2 weeks after discontinuing the drug; and aortic wall, but not plasma ACE activity, remained inhibited during drug withdrawal (Unger et al., 1985). More recently, an ACE inhibitor, in a dose that neither reduced arterial pressure nor plasma ACE activity, prevented LVH and myocardial fibrosis in rat hypertensive model of aortic banding (Linz et al., 1992). Moreover, ACE inhibitors effectively reduced elevated arterial pressure in genetic hypertensive model and in patients with essential hypertension with normal or low plasma renin activity. These findings suggested that the effect was independent of circulating Ang II levels, although normal plasma renin activity in the face of elevated arterial pressure may be considered as an 'inappropriately' elevated activity. Nevertheless, increased cardiac ACE activity (Diez et al., 1997) and AT_1 receptor expression (Suzuki et al., 1993) in SHR with LVH as compared with normotensive rats most likely reflect increased participation of local RAS in variety of hypertension-associated cardiovascular alteration. For example, increased ACE activity has been related to increased cardiomyocyte apoptosis and reparative myocardial fibrosis (Diez et al., 1997). Surprisingly, cardiac Ang II level in SHR and their normotensive controls was found to be similar (Campbell et al., 1995). While those observations seem to be contradictory with the concept of activated RAS in this experimental model, one must bear in mind several possible explanations. First, how sensitive the necessary method must be to be able to distinguish slight changes in Ang II concentration necessary to elicit paracrine or autocrine mechanisms. Second, an increased number of AT_1 receptors (or an alteration of the AT_1/AT_2 ratio) even with unchanged cardiac Ang II concentration may lead to augmented action of the effector peptide. Third, upregulation of ACE mRNA and activity may be related to the detrimental effects of decreased activity of other paracrine-acting hormonal systems (e.g., bradykinin) that interact with local RAS. Thus, ability of different drugs that interfere with RAS to reduce LV mass, excessive accumulation of extracellular matrix proteins as well as impairment in coronary hemodynamics and ventricular function in experimental and clinical hypertension may at least, in part, rely on their ability to blockade detrimental effects of local cardiac Ang II. The same arguments may be applied to the beneficial effects of RAS inhibition achieved in patients with CHF (SOLVD Investigators, 1991; Greenberg, 2002). Moreover, we and others have repeatedly reported cardioprotective effects of RAS blockade independent of its antihypertensive effect (Kaneko et al., 1997; Brilla et al., 2000; Lopez et al., 2001). The findings that more complete inhibition of local cardiac Ang II actions (including inhibition of nonrenin-, nonACE-dependent Ang II synthesis) by a combination therapy of an ACE inhibitor and an AT_1 receptor antagonist provides greater benefit than either drug alone in SHR are even more promising (Nunez et al., 1997), although the clinical benefit of the combination in the patients with CHF was not as profound (Val-HeFT Trial, 2000). Thus, tremendous research progress over the past decades has resulted in better understanding the impact activated RAS (circulating as well as locally generated) makes in development of HHD. Besides vasoconstrictor potency, Ang II exerts mitogenic, growth and apoptotic effects on cardiac and vascular myocytes and fibroblasts and thereby stimulates the process and exacerbation of LV hypertrophy. Conversely, numerous experimental and clinical studies of RAS blockade have demonstrated cardiovascular benefits over the benefits of lowering elevated arterial pressure only thereby supporting our expectation that we will be able to treat better or even to prevent HHD and its major complication CHF in near future.

Acknowledgments

This work was supported in part by an award from American Heart Association Southeast Affiliate.

References

Admiraal PJ, van Kesteren CA, Danser AH, et al. (1999) Uptake and proteolytic activation of prorenin by cultured human endothelial cells. *Journal of Hypertension* **17**, 621–629.

Alpert NR and Mulieri LA (1982) Increased myothermal economy of isometric force generation in compensated cardiac hypertrophy induced by pulmonary artery constriction in the rabbit. A characterization of heat liberation in normal and hypertrophied right ventricular papillary muscles. *Circulatory Research* **50**, 491–500.

Ando K, Frohlich ED, Chien Y and Pegram BL (1991) Effects of quinapril on systemic and regional hemodynamics and cardiac mass in spontaneously hypertensive and Wistar-Kyoto rats. *Journal of Vascular Medicine and Biology* **3**, 117–123.

Baker KM and Aceto JF (1990) Angiotensin II stimulation of protein synthesis and cell growth in chick heart cells. *American Journal of Physiology* **259**, H610–H618.

Balcells E, Meng QC, Johnson WH, Jr, et al. (1997) Angiotensin II formation from ACE and chymase in human and animal hearts: methods and species considerations. *American Journal of Physiology* **273**, H1769–H1774.

Barlucchi L, Leri A, Dostal DE, et al. (2001) Canine ventricular myocytes possess a renin–angiotensin system that is upregulated with heart failure. *Circulation Research* **88**, 298–304.

Bartunek J, Weinberg EO, Tajima M, et al. (1999) Angiotensin II type 2 receptor blockade amplifies the early signals of cardiac growth response to angiotensin II in hypertrophied hearts. *Circulation* **99**, 22–25.

Braun-Mendez E and Page IH (1958) Suggested revision of nomenclature: angiotensin. *Science* **127**, 242.

Brilla CG, Pick R, Tan LB, et al. (1990) Remodeling of the rat right and left ventricles in experimental hypertension. *Circulation Research* **67**, 1355–1364.

Brilla CG, Janicki JS and Weber KT (1991a) Cardioreparative effects of lisinopril in rats with genetic hypertension and left ventricular hypertrophy. *Circulation* **83**, 1771–1779.

Brilla CG, Janicki JS and Weber KT (1991b) Impaired diastolic function and coronary reserve in enetic hypertension. Role of interstitial fibrosis and medial thickening of intramyocardial coronary arteries. *Circulation Research* **69**, 107–115.

Brilla CG, Zhou G, Matsubara L and Weber KT (1994) Collagen metabolism in cultured adult rat cardiac fibroblasts: response to angiotensin II and aldosterone. *Journal of Molecular and Cellular Cardiology* **26**, 809–820.

Brilla CG, Funck RC and Rupp H (2000) Lisinopril-mediated regression of myocardial fibrosis in patients with hypertensive heart disease. *Circulation* **102**, 1388–1393.

Britton S and Di Salvo J (1973) Effects of angiotensin I and angiotensin II on hindlimb and coronary vascular resistance. *American Journal of Physiology* **225**, 1226–1231.

Campbell DJ, Duncan A-M, Kladis A and Harrap SB (1995) Angiotensin peptides in spontaneously hypertensive and normotensive Donryu rats. *Hypertension* **25**, 928–934.

Collins R, Peto R, MacMahon S, et al. (1990) Blood pressure, stroke, and coronary heart disease. Part 2, Short-term reductions in blood pressure: overview of randomised drug trials in their epidemiological context. *Lancet* **335**, 827–838.

Crawford DC, Chobanian AV and Brecher P (1994) Angiotensin II induces fibronectin expression associated with cardiac fibrosis in the rat. *Circulation Research* **74**, 727–739.

Danser AH, van Kats JP, Admiraal PJ, *et al.* (1994) Cardiac renin and angiotensins: uptake from plasma versus *in situ* synthesis. *Hypertension* **24**, 37–48.

Delcayre C, Silvestre JS, Garnier A, *et al.* (2000) Cardiac aldosterone production and ventricular remodeling. *Kidney International* **57**, 1346–1351.

Diez J, Panizo A, Hernandez M, *et al.* (1997) Cardiomyocyte apoptosis and cardiac angiotensin-converting enzyme in spontaneously hypertensive rats. *Hypertension* **30**, 1029–1034.

Dostal DE, Rothblum KN, Chernin MI, *et al.* (1992a) Intracardiac detection of angiotensinogen and renin: a localized renin–angiotensin system in neonatal rat heart. *American Journal of Physiology* **263**, C838–C850.

Dostal DE, Rothblum KN, Conrad KM, *et al.* (1992b) Detection of angiotensin I and II in cultured rat cardiac myocytes and fibroblasts. *American Journal of Physiology* **263**, C851–C863.

Dostal DE, Rothblum KN and Baker KM (1994) An improved method for absolute quantification of mRNA using multiplex polymerase chain reaction: determination of renin and angiotensinogen mRNA levels in various tissues. *Analytical Biochemistry* **223**, 239–250.

Dostal DE, Booz GW and Baker KM (2000) Regulation of angiotensinogen gene expression and protein in neonatal rat cardiac fibroblasts by glucocorticoid, and beta-adrenergic stimulation. *Basic Research in Cardiology* **95**, 485–490.

Du Cailar G, Ribstein J, Grolleau R and Mimaran A (1989) Influence of sodium intake on left ventricular structure in untreated essential hypertensives. *Journal of Hypertension* **7**, S258–S259.

Dzau VJ (1988) Circulating versus local renin–angiotensin system in cardiovascular homeostasis. *Circulation* **77**, I4–I13.

Dzau VJ and Re RN (1987) Evidence for the existence of renin in the heart. *Circulation* **75**, I134–I136.

Dzau VJ, Sasamura H and Hein L (1993) Heterogeneity of angiotensin synthetic pathways and receptor subtypes: physiological and pharmacological implications. *Journal of Hypertension* **11** (Suppl 3), S13–S18.

Endo-Mochizuki Y, Mochizuki N, Sawa H, *et al.* (1995) Expression of renin and angiotensin-converting enzyme inhuman hearts. *Heart Vessels* **10**, 285–293.

Falkenhahn M, Franke F, Bohle RM, *et al.* (1995) Cellular distribution of angiotensin-converted enzyme after myocardial infarction. *Hypertension* **25**, 219–226.

Feletou M and Vanhoutte PM (1999) The third pathway: endothelium-dependent hyperpolarization. *Journal of Physiology and Pharmacology* **50**, 525–534.

Fischer TA, Ungureanu-Longrois D, Singh K, *et al.* (1997) Regulation of bFGF expression and Ang II secretion in cardiac myocytes and microvascular endothelial cells. *American Journal of Physiology* **272**, H958–H968.

Folkow B (1993) Early structural changes in hypertension: pathophysiology and clinical consequences. *Journal of Cardiovascular Pharmacology* **22** (Suppl 1), S1–S6.

Fortuno MA, Ravassa S, Fortuno A, *et al.* (2001) Cardiomyocyte apoptotic cell death in arterial hypertension: mechanisms and potential management. *Hypertension* **38**, 1406–1412.

Fortuno MA, Gonzalez A, Ravassa S, *et al.* (2003) Clinical implications of apoptosis in hypertensive heart disease. *American Journal of Physiology* **284**, H1495–H1506.

Frohlich ED (1999) Risk mechanisms in hypertensive heart disease. *Hypertension* **34**, 782–789.

Frohlich ED, Apstein C, Chobanian AV, et al. (1992) The heart in hypertension. *New England Journal of Medicine* **327**, 998–1008.

Frohlich ED, Chien Y, Sesoko S and Pegram B (1993) Relationship between dietary sodium intake, hemodynamics, and cardiac mass in SHR and WKY rats. *American Journal of Physiology* **264**, R30–R34.

Fu ML, Schulze W, Wallukat G, et al. (1998) Immunochemical localization of angiotensin II receptor (AT$_1$) in the heart with anti-peptide antibodies showing a positive chronotropic effect. *Receptors Channels* **6**, 99–111.

Gohlke P, Pees C and Unger T (1998) AT$_2$ receptor stimulation increase aortic GMP in SHRSP by kinin-dependent mechanisms. *Hypertension* **31**, 349–355.

Greenberg BH (2002) Effects of angiotensin converting enzyme inhibitors on remodeling in clinical trials. *Journal of Cardiac Failure* **8** (Suppl 6), S486–S490.

Hamasaki S, Al Suwaidi J, Higano ST, et al. (2000) Attenuated coronary flow reserve and vascular remodeling in patients with hypertension and left ventricular hypertrophy. *Journal of the American College of Cardiology* **35**, 1654–1660.

Heller LJ, Opsahl JA, Wernsing SE, et al. (1998) Myocardial and plasma renin–angiotensinogen dynamics during pressure-induced cardiac hypertrophy. *American Journal of Physiology* **274**, R849–R856.

Hodge G, Ye VZ and Duggan KA (2002) Dysregulation of angiotensin II is associated with salt sensitivity in the spontaneous hypertensive rat. *Acta Physiologica Scandinavica* **174**, 209–215.

Hokimoto S, Yasue H, Fujimoto K, et al. (1996) Expression of angiotensin-converting enzyme in remaining viable myocytes of human ventricles after myocardial infarction. *Circulation* **94**, 1513–1518.

Iwai N, Shimoike H and Kinoshita M (1995) Cardiac renin–angiotensin system in the hypertrophied heart. *Circulation* **92**, 2690–2696.

Janiak P, Pillon A, Prost JF and Vilaine JP (1992) Role of the angiotensin subtype 2 receptor in neointima formation after vascular injury. *Hypertension* **20**, 737–745.

Kaneko K, Susic D, Nunez E and Frohlich ED (1996) Losartan reduces cardiac mass and improves coronary flow reserve in the spontaneously hypertensive rat. *Journal of Hypertension* **14**, 645–653.

Kaneko K, Susic D, Nunez E and Frohlich ED (1997) ACE inhibition reduces left ventricular mass independent of pressure without affecting coronary flow and flow reserve in spontaneously hypertensive rats. *American Journal of Medical Science* **314**, 21–27.

Kannel WB, Castelli WP, McNamara PM, et al. (1972) Role of blood pressure in the development of congestive heart failure. The Framingham study. *New England Journal of Medicine* **287**, 781–787.

Katwa LC, Campbell SC, Tyagi SC, et al. (1997) Cultured myofibroblasts generate angiotensin peptides *de novo*. *Journal of Molecular and Cellular Cardiology* **29**, 1375–1386.

Kawaguchi H and Kitabatake A (1996) Altered signal transduction system in hypertrophied myocardium: angiotensin II stimulates collagen synthesis in hypertrophied hearts. *Journal of Cardiac Failure* **2** (Suppl 4), S13–S19.

Kelm M, Preik M, Hafner D and Strauer B (1996) Evidence for a multifactorial process involved in the impaired flow response in hypertensive patients with endothelial dysfunction. *Hypertension* **27**, 346–353.

van Kesteren CA, Danser AH, Derkx FH, et al. (1997a) Mannose 6-phosphate receptor-mediated internalization and activation of prorenin by cardiac cells. *Hypertension* **30**, 1389–1396.
van Kesteren CA, van Heugten HA, Lamers JM, et al. (1997b) Angiotensin II-mediated growth and antigrowth effects in cultured neonatal rat cardiac myocytes and fibroblasts. *Journal of Molecular and Cellular Cardiology* **29**, 2147–2157.
van Kesteren CA, Saris JJ, Dekkers DH, et al. (1999) Cultured neonatal cardiac myocytes and fibroblasts do not synthesize renin or angiotensinogen: evidence for stretch-induced cardiomyocyte hypertrophy independent of angiotensin II. *Cardiovascular Research* **43**, 148–156.
Kim S, Ohta K, Hamaguchi A, et al. (1995) Angiotensin II induces cardiac phenotypic modulation and remodeling *in vivo* in rats. *Hypertension* **25**, 1252–1259.
Kozakova M, Galetta F, Gregorini L, et al. (2000) Coronary vasodilator capacity and epicardial vessel remodeling in physiological and hypertensive hypertrophy. *Hypertension* **36**, 343–349.
Kreutz R, Fernandez-Alfonso MS, Liu Y, et al. (1995) Induction of cardiac angiotensin I-converting enzyme with dietary NaCl-loading in genetically hypertensive and normotensive rats. *Journal of Molecular Medicine* **73**, 243–248.
Kudoh S, Komuro I, Mizuno T, et al. (1997) Angiotensin II stimulates c-Jun NH_2-terminal kinase in cultured cardiac myocytes of neonatal rats. *Circulation Research* **80**, 139–146.
Lee YA, Liang CS, Lee MA and Lindpaintner K (1996) Local stress, not systemic factors, regulate gene expression of the cardiac renin–angiotensin system *in vivo*: a comprehensive study of all its components in the dog. *Proceedings of the National Academy of Sciences of the United States of America* **93**, 11035–11040.
Leenen FHH and Yuan B (1998) Dietary-sodium-induced cardiac remodeling in spontaneously hypertensive rat versus Wistar-Kyoto rat. *Journal of Hypertension* **16**, 885–892.
Linz W, Schaper J, Wiemer G, et al. (1992) Ramipril prevents left ventricular hypertrophy with myocardial fibrosis without blood pressure reduction: a one year study in rats. *British Journal of Pharmacology* **107**, 970–975.
Linz W, Wiemer G, Gohlke P, et al. (1995) Contribution of kinins to the cardiovascular actions of angiotensin-converting enzyme inhibitors. *Pharmacology Reviews* **47**, 25–49.
Liu YH, Yang XP, Sharov VG, et al. (1997) Effects of angiotensin-converting enzyme inhibitors and angiotensin II type 1 receptor antagonists in rats with heart failure. Role of kinins and angiotensin II type 2 receptors. *Journal of Clinical Investigation* **99**, 1926–1935.
Lopez B, Querejeta R, Varo N, et al. (2001) Usefulness of serum carboxy-terminal propeptide of procollagen type I in assessment of the cardioreparative ability of antihypertensive treatment in hypertensive patients. *Circulation* **104**, 286–291.
Lopez JJ, Lorell BH, Ingelfinger JR, et al. (1994) Distribution and function of cardiac AT_1 and AT_2 receptors subtypes in hypertrophied rat hearts. *American Journal of Physiology* **267**, H844–H852.
Malmqvist K, Kahan T, Edner M, et al. (2001) Regression of left ventricular hypertrophy in human hypertension with irbesartan. *Journal of Hypertension* **19**, 1167–1176.
De Marchi SF, Allemann Y and Seiler C (2000) Relaxation in hypertrophic cardiomyopathy and hypertensive heart disease: relations between hypertrophy and diastolic function. *Heart* **83**, 678–684.

Marcus ML, Mueller TM and Eastham CL (1981) Effects of short- and long-term left ventricular hypertrophy on coronary circulation. *American Journal of Physiology* **241**, H358–H362.

Mazzolai L, Pedrazzini T, Nicoud F, *et al*. (2000) Increased cardiac angiotensin II levels induce right and left ventricular hypertrophy in normotensive mice. *Hypertension* **35**, 985–991.

Miyata S and Haneda T (1994) Hypertrophic growth of cultured neonatal rat heart cells mediated by type 1 angiotensin II receptor. *American Journal of Physiology* **266**, H2443–H2451.

Miyata S, Haneda T, Osaki J and Kikuchi K (1996) Renin–angiotensin system in stretch-induced hypertrophy of cultured neonatal rat heart cells. *European Journal of Pharmacology* **307**, 81–88.

Motz W and Strauer BE (1996) Improvement of coronary flow reserve after long-term therapy with enalapril. *Hypertension* **27**, 1031–1038.

Mukherjee D and Sen S (1990) Collagen phenotypes during development and regression of myocardial hypertrophy in spontaneously hypertensive rats. *Circulation Research* **67**, 1474–1480.

Narayan S, Janicki JS, Shroff SG, *et al*. (1989) Myocardial collagen and mechanics after preventing hypertrophy in hypertensive rats. *American Journal of Hypertension* **2**, 675–682.

Neri Serneri GG, Boddi M, Coppo M, *et al*. (1996) Evidence for the existence of a functional cardiac renin–angiotensin system in humans. *Circulation* **94**, 1886–1893.

Nunez E, Hosoya K, Sussic D and Frohlich ED (1997) Enalapril and losartan reduced cardiac mass and improved coronary hemodynamics in SHR. *Hypertension* **29**, 519–524.

Ohkubo N, Matsubara H, Nozawa Y, *et al*. (1997) Angiotensin type 2 receptors are re-expressed by cardiac fibroblasts from failing myopathic hamster hearts and inhibit cell growth and fibrilar collagen metabolism. *Circulation* **96**, 3954–3962.

Pahor M, Bernabei R, Sgadari A, *et al*. (1991) Enalapril prevents cardiac fibrosis and arrhythmias in hypertensive rats. *Hypertension* **18**, 148–157.

Pan J, Fukuda K, Kodama H, *et al*. (1997) Role of angiotensin II in activation of the Jak/STAT pathway induced by acute pressure overload in the rat heart. *Circulation Research* **81**, 611–617.

Pieruzzi F, Abassi ZA and Keiser HR (1995) Expression of renin–angiotensin system components in the heart, kidneys, and lungs of rats with experimental heart failure. *Circulation* **92**, 3105–3112.

Rajagopalan S, Kurz S, Munzel T, *et al*. (1996) Angiotensin II-mediated hypertension in the rat increases vascular superoxide production via membrane NADH/NADPH oxidase activation. Contribution to alterations of vasomotor tone. *Journal of Clinical Investigation* **97**, 1916–1923.

Re R (2001) The clinical implication of tissue renin angiotensin system. *Current Opinion in Cardiology* **6**, 317–327.

Rothermund L, Pinto YM, Vetter R, *et al*. (2001) Effects of angiotensin II subtype 1 receptor blockade on cardiac fibrosis and sarcoplasmic reticulum Ca^{2+} handling in hypertensive transgenic rats overexpressing the ren2 gene. *Journal of Hypertension* **19**, 1465–1472.

Sadoshima J, Xu Y, Slayter HS and Izumo S (1993) Autocrine release of angiotensin II mediates stretch-induced hypertrophy of cardiac myocytes *in vitro*. *Cell* **75**, 977–984.

Sawa H, Tokuchi F, Mochizuki N, *et al.* (1992) Expression of the angiotensinogen gene and localization of its protein in the human heart. *Circulation* **86**, 138–146.

Scheler S, Motz W and Strauer BE (1994) Mechanism of angina pectoris in patients with systemic hypertension and normal epicardial coronary arteries by arteriogram. *American Journal of Cardiology* **73**, 478–482.

Schiffrin EL, Deng LY and Larochelle P (1994) Effects of beta-blocker or a converting enzyme inhibitor on resistance arteries in essential hypertension. *Hypertension* **23**, 83–91.

Schmieder RE, Langenfeld MRW, Friedrich A, *et al.* (1996) Angiotensin II related to sodium excretion modulates left ventricular structure in human essential patients. *Circulation* **94**, 1304–1309.

Schunkert H, Dzau VJ, Tang SS, *et al.* (1990) Increased rat cardiac angiotensin converting enzyme activity and mRNA expression in pressure overload left ventricular hypertrophy. Effects on coronary resistance, contractility, and relaxation. *Journal of Clinical Investigation* **86**, 1913–1920.

Schwartzkopff B, Brehem M, Mundhenke M and Strauer B (2000) Repair of coronary arterioles after treatment with perindopril in hypertensive heart disease. *Hypertension* **36**, 220–225.

Senni M, Tribouilloy CM, Rodeheffer RJ, *et al.* (1999) Congestive heart failure in the community: trends in incidence and survival in a 10-year period. *Archives of Internal Medicine* **159**, 29–34.

Serneri GGN, Boddi M, Cecioni I, *et al.* (2001) Cardiac angiotensin II formation in the clinical course of heart failure and its relationship with left ventricular function. *Circulation Research* **88**, 961–968.

Shyu KG, Chen JJ, Shih NL, *et al.* (1995) Angiotensinogen gene expression is induced by cyclical mechanical stretch in cultured rat cardiomyocytes. *Biochemical and Biophysical Research Communications* **211**, 241–248.

SOLVD Investigators (1991) Effect of enalapril on survival in patients with reduced left ventricular ejection fractions and congestive heart failure. *New England Journal of Medicine* **325**, 293–301.

Spieker LE, Noll G, Ruschitzka FT, *et al.* (2000) Working under pressure: the vascular endothelium in arterial hypertension. *Journal of Human Hypertension* **14**, 617–630.

Strauer BE and Schwartzkopff B (1998) Objectives of high blood pressure treatment: left ventricular hypertrophy, diastolic function, and coronary reserve. *American Journal of Hypertension* **11**, 879–881.

Sun Y, Zhang J, Zhang JQ and Weber KT (2001) Renin expression at sites of repair in the infracted rat heart. *Journal of Molecular and Cellular Cardiology* **33**, 995–1003.

Susic D and Frohlich ED (1993) Left ventricular hypertrophy: a pathophysiological and molecular biological perspective. *Hypertension Research* **16**, 163–177.

Susic D, Nunez E, Frohlich ED and Prakash O (1996) Angiotensin II increases left ventricular mass without affecting myosin isoform mRNAs. *Hypertension* **28**, 265–268.

Susic D, Nunez E, Hosoya K and Frohlich ED (1998) Coronary hemodynamics in aging spontaneously hypertensive and normotensive Wistar-Kyoto rats. *Journal of Hypertension* **16**, 231–237.

Susic D, Varagic J and Frohlich ED (1999) Pharmacologic agents on cardiovascular mass, coronary dynamics and collagen in aged spontaneously hypertensive rats. *Journal of Hypertension* **17**, 1209–1215.

Suzuki J, Matsubara H, Urakami M and Inada M (1993) Rat angiotensin II (type 1A) receptor mRNA regulation and subtype expression in myocardial growth and hypertrophy. *Circulation Research* **73**, 439–447.

Swynghedauw B (1999) Molecular mechanisms of myocardial remodeling. *Physiological Reviews* **79**, 215–262.

Takeda Y, Yoneda T, Demura M, *et al.* (2001) Effects of high sodium intake on cardiovascular aldosterone synthesis in stroke-prone spontaneously hypertensive rats. *Journal of Hypertension* **19**, 635–639.

Thijs L, Fagard R, Lijnen P, *et al.* (1992) A meta-analysis of outcome trials in elderly hypertensives. *Journal of Hypertension* **10**, 1103–1109.

Thybo MK, Stephens N, Cooper A, *et al.* (1995) Effect of hypertensive treatment on small arteries of patients with previously untreated hypertension. *Hypertension* **25**, 474–481.

Unger T, Ganten D, Lang RE and Scholkens BA (1985) Persistent tissue converting enzyme inhibition following chronic treatment with HOE498 and MK421 in spontaneously hypertensive rats. *Journal of Cardiovascular Pharmacology* **7**, 36–41.

Val-HeFT Trial (2000) Presented at the Annual Meeting of the American Heart Association, New Orleans, LA, November.

Varagic J, Dusuc D and Frohlich ED (2001a) Coronary hemodynamic and ventricular responses to AT_1 receptor inhibition in SHR: interaction with AT_2 receptors. *Hypertension* **37**, 1399–1403.

Varagic J, Susic D and Frohlich ED (2001b) Low-dose ACE with alpha- or beta-adrenergic receptor inhibitors have beneficial SHR cardiovascular effects. *Journal of Cardiovascular Pharmacology and Therapeutics* **6**, 57–63.

Varo N, Etayo JC, Zalba G, *et al.* (1999) Losartan inhibits the post-transcriptional synthesis of collagen type I and reverses left ventricular fibrosis in spontaneously hypertensive rats. *Journal of Hypertension* **17**, 107–114.

Varo N, Iraburu MJ, Varela M, *et al.* (2000) Chronic AT (1) blockade stimulates extracellular collagen type I degradation and reverses myocardial fibrosis in spontaneously hypertensive rats. *Hypertension* **35**, 1197–1202.

Vasan RS and Levy D (1996) The role of hypertension in the pathogenesis of heart failure: a clinical mechanistic overview. *Archives of Internal Medicine* **156**, 1789–1796.

Vasan RS, Benjamin EJ and Levy D (1995) Prevalence, clinical features and prognosis of diastolic heart failure: an epidemiologic perspective. *Journal of the American College of Cardiology* **26**, 1565–1574.

Weber KT (2000) Fibrosis and hypertensive heart disease. *Current Opinion in Cardiology* **15**, 264–272.

Whelan RF, Scroop GC and Walsh JA (1969) Cardiovascular actions of angiotensin in man. *American Heart Journal* **77**, 546–565.

Yamamoto K, Masuyama T, Sakata Y, *et al.* (2000) Roles of renin–angiotensin and endothelin systems in development of diastolic heart failure in hypertensive hearts. *Cardiovascular Research* **47**, 274–283.

Yamazaki T, Shiojima I, Komuro I, *et al.* (1994) Involvement of the renin–angiotensin system in the development of left ventricular hypertrophy and dysfunction. *Journal of Hypertension Supplement* **12**, S153–S157.

Yamazaki T, Komuro I and Yazaki Y (1999) Role of the renin–angiotensin system in cardiac hypertrophy. *American Journal of Cardiology* **83**, 53H–57H.

Yu HC, Burrell LM, Black MJ, *et al.* (1998) Salt induces myocardial and renal fibrosis in normotensive and hypertensive rats. *Circulation* **98**, 2621–2628.

Yuan B and Leenen FHH (1991) Dietary sodium intake and left ventricular hypertrophy in normotensive rats. *American Journal of Physiology* **261**, H1397–H1401.

Zhang X, Dostal DE, Reiss K, *et al.* (1995) Identification and activation of autocrine renin–angiotensin system in adult ventricular myocytes. *American Journal of Physiology* **269**, H1791–H1802.

Zhao X, White R, Van Huysse J and Leenen FH (2000) Cardiac hypertrophy and cardiac renin–angiotensin system in Dahl rats on high salt intake. *Journal of Hypertension* **18**, 1319–1326.

Index

ACE-labeled fibroblasts   145
ACE2   125–7, 131–2
  knockout mouse   128
  role in counter-regulatory response to heart failure   119–35
ACE2-mediated Ang-(1–7) formation   129
ACE2-mediated hydrolysis of biological peptides   127
ACE2-specific inhibitors, design and characteristics   128–9
ACEH   119, 125, 127
ACEI   167
ACTH   170
N-acyl-D-glucosamine 2-epimerase   34, 76
adrenal cortex   67
adrenal gland   111
adrenal mitochondria   70
adrenal renin   181
α-adrenergic receptors   50
β-adrenergic receptors   50
adrenergic system   120
adrenomedullin   163
adventitia of aorta   138
alanine   24
aldosterone   54, 111–12, 141, 143–4, 151
  infusion   166
  intracardiac production   161
  mechanisms of action   163
  metabolism   162
  modulates effect of Ang II   111–12
  renal effects of   162–3
  role in vascular injury   169
  tissue concentration   171
  trophic effects   163–7
aldosterone antagonists   207
aldosterone blockade
  mechanisms of action   168–9
  trials with   167–8
aldosterone-induced fibrosis   164–6, 168
aldosterone production   70, 145, 181
  cardiac remodeling   161
  heart failure   173–5
  normal heart   170–2
  transgenic models   173
aldosterone receptor   137, 161, 163
  antagonism   148
  up-regulation   166
aldosterone-salt treatment   168
aldosterone specific binding   164
aldosterone synthase   70, 143
aldosterone synthesis   169, 171, 187
  myocardial infarction   172
aldosteronism   151
amino acids   24
aminopeptidases   122
amlodipine   198
aneurysmectomy   146
Ang I   75, 101, 120
  cardiac levels   102
  co-converting enzyme (ACE) inhibitors   31
  generation   63, 75
  intracellular   40–1
  pituitary   25
Ang II   1, 26, 75, 101, 107, 120–1, 131–2, 137, 140, 144–7, 150–1, 161, 166, 180
  aldosterone modulation of effect of   111–12
  and cardiac hypertrophy   51
  application   41
  cardiac concentration   2
  cardiac levels   102
  cardiac remodeling by   2–3
  circulating levels   2
  extracellular   40, 112–13
  formation of   108–9, 111
  generation   31, 75, 77, 79–80, 103, 147, 149
  in cardiac remodeling   2–3, 193–4
  in myocardial fibrosis   196–8
    animal models   196–7
    cellular and molecular mechanisms   199–203
    clinical consequences   203–6
    clinical findings   198
    experimental findings   197–8
    in vivo evidence   196–7
    pharmacological studies   197–8

therapeutic implications 207
infusion model 197
intracellular 41, 108–9, 112–13
intracellular dialysis 108
intracrine actions 10–11
paracrine/autocrine actions 10
synthesis 167
Ang II-dependent cardiac hypertrophy 197
Ang II-dependent effects 41
Ang II-induced cardiac hypertrophy 50
Ang II-induced cardiomyocyte hypertrophy 8
Ang II-induced hypertrophy 5
Ang II-mediated signal transduction 131–2
Ang II peptide 11
Ang II receptor 22, 108, 138, 140, 145
Ang III 123
Ang IV 123
Ang-(1–7) 121–3, 132
 formation and total angiotensin receptor membrane concentration 132
 formation in heart failure 129–31
angiogenesis and nuclear binding 188
angiogenin 186
angiotensin
 binding 108, 180
 generation 66, 71
  in the heart 41
  intracellular versus extracellular 40–1
 intracellular 77, 179–92
 intracrine 180–3
 metabolism, pathways for 123
 metabolites 121–4
 see also Ang I; Ang II
angiotensin-converting enzyme (ACE) 47, 51, 75, 101, 108, 119, 122, 131–2, 137–8, 140, 144, 147, 151, 166
 as angiotensinase 125–7
 as carboxypeptidase 125–7
 autiradiographic binding 140
 binding 141, 143, 146
 constitutive 174
 fibrous vs. nonfibrous tissue 146–7
 forms of 127, 174
 inhibitors 2, 22, 49, 52, 76, 89, 107, 109, 121, 137, 149–50, 197–8, 206–7, 219–20, 225–6
 recruitable 174
angiotensin peptides 47

angiotensin receptors 180
angiotensinase, ACE as 125–7
angiotensinase C 123
angiotensinogen 25, 80, 102, 140, 180
 internalization 40
 see also AOGEN
angiotensinogen–green fluorescent protein fusion constructs 182
animal models
 Ang II and myocardial fibrosis 196–7
 infarction 2
 transgenic 19–30, 51, 122
α_1-antitrypsin promotor 25
antennopedia 187
AOGEN 47–51
aorta–coronary sinus 140
aortic-pulmonary banding 25
AP-13
β-arrestins 9
arterial hypertension 203
AS 173
Asp–Arg bond 122
aspartyl proteases 122
AT receptor 41
AT_1 47, 107, 1, 197
AT_1
 activation 2–3
 and cardiac fibrosis 52–3
 and cardiac hypertrophy 49–52
 antagonists 49, 51
 antisense therapy 22
 receptor blockers 31
AT_1-induced hypertrophy 3
AT_1-mediated intracellular signaling 3–4
AT_1 receptor 22, 47–51, 53, 131, 145, 148–50, 180, 218, 221
 crosstalk of signaling 85–7
 signaling mechanisms 86
 three-dimensional structure 88
AT_1 receptor antagonist 2, 207, 220
AT_1 receptor blockade 85–9
AT_1 receptor blocker, binding characteristics 87–9
AT_1 receptor-elicited growth 86
AT_1 receptor-mediated event 138
AT_{1A} 1–2, 25
AT_{1B} 1–2
AT_2 47
 antagonists 53
 in cardiac fibrosis 53–4
 in cardiac hypertrophy 53–4

INDEX

AT$_2$ receptor 9, 47–8, 53–4, 121–2, 145
  and cardiac apoptosis 92–3
  and cardiac fibrosis 93–4
  and cardiac function 85–99
  and cardiac growth 90–2
  crosstalk of signaling 85–7
  expression in cardiac tissue 89–90
  growth inhibitory effects 86
  pathophysiological roles 91
  role in cardiac structure and function 90–5
  signaling mechanisms 86
  stimulation 85–9
AT$_2$-transfected adult rat VSMC 92
AT$_4$ receptor 122
atherosclerosis 76, 80
ATP synthesis 68
atrial fibrillation 217
autocrine/paracrine cascade 26
autocrine/paracrine system 120
autoradiographic ACE binding 140
autoradiography 138
AvrXa7 188

bacterial virulence factors 188
baroreflex 48
basic fibroblast growth factor (bFGF) 107
bilateral nephrectomy 31, 70–1
blood pressure 22, 31, 34, 49, 63, 75–6, 103, 162, 165, 179, 198, 205
bovine rhodopsin 87
bradykinin 226
bradykinin B$_2$ 9
bradykinin receptor 166
bradykinin type 2 receptor 122
BTEB2 200

Ca^{2+} 11
calcifications 105
calcium 92
calcium channels 166, 181
calcium current 112
calcium-dependent DNase 193
cancer cells 107
candesarton CV11971 182
canonical signaling 4–10
captopril 125, 149–50
carbenoxolone 169
carboxyl terminal-dependent signaling 9–10
carboxypeptidase 122, 124
  ACE as 125–7

cardiac apoptosis and AT$_2$ receptor 92–3
cardiac-based renin angiotensin system (RAS), transgenic evidence of 21–2
cardiac damage 66
  renin angiotensin system (RAS) role in 47–62
cardiac fibroblasts 4, 7, 52, 64
cardiac fibrosis 141, 168–9, 173, 197
  and AT$_1$ 52–3
  and AT$_2$ 53–4
  and AT$_2$ receptor 93–4
cardiac function, and AT$_2$ receptor 85–99
cardiac gene expression 112
cardiac growth and AT$_2$ receptor 90–2
cardiac hypertrophy 2, 9, 11, 19, 22, 24–6, 66–7, 76, 164
  and AT$_1$ 49–52
  and AT$_2$ 53–4
  Ang II-induced 50
cardiac muscle 103, 108
cardiac myocytes 5, 32, 77, 103
  necrosis 141
cardiac remodeling 95, 161, 165, 193
  aldosterone production in 161
  Ang II in 2–3, 193–4
  cell types principally involved in 3
cardiac renin
  levels 33
  membrane association 34
  transgenic evidence of uptake 23–4
cardiac sequestration of circulating (pro)renin 33–4
cardiac-specific transgene expression 20
cardiac structure and function, AT$_2$ receptor role in 90–5
cardiomycocytes 108
cardiomyocytes 9, 23, 40, 50–1, 107, 140
  growth 50
  hypertrophy 193, 218–19
cardioreparative concept 207
cardiotrophin-13
cardiovascular diseases 81
  pathogenesis 80
cardiovascular disorders 137
cardiovascular homeostasis 137
cardiovascular system 92
cardiovasculature, structural remodeling 151
catecholamines 140
cathepsin A 124
cell hypertrophy 164

cell surface angiotensin generation 41
cell-to-cell communication 107
cell-to-cell coupling 111
cellular memory/differentiation 189
cerebrovascular injury 149
3CH134 86
chemical cross-linking 35
Chinese hamster ovary cells 86
p-chloromercuriphenylsulfonate (P-CMPS) 124
chromatin 180
chymase 75
circulating (pro)renin, cardiac sequestration of 33–4
circulating RAS 71
circulating renin angiotensin aldosterone system (cRAAS) 137
collagen 165
  accumulation 165, 205
  degradation inhibition 201
  deposition 174
  formation inhibition 151
  metabolism 164–6
  synthesis 151, 194–5
    stimulation of 200–1
  turnover 137, 143, 151, 194
  type I 138, 143, 148, 150, 194, 196–7, 200–3, 217
  type III 148, 150, 194, 196–7, 200, 217
  see also fibrillar collagen; procollagen
collagenase 195
collectrin 127–8
colloidal gold-tagged anti-angiotensin antibody 180
column chromatography 129
congestive heart failure (CHF) 173, 215–16, 221, 223, 226
connective tissue growth factor (CTGF) 200
connexin 43 105–7
connexin molecule 104
contractile dysfunction 19
coronary artery ligation 141
coronary blood flow 216–17
coronary hemodynamics 216, 219
coronary insufficiency 219–20
coronary reserve 205–6
coronary vasculature 216
corticosterone 166, 170
  intracardiac production 161
cortisone 151
costimulation 86
Cox-2 169

croton oil 141, 150
C-terminal amino acid 124
C-terminal telopeptide (CITP) 202–3
C-terminal transmembrane 111
CVF 202–6
cyclosporine 150
Cyp11b1 69
Cyp11b2 69, 143–4
cysteine proteases 122
cytokines 48, 107

death 76
deoxycorticosterone 169–70
desmin-deficient cardiomyopathy 141
diabetes 80
diabetic cardiomyopathy 196
diacylglycerol (DAG) 3–4
diastolic dysfunction 221–2
DNA, irreversible double-strand cleavage 92
DNA binding proteins 187
DNA encoding 20
DNA proteins 187
DNA sequences 6
DNA synthesis 49
DNA synthesis rates vs. medium and cellular Ang II levels 39
Drosophila 127

EDTA 125
electrolyte balance 63
electron microscopy 87
embryonic stem cells (ES cells) 20
enalapril 149
enalaprilat 109–10, 125
endocardial fibrosis 145, 149
endocrine vs. paracrine/autocrine/intracrine RAS 222–4
endogenous Ang II in heart cell communication 108–11
endopeptidases 122
endoplasmatic reticulum (ER) 67
endothelial cells 65, 77
endothelin 26, 48, 50, 52, 54, 120, 166
endothelin-1 (ET1) 5, 124, 140, 200
endothelin-converting enzyme (ECE) 122, 124
endothelin receptors 207
endothelium 138
Engrailed 185, 187
EPHESUS 167, 174
epidermal growth factor (EGF) 8, 50, 53, 107

epithelial tissue 164
eplerenone 151, 167
eprosartan 39
essential hypertension 198
exogenous cAMP 112
exon 1 renin 68
exon 1A renin 70–1
　possible functions 70
　transcripts 69
exon 1C renin 68
exon 2 renin 68
extracellular Ang II 40, 112–13
extracellular matrix (ECM) 2–3, 12, 52, 121, 138
extracellular RAS 65
extracellular signal-regulated kinase see ERK

Fas receptor 9
Fas/Fas ligand system 9
fetal VSMC 92
fibrillar collagen 194, 196, 217
　metabolism 199
　network 141
　scaffolding 138
fibroblast growth factor-250
fibroblast proliferation, stimulation of 199–200
fibroblasts 32, 108
fibronectin 168
fibrosis 25–6, 80
fibrous tissue formation 138
fluorescent proteins 21
foreign-body fibrosis 145
furin convertases 122

β-galactosidase 21
gap junction
　communication 107
　conductance 104
　proteins 106
GATA4 3
gene-targeted mice 21
glomerular mesangial cells 36
glucocorticoid receptors 166
glucocorticoids 106, 144, 164
glucoreceptor 173
glycogen synthase kinase 3β (GSK3β) 9
G-protein 10, 87
G-protein-coupled receptor (GPCR) 47, 85–7
growth and cell coupling 107
growth factors 107

growth-stimulatory responses 37
GTP-binding proteins 49

[^{3}H]-thymidine 39, 77
heart as target for RAS 101–17
heart cell communication, endogenous Ang II in 108–11
heart failure 31, 95, 104–6, 161–2, 196
　aldosterone production in 173–5
　Ang-(1–7) formation in 129–31
　events involved in 113
　general model of 120
　paradigm of 120–1
　pathophysiology of 119
　results from clinical trials 167–9
　see also ACE2
heart valve leaflets 138–9
hepatic growth factor (PDGF) 107
herpes virus protein VP 22 188
HEXXH motif 125
high-affinity renin-binding sites/receptors 36
high-mobility group protein B1 (HMGB1) 185
His–Leu bond 125
HOE140 94
homeobox transcription factors 185
homeodomain transcription factor fusion proteins 188
hormonal action 103, 107
hormonal system, intracrine 103
hormones, intracrine 179–92
HOXA5 185, 187
11-β-HSD1 169
11-β-HSD1/2 169
hydralazine 146, 197
hydrochlorothiazide 198
11-β-hydroxylase 173
hydroxyproline 151
11-β-hydroxysteroid-dehydrogenase 144
　type 2 164
hyperkalemia 162
hypertension 19, 22–4, 66, 80, 146
hypertensive heart disease (HHD) 196, 198, 202–8, 215–34
　contribution of Ang II cardiac effects 218
　RAS in 215–34
　　experimental and clinical evidence 222–5
　　pharmacological blockade 225–6
　structural and functional alterations 216

hypertensive LVH   217
hypertensive ren2 rat   197
hypertrophic cardiomyopathy   196
hypokalemia   165

^{125}I-Ang I infusions   41
IGFII   37
3-indol-carabinol plasma ren-2-derived prorenin   66
IKLF   200
immune disease   80
impulse propagation   105
infarcted rat heart   143
inflammation   76, 80
inflammation markers   165, 169
inositol 1,4,5-trisphosphate (IPU3u)   4
insulin-like growth factor-1   11
intercellular communication   104
intercellular signaling   189
  and RAS   103-7
interlukin (IL)-1β   3
interstitial fibrosis   19, 105, 196
interstitial fluids   79
interstitial pulmonary fibrosis   150
interventricular septal specimen biopsies   195
intracellular Ang I   40-1
intracellular Ang II   41, 108-9, 112-13
intracellular angiotensin   77, 179-92
  clinical implications   184
intracellular calcium channels   181
intracellular dialysis of Ang II   108
intracellular orangelles   67
intracellular RAS, evidence for   107-8
intracellular signaling   1-17
  AT$_1$-mediated   3-4
intracrine, use of term   179, 184-5
intracrine action   179-80, 184
  and nucleolar function   188
  associated with homeodomain transcription factors   187
  theory   188-9
intracrine angiotensin   180-3
intracrine biology and nucleolus   188
intracrine genes   189
intracrine hormonal system   103
intracrine hormones   179-92
intracrine memory hypothesis   189
intracrine origin hypothesis   189
intracrine physiology   184-8
intracrine renin   183-4
  clinical implications   184
intracrine signaling   189
intracrine system, evidence of   101-17

intracrines
  as transcription factors   189
  directly interacting with rDNA   188
  renin and prorenin as   186-7
  selection of   185-6
  trafficking to nucleolus   188
  transcription factors as   188
intramitochondrial cholesterol transfer   171
intramural coronary arteries   138
in vitro emulsion autoradiography   145
in vitro studies   92
in vivo studies   90
inward calcium current   112-13
irradiation   150
ischemic cardiomyopathy   196
ischemic vs. nonischemic injury   141
isoproterenol   49, 112, 141

Jak1   6
Jak2   6
Jak/STAT   6-7, 51-2
JNK   4-5

kidney   65
KNOTTED   188
Krüppel-like zinc-finger transcription factor 5 (KLF5)   200

LEAFY   188
left ventricular hypertrophy (LVH)   25, 215, 217-18, 225
left ventricular (LV) apoptosis   217
left ventricular (LV) performance   215
ligand-induced receptor oligomerization   6
lisinopril   125, 198
L-NAME   94
losartan   93, 109-10, 145, 149, 161, 172-4, 181-2, 198
lysine   24
lysosomal degradation   71
lysosomal enzymes   65
lysosomal pathway   65

M6P   36, 39
M6P-containing prorenin   36
M6P-containing proteins   37
M6P/IGFII receptor   36-7, 40, 183-4
  recycling   38
M6P/IGFII receptor-induced internalization   35
M6P/IGFII receptor-mediated (pro)renin binding   37-8

M6P/IGFII receptor-mediated (pro)renin internalization 38
M6P/IGFII receptor-specific binding 38
M6P-receptor 64, 66, 77
M6P-receptor-independent uptake of renin 71
M8-9 protein 36
macrophages 64, 144
malate dehydrogenase 67
mannose 6-phosphate see M6P
MAP kinase 36, 49, 107
  activation 5–6
  e/ER pathway 200
  ERK 4–6, 86–7, 92, 218
  ERK1 78
  ERK1/2 79
  ERK1/ERK2 80
  signaling cascades 4–5
MAP kinase phosphatase-1 (MKP-1) 86
marker molecule 21
matrix metalloproteinase (MMP) family of zinc-containing endoproteinases 195
MCP-1 169
mechanical stretch 50–2, 54
membrane proteins 87
membranes 36
mesangial cells 36
messenger RNA 49, 66, 68–9, 78, 89, 103, 106, 123, 131, 140–1, 143, 145, 150, 166, 170, 197
metabolic/genetic regulation 189
metallocarboxypeptidases 124
metalloproteases 122
metazoans 189
α-MHC promotor 20, 22–3
MHChAgt-2 102
Michaelis–Menten kinetics 127
mineralocorticoid receptor 144
mineraloreceptor 163, 173
mitochondria 180–1
mitochondrial fraction 67
mitochondrial P-450 aldosterone-synthase 170
mitogen-activated protein kinase see MAP kinase
monocrotaline-induced pulmonary injury 141
mural thrombus 141
myocardial aldosterone synthase mRNA concentration 170
myocardial fibers 103
myocardial fibrinoid necrosis 165
myocardial fibrosis 49, 193–213

Ang II in 196–8
  animal models 196–7
  cellular and molecular mechanisms 199–203
  clinical consequences 203–6
  clinical findings 198
  experimental findings 197–8
  in vivo evidence 196–7
  pharmacological studies 197–8
  therapeutic implications 207
factors involved 194
general aspects of 194–6
myocardial infarction 54, 67, 70–1, 76, 90, 95, 103, 138, 140, 143, 147–9, 161–2, 173–4
  aldosterone synthesis 172
  animal models of 2
myocardial ischemia 140
myocardium 50, 54, 90, 120, 138, 141
myoFb 144–5, 148, 151
α-myosin-heavy chain promoter 51

N1E-115 neuroblastoma cells 86
NaS + s/KS + s-ATPase 164, 166
NAD(P)H-mediated ROS generation 5
NAD(P)H oxidase 3, 5–6, 50, 53
Na–K pump 111
necrosis 105
neonatal cardiomyocytes 66
nested reverse transcriptase–polymerase chain reaction 69
neurohormonal systems 120–1
neuroleukin 186
neutral endopeptidase (NEP) 122, 124, 129, 131
nonAng I/nonAng II fragments 123
noncardiomyocyte cells 140
nonepithelial cells 164
nonepithelial tissue 164
nonproteolytic activation 33
norepinephrine 50
novel signaling 5
nuclear binding and angiogenesis 188
nuclear factor (NF)-kB 3
nuclear magnetic resonance spectroscopy 87
nucleolar function and intracrine action 188
nucleolus
  and intracrine biology 188
  intracrines trafficking to 188

obesity 80
osteopontin 169

osteoporosis 151
oxidative stress 48

p38 4–5
p53 50
P450scc 69
papaverine 140
PC12W 86, 92
PD123177 91, 145
PD123319 93–4
peptidases, overview 122–4
pericardial fibrosis 145, 150
perivascular fibrosis 94, 196
pH effects 33
pH environment 35
phosphatase 2A (PP2A) activation 86
phosphoglucose isomerase 186
phosphoinositide 3-kinase (PI3K) 3
phospholipase C-β (PLCβ) 3
phospholipases 3
phosphomannosylated glycoforms 36
phosphomannosylated proteins 37
pig, origin of cardiac angiotensin in 32
pituitary Ang I 25
plant transcription factors 188
plasma and cardiac renin correlation 32
plasma RAS 106
plasma renin, contribution to cardiac renin 102
plasminogen activator inhibitor-1 (PAI-1) 201
platelet-derived growth factor (PDGF) 107, 180, 182–3, 199
PLC activation 7, 9
PMKRL 24–5
post-infarction myocytes 91
post-myocardial infarction remodelling 19, 22
potassium sparing 165
prazosin 197
preprohormone angiotensinogen 120
preprorenin
  differential expression 69
  transcripts 70–1
primary pulmonary hypertension (PPH) 131–2
procathepsin D 37
procollagen
  type I 201
  type I carboxy-terminal propeptide (PIP) 202
  type III aminoterminal peptide 143
prolylendopeptidases (PEPs) 123

prolyl-4-hydroxylase 201
pro-mitogenic effects 92
Pro–Phe bond 123
propranolol 150
prorenin 26
  activation 37–8
  activity 24–5
  binding 77, 79, 183
  clearance 38
  closed and open conformation 33
  glycosylated and nonglycosylated 65
  in interstitial space 75
  internalization 35, 108
  mannose-6-phosphate receptor mediated internalization 65
  ren-2 derived 65
  uptake 31–45
  uptake by tissues 33
prorenin-induced effects in the heart 35
prorenin-induced mycocyte proliferation 40
prorenin-mediated direct effects 38–40
prorenin receptors 34–6, 75
protease cleavage 70
protein kinase C (PKC) 4–5, 7, 49, 106–7, 112
protein tyrosine phosphatases (PTPase) 86
pulmonary artery 138
PYK2 8

quantitative RT–PCR 170
quinapril 146

R3T3 mouse fibroblasts 92
5′-RACE 68
Randomized Aldactone Evaluation Study (RALES) 151, 161, 167–8
RAS see renin angiotensin system (RAS)
rat renin gene, discovery of second transcript 67–9
rDNA 188
reactive oxygen species (ROS) 6, 50, 54
receptor transactivations/interactions 7–9
remodeling 76, 90
ren-2d 25
ren-2 gene 66
renal effects of aldosterone 162–3
renal infarction 145
renal renin granules 65
renin 48, 75, 140, 180
  binding 78–80
  cardiac expression 66–7

cardiac tissue levels   32
cardiac-specific regulation   63
de novo synthesis and uptake   63–73
degradation   77
formation   108
internalization   71
intracellular location   67
intracrine   183–4
M6P-receptor-independent uptake   71
mannose-6-phospate receptor-independent uptake of   71
presence in the heart   64
synthesis   187
uptake and expression, significance of   70–1
uptake into the heart   64–6
renin angiotensin aldosterone system (RAAS)   162, 167, 172
see also tRAAS
renin angiotensin system (RAS)   1–17, 19, 63, 75, 120
activation   23, 121
and intercellular signaling   103–7
circulating   71
components   1
synthesis of   102
dysfunction, transgenic models of   26
extracellular   65
heart as target for   101–17
in cardiac hypertrophy and fibrosis   25–6
in HHD   215–34
experimental and clinical evidence   222–5
pharmacological blockade   225–6
intracellular, evidence for   107–8
major role   76
plasma   106
role in cardiac damage   47–62
transgenic evidence of cardiac-based   21–2
renin-binding protein (RnBP)   34, 76–8
renin-binding sites/receptors, high-affinity   36
renin exon 1A   181
renin gene transcription start site   102
renin mRNA levels   31
renin receptors   75–83
renin transcripts   67
retinoids   107

serine kinase   92
serine proteases   122

serotonin   140
SHP-1   86
SHP-2   7
signal transduction   106
Ang II-mediated   131–2
α-smooth muscle actin (α-SMA)   140
positive myoFb phenotype   144
smooth muscle cells   36
sodium dodecyl sulfate–polyacrylamide gel electrophoresis   123
sodium homeostasis   162
sodium pump subunits   166
sodium supplementation   165
spironolactone   151, 165, 168–9, 172, 174
spontaneously hypertensive rats (SHR)   93, 219, 224–5
STAT1   7, 86–7
STAT2   86
STAT3   6–7, 86–7
STAT6   7
STATs   50
steroidogenesis   181
steroidogenic acute regulatory (StAR) protein   171
stroke   150
subcellular fractionation techniques   67
systolic dysfunction   163

T cell PEP   123
T cells   188
tACE   127
Tat protein   188
TCV116   93, 218–19
TGRcyp1a1ren2   23, 25
TGRhAT-rpR   24–5
TGRmren2–27   25, 66
threonine kinase   92
thromboembolic renal infarction   141
thrombosis   76
tissue inhibitors of MMPs (TIMPs)   195
tissue renin angiotensin aldosterone system *see* tRAAS
tissue repair   137, 147
toxic nephropathy   150
tRAAS   137–60, 172
and wound healing   146–51
diseased hearts and cardiovasculature   146–51
normal heart   146
tRAAS expression   138–45
diseased hearts   140–5
normal heart   138–44

transforming growth factor-β (TGF-β) 3, 11, 37, 48, 50, 53–4, 145
transforming growth factor-β1 (TGF-β1) 5, 26, 138, 140–1, 143–5, 147, 151, 197, 200–1
transgenesis, overview 20–1
transgenic animal models 19–30, 51, 102
transgenic evidence of cardiac renin uptake 23–4
transgenic evidence of cardiac-based renin angiotensin system (RAS) 21–2
transgenic models 224–5
  aldosterone production 173
  RAS dysfunction 26
transmembrane action potentials 104
tRNA 188
trophic effects of aldosterone 163–7
TTRhren-A3 102
tubulointerstitial fibrosis 150
tumor necrosis factor-α (TNF-α) 3
Tyk2 6
tyrosine kinase 106
tyrosine phosphorylation 106–7

unglycosylated (pro)renin 77
unilateral ureteral obstruction 150
uninephrectomy 164
urinary hydroxyproline excretion 151
urinary sodium:potassium ratio 163

valsartan 94
vascular barotrauma 148
vascular disease 76
vascular hypertrophy 76
vascular injury 19
vascular remodeling 216
vascular RnBPs 35
vascular smooth-muscle cells 80, 169
vasopressin 163
  secretion 48
ventricular arrhythmias 150, 206
ventricular dysfunction 120, 174, 203–5
ventricular fibrosis 173, 220–1
ventricular hypertrophy 103, 107
ventricular muscle 111
ventricular remodeling 112
ventricular stiffness 150
ventricular tachycardia 168
vimentin-positive myoFb 145
VSMC 92

wild-type gene 21
wound healing 137, 146–51

X chromosome 127
X-ray crystallography 87

Y319 8
Y319F 8
YIPP motif 6, 8–9

zinc-containing endoproteinases, matrix metalloproteinase (MMMP) family of 195
Z-Pro-Prolinal 124